PHLEBOTOMY EXAM REVIEW

second edition

Ruth E. McCall, BS, MT(ASCP)
Director of Phlebotomy and Clinical Laboratory Assistant Programs
TVI Community College
Albuquerque, New Mexico

Cathee M. Tankersley, BS, MT(ASCP), CLS (NCA)
Director of Phlebotomy Program
Phoenix College, Phoenix, Arizona
Clinical Educational Specialist
HemoCue, Inc., Mission Viejo, California
Laboratory Technical Supervisor
Valley Integrative Physicians, Phoenix, Arizona

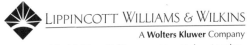

LIPPINCOTT WILLIAMS & WILKINS
A **Wolters Kluwer** Company
Philadelphia • Baltimore • New York • London
Buenos Aires • Hong Kong • Sydney • Tokyo

Executive Editor: John Goucher
Managing Editor: Emilie Linkins
Production Editor: Karen Ruppert
Marketing Manager: Mary Martin
Designer: Risa Clow
Compositor: Graphic World
Printer: Quebecor

351 West Camden Street
Baltimore, MD 21201
530 Walnut St.
Philadelphia, PA 19106

Printed in the United States of America
First Edition, 1997
Library of Congress Cataloging-in-Publication Data
McCall, Ruth E.
   Phlebotomy exam review / Ruth E. McCall, Cathee M. Tankersley.--2nd ed.
      p. cm.
   Includes index.
   ISBN 0-7817-3354-5
      1. Phlebotomy--Examinations, questions, etc. I. Tankersley, Cathee M. II Title.

RB45.15.M332 2003
616.07'561--dc21

                                                                    2003040114

To purchase additional copies of this book, call our customer service department at **(800) 638-3030** or fax orders to **(301) 824-7390**. International customers should call **(301) 714-2324.**

Visit Lippincott Williams & Wilkins on the Internet: http://www.LWW.com. Lippincott Williams & Wilkins customer service representatives are available from 8:30 am to 6:00 pm, EST.

06 07 08
5 6 7 8 9 10

To my husband, John; my sons, Chris and Scott; my daughter-in-law, Tracy; and my parents, Charles and Marie Ruppert, for their encouragement, patience, and support; and to my grandchildren, Katie and Ryan, for regular doses of pure joy that kept me motivated.

RUTH E. McCALL

To my children, Todd and Jaime, and sisters, Dorothy Carney and Judy Hightower, for their sensitivity and loving support.

CATHEE M. TANKERSLEY

PREFACE

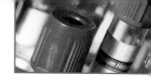

The demand for phlebotomists and other allied health workers who perform phlebotomy to demonstrate competency through national certification has increased in light of recent federal safety requirements and healthcare accrediting agency requirements for quality assurance. In addition, some states, such as California, require national certification by an approved certification agency as a condition of obtaining licensure.

Phlebotomy Exam Review, 2nd edition continues the tradition of the first edition by providing a comprehensive review of current phlebotomy theory and offers an ideal way to study for phlebotomy licensing or national certification exams. It also makes an excellent study guide for students taking formal phlebotomy training programs.

Answering the questions in this review provides the user an opportunity to test his or her knowledge and application of current phlebotomy theory. Theory questions address recent federal safety standards, National Committee for Clinical Laboratory Standards (NCCLS) guidelines, and the newly updated National Accrediting Agency for Clinical Laboratory Sciences (NAACLS) phlebotomist competencies when applicable. Questions include standard multiple-choice format used on national exams as well as matching exercises to quickly master key terms.

The format of the question section of the book follows that of the companion textbook, *Phlebotomy Essentials,* 3rd edition by the same authors. This format makes it an ideal chapter-to-chapter study reference when used in conjunction with the textbook in phlebotomy training programs.

Outstanding features:

- Current information on the various exams, including names and contact information for 10 organizations that offer phlebotomy certification exams
- A section on study and test-taking skills to help ensure success on the exam
- More than 1000 multiple choice questions with correct answers and detailed explanations
- New key term matching exercises
- Two comprehensive mock exams, one traditional (pencil and paper) and one computer-based

This book is designed to help the user identify areas of strength and weakness in his or her phlebotomy knowledge. It is not intended to replace formal education in phlebotomy theory, nor is there any guarantee that using this examination review will ensure passage of any certification or licensing exam.

The authors wish to express their gratitude to all who assisted and supported this effort.

TABLE OF CONTENTS

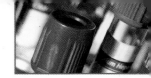

INTRODUCTION

CERTIFICATION

Certification is a process in which a national nongovernmental organization recognizes the competence of an individual in a particular profession or discipline. In today's healthcare climate, recognition through certification is becoming more popular because of the need for healthcare professionals to show evidence of proficiency in many different areas of practice. Because the majority of laboratory errors occur in the preanalytical phase, it is essential that all healthcare workers who collect blood specimens prove their competence in an effort to ensure quality patient care. In addition, national certification in phlebotomy is required by many institutions to address federal safety and QA requirements and to meet licensing requirements in some states.

Proof of certification is provided by credentials awarded to candidates who have met the educational or experiential requirements of a certifying organization and have successfully passed the organization's certification exam. Certification credentials provide evidence that the individual has mastered fundamental competencies in the profession. Certification credentials indicate competence at the time of the examination, and recertification is a mechanism used to demonstrate continued

competence either through reexamination or continuing education.

Eligibility requirements for obtaining certification vary according to the certifying organization; however, most certifying organizations recognize several eligibility routes. Eligibility routes typically include graduation from an approved educational program, other specific education requirements, or work experience. Requirements to maintain or renew certification also vary, from no requirements (meaning once certified, always certified) to submitting proof of a minimum number of hours of continuing education and payment of a renewal fee.

Currently, at least 10 organizations offer certification in phlebotomy. Generally speaking, employers do not favor any single certifying organization, but the applicant may find that one exam better suits his or her needs than another. In making a selection, the applicant may choose from any of the organizations listed in Table I-1, Phlebotomy Certification Organizations. All these organizations have exam sites throughout the United States. Several of them also offer exams in United States territories, such as Puerto Rico, and in other countries such as Canada.

Although some certification exams are still traditional hard copy exams taken with pencil

Table I-1

Phlebotomy Certification Organizations

Organization	Address	Website	Contact Person
American Certification Agency (ACA)	P.O. Box 58 Osceola, IN 46561	acacert.com	Shirley Evans Carole Mullins
American Medical Technologists (AMT)	710 Higgins Road Park Ridge, IL 60068	amt1.com	Geri Mulcahy Sharon Gautschy Chris Damon Dr. James Fidler
American Society of Clinical Pathologists (ASCP)	2100 W. Harrison Street Chicago, IL 60612	ascp.org/org	Geraldine Piskorski Kory Ward-Cook
American Society of Phlebotomy Technicians (ASPT)	P.O. Box 1831 Hickory, NC 28603	aspt.org	Helen Maxwell Ralph Maxwell
International Academy Phlebotomy Sciences, Inc. (IAPA)	631 D'Lyn Street Columbus, OH 43228	Not available	Sue Hyatt
National Association of Health Professionals (NAHP)	P.O. Box 459 Gardner, KS 66030	nahpusa.com	Connie Wright Robin McDowell
National Credentialing Agency (NCA)	P.O. Box 15945-289 Lenexa, KS 66285	nca-info.org	Sheila O'Neal Janene Dawson
National Center for Competency Testing (NCCT)	7007 College Blvd., Suite 250 Overland Park, KS 66211	Ncctinc.com	Stan Adams Bruce Brackett Nancy Graham
National Healthcareer Association (NHA)	134 Evergreen Place, 9th Floor East Orange, NJ 07018	nhanow.com	Jon Brandt Olga Suau, RN
National Phlebotomy Association (NPA)	1901 Brightseat Road Landover, MD 20785	scpt.com	Altonese Reese

and paper, many certification organizations administer exams by computer. Computer exams often use "computer adaptive testing (CAT)," in which the computer selects sets of questions based on the performance of the exam candidate on previous questions. For example, if the candidate does well on a set of intermediate-level questions, the next set of questions selected by the computer will be more advanced questions. Conversely, if the candidate does poorly on the intermediate-level questions, the next set of questions selected by the computer will be novice-level questions. CAT testing attempts to establish an appropriate level of performance and stops the test once the candidate's performance is determined to be at the highest sustainable level. Because CAT scoring takes into account *which* questions were correctly answered as well as how many, candidates who answer more diffi-

Telephone	E-mail	Fax	Testing Period	Testing Site
574-277-4538	info@acacert.com	574-277-4624	Open as needed	Available on site
800-275-1268 847-823-5169, X222	mail@amt1.com geri.mulcahy@amt1.com	847-823-0458	Self-scheduled; open all year	300 sites @ Sylvan Prometric www.2test.com
312-738-1336	bor@ascp.org	312-738-5808	Jan.– Mar. April–June July–Sept. Oct.–Nov.	200 test centers across the U.S.
828-294-0078	asptInc@msn.com asptInc@aol.com	828-327-2969	Contact office for times	Contact officer for sites
614-878-7751	Not available	Not available	Upon invitation	Hospitals, accredited clinical labs, educational institutions
800-444-0839 913-884-5744 888-267-4090	nahtr@worldnet.att.net	913-856-6125	As scheduled by schools	Post-secondary colleges
913-438-5110	soneal@goamp.com nca-info@goamp.com	913-541-0156	5 days/week 52 wks/year No application deadline	100+ nationally located assessment centers
800-875-4404	mmpa@planetkc.com cindy@ncctinc.com	913-498-1243	As determined by testing site	390 sites in 43 states Can be offered in any lab in the U.S.
800-499-9092 973-678-9100	jb@nhanow.com info@nhanow.com	973-678-7305	Offered monthly	Across the U.S.
301-386-4200	naltphle@aol.com	301-386-4203	As scheduled	Where requested

cult questions correctly obtain higher scores than those who correctly answer easier questions.

Regardless of the format, currently available exams are based on similar versions of accepted competencies for entry-level phlebotomists. Most often these competencies are determined through job/task analysis surveys. The National Accrediting Agency for Clinical Laboratory Sciences (NAACLS) outlines com-

petencies for phlebotomy programs approved by their organization. Outlines reflecting exam content and references used in developing questions are available from most certifying organizations and are usually sent automatically to applicants. Exam questions typically are based on standards for venipuncture, skin puncture, and other phlebotomy procedures developed by the National Committee for Clinical Laboratory Standards (NCCLS). The number of questions varies from 80 to 250, depending on the offering agency.

Application deadlines for examinations offered during a particular period vary according to organization policies. Applications can generally be submitted at any time throughout the year but will typically apply to the examination offering that corresponds with the deadline closest to the date that the application is received. Applications can be submitted by mail or on-line, depending on the organization.

STUDYING AND TEST-TAKING TIPS

Regardless of the type of test you are preparing for, there are numerous techniques that you can use to study and review effectively and improve your test-taking ability. The following information is designed to help you develop a study plan, control the study and test-taking environment, and learn key ways to retain information while studying. The desired result is to be able to effectively express your knowledge of a subject while taking a test.

How To Prepare To Study

Cultivate a Positive Attitude

The old adage, "You can do anything if you set your mind to it," makes a lot of sense. Those who think they can succeed at something and have a plan to achieve it are usually successful. Those who think they will fail usually do. If your goal is to pass a national certification exam, your belief that you will be able to successfully pass that exam actually helps you achieve that goal. In addition, your attitude plays an important role in determining how you approach preparation for an exam and ultimately how well you do on the actual exam. A positive attitude during the study process will result in more effective studying and increase learning and retention. Bringing a positive attitude to the test will help relieve the

stress associated with the testing process and leave your mind free to think logically and make you a more successful test-taker.

Plan To Study

A key element of effective studying is the ability to manage your study or review time. Plan to study. Develop a routine by establishing a particular time and place to study. Committing yourself to a regular routine eliminates the continual need to decide when and where to study. This keeps you in control and helps eliminate procrastination.

Establish a Consistent Study Setting

Choose a site that is compatible with study activities, such as a desk or table. Make sure the site is comfortable and has adequate lighting to minimize eye strain and fatigue. Resist the temptation to get too comfortable, however. Avoid beds or couches where you may become too relaxed and fall asleep.

Limit Distractions

Select a place to study where you are less likely to be disturbed by family members, roommates, pets, TV, phones, etc.

Do not answer the phone. If you do not have an answering machine, unplug the phone.

Limit Commitments

Do not disrupt your study schedule unless it is really important. Learn to say "no." Put a "Do Not Disturb" sign on the door.

When To Study

Study When You Are Rested

You are more alert when you are rested. Do not study when you are already physically or emotionally tired, and never study to the point of exhaustion.

Follow Your Daily Biorhythm

If possible, study during a time of day when you are most alert and efficient. For example, if you are a morning person, try to arrange study time in the morning.

How To Study

Have a Review Strategy

Decide in advance how you will review the material and allow adequate time to accomplish everything you want to do. Use whatever method works best for you.

Effective study strategies include reviewing your notes, textbook, and study questions and taking practice tests or mock exams.

Consider Forming a Study Group

Set aside some time to study with other students or peers who are also preparing to take the same exam. Members of study groups tend to motivate each other. Members can also share study tips and techniques that work well for them.

Establish a Realistic Study Schedule

Avoid resorting to marathon study sessions. Short 1- to 3-hour study sessions on a regular basis are usually more beneficial than an occasional long, drawn-out session.

Use Time Effectively

Copy information that needs to be memorized into a small notebook or on note cards and carry them with you. That way you can study small amounts while waiting in line, riding the bus, or waiting for appointments. Note cards can also be taped on mirrors, cupboards, etc. for quick reviews in between other chores or activities.

Take Breaks

Do not forget the old saying, "All work and no play makes Jack a dull boy." You by no means want to be "dull" on test day. Schedule breaks into your allotted study time. The ideal break should be short enough to relieve stress but not so extended that you lose focus, interest, or rhythm.

Watch the Time

Keep track of the time and do not waste it. If you get frustrated or your attention starts to wander, take a break.

What To Study

Study difficult or boring concepts or topics first.

Do Not Try To Study Everything At Once

Think about the answer to the joke, "How do you eat an elephant?" Answer: "One bite at a time!" Divide extensive topics into smaller portions.

Study What Is Appropriate

Try not to overstudy or do more than necessary. Do not repeatedly go over material you already know. Review it every so often to make certain you still remember it, but do not spend a great deal of time on it. For example, it would be a waste of time to read the textbook or your class notes over and over. A more effective method would be to review your notes and refer to the textbook to clarify concepts or information you have forgotten or do not completely understand.

Use the Exam Review Effectively

Once you feel that you are familiar with the material, try to answer the questions from this exam review. Refer to the textbook for information if you cannot answer a question or still need to clarify material after you read the explanation for the correct answer.

Take the Mock Exams

When you feel you have a good grasp of the material, you are ready to take the mock exams. Again, refer to the text or class notes when you cannot answer a question. Never attempt to memorize questions and answers. The intent of the study questions and mock exams is to help you identify areas in which your knowledge is weak. In addition, taking the computer mock exam will help you feel more comfortable taking a computer exam in the future.

How To Improve Your Thinking Skills

Multiple-choice questions usually cover six commonly recognized thinking levels. From lowest to highest they are: memory, comprehension, application, analysis, synthesis, and evaluation. When studying for multiple-choice tests, many students mistakenly spend their study time learning at the lowest level, memorizing facts without understanding how to analyze and apply the information. Learning how to identify the various thinking levels and using the skills associated with them as you study should help to enhance your knowledge of the subject and help you be a successful test-taker.

Memory Skills

Memory questions require the lowest level of thinking and involve the ability to recall specific information such as terminology, struc-
tures, classifications, facts, or concepts. Information of this type is most commonly memorized using techniques involving constant repetition. Examples of memorization techniques include reciting information aloud, listing information, and using flash cards. Information learned this way is committed to short-term memory and may be forgotten unless reinforced using other study methods or practical application.

The following are ways to assist in the memorization of information and enhance recall.

ABCS

Associating information with letters of the alphabet is an effective means of recalling information. Each letter of the alphabet acts as a cue or hint to recall information. You can make up your own ABCs to remember information and use established ones such as the following: the ABCs of cardiopulmonary resuscitation are A = airway, open the airway; B = breathing, perform rescue breathing; and C = circulation, initiate chest compressions.

ACRONYMS

Another helpful technique used to recall information is the use of acronyms or words formed by the first letter of a series of statements or facts. Each letter of the word jogs the memory to recall previously learned information. An example is the acronym RACE, used to remember action to take in the event of a fire: R = rescue, A = alarm, C = confine, E = extinguish.

ACROSTICS

Acrostics are catchy phrases or jingles in which the first letter of each word helps you to remember certain information. An example is the jingle used to help remember the order of draw for the evacuated tube method of venipuncture: Stop, red light, stay put, green light, go. S = sterile tubes, R = red (nonadditive) tubes, L = light blue tubes, S = serum separator tubes (SSTs), P = plasma separator tubes (PSTs), G = green tubes, L = lavender tubes, G = gray tubes.

IMAGING

Forming a mental picture associated with the information is another technique used to recall information. For example, one way to remember that a lipemic specimen is caused by fatty substances in the blood that make the serum appear cloudy or milky looking is to visualize a fat, white cloud when thinking about or saying the term "lipemic."

Comprehension Skills

Comprehension questions test your ability to understand information. To answer comprehension questions, you must not only recall information but also be able to understand the significance of the information. Comprehension questions test your ability to interpret information to draw conclusions or determine consequences, effects, or implications. A good way to enhance comprehension of material is to ask yourself, "What is the significance of this information—how or why is this information useful?" Again, using the term "lipemic" as an example, once we know what the term lipemic means and what a lipemic specimen looks like, we can now ask ourselves, "What is the significance of a lipemic specimen? Why or how is this information useful?" One answer is that a lipemic specimen is a clue that the patient was not fasting. This is significant if the test was ordered fasting. Lipemia also interferes with the testing process for some chemistry tests. Now we not only can recall facts but also are learning to comprehend the significance of these facts.

Application Skills

Application questions test your ability to use information. Answering application questions requires that you not only remember and comprehend information but are also able to relate that information to a real-life situation. Again, using the example of the term "lipemic," an application question might be: "When processing a specimen for a fasting glucose test, you notice that the specimen is lipemic. What does this tell you about the specimen?" Thought process: Lipemia can occur after eating fatty foods. If the specimen is lipemic, the patient must have eaten recently, which means the specimen is probably not a fasting specimen.

Analysis Skills

Analysis questions test your ability to analyze or evaluate information. Analysis questions often require you to evaluate several options to reach an answer. You must be able to recognize differences and determine the significance of several choices before arriving at your answer. Example: Which of the following specimens would most likely be rejected for testing?

a. lipemic specimen submitted for glucose testing
b. platelet count collected in an EDTA tube
c. routine UA in an unsterile container
d. specimen for potassium testing that is hemolyzed

The following is a typical thought process used to analyze the choices for the question above and determine the correct answer:
A lipemic specimen is an indication that the patient was not fasting, but it does not say it was a fasting glucose. In addition, a few people have lipemic serum for other reasons, so the specimen would not necessarily be rejected.

A platelet count **should** be collected in EDTA, so it would not be rejected for that reason.

A urine C&S must be collected in a sterile container, but a routine UA **does not have to be,** so an unsterile container would not cause it to be rejected.

Lastly, hemolysis liberates potassium from the red blood cells. That means a hemolyzed potassium specimen would most likely be rejected. The correct answer is "d."

How To Answer Multiple-Choice Questions

- For written examinations, jot down memory aids in the margins if you are allowed.
- Read the question carefully.
- Do not assume information that is not given.
- Eliminate choices that are clearly incorrect.
- Answer the easy questions first.
- Do not spend a great deal of time on questions you cannot answer.
- If you do not know the answer, skip the question and come back later. Information in other questions may remind you of the correct answer. If you still do not know the answer, try to make an educated guess.
- Do not change answers without a good reason. Your first guess is usually your best unless other questions remind you of the correct response.

TIPS FOR TEST DAY

Get a good night's sleep before the test.

Collect the items that you must bring to the test, such as identification and test documents, ID, calculator, pencils, etc., ahead of time so that you will not be scrambling to find them at the last minute.

Wear comfortable clothes to the exam. Dress in layers so that you can adapt in case the room is too cold or too warm.

Know your test site. If the test is in a location with which you are unfamiliar, drive by the testing site a day or two before the exam. If possible, travel during the same time of day as when you will be traveling to take the actual test. Allow yourself extra travel time the day of the test in case there are unexpected delays.

Arrive early for the test. That way you can get yourself situated and mentally prepared. You also have the opportunity to situate yourself in a location that is comfortable for you and suits your needs, rather than having to choose quickly from the seats that are left.

Listen carefully while test directions are given. Ask for clarification from the proctor if you do not understand something.

Try to relax. Pause to take a deep breath and stretch now and then.

OVERCOMING TEST ANXIETY

Being well-prepared is an excellent way to reduce test anxiety. Familiarity with the material builds confidence. The more familiar you are with the material, the more confident you will be. The more confident you are, the better you will do on the exam. Confidence in your ability and a positive attitude about your chances of success go a long way toward relieving stress or anxiety about the testing process.

Exam Review

1

PHLEBOTOMY: PAST AND PRESENT AND THE HEALTHCARE SETTING

d) Serology or immunology
e) Urinalysis
f) Microbiology
g) Blood bank or immunohematology
2) Anatomic and Surgical Pathology
a) Histology
b) Cytology
c) Cytogenetics
b. STAT Labs
c. Reference Laboratories

5. Clinical Laboratory Personnel
a. Laboratory Director/Pathologist
b. Laboratory Administrator/Laboratory Manager
c. Technical Supervisors
d. Medical Technologist/Clinical Laboratory Scientist
e. Medical Laboratory Technicians/Clinical Laboratory Technicians
f. Phlebotomist
g. Other Laboratory Personnel
6. Clinical Laboratory Improvement Act

REVIEW QUESTIONS

Match the term with the BEST description.

1. ____ barriers
2. ____ certification
3. ____ CEUs
4. ____ exsanguinate
5. ____ hemochromatosis
6. ____ ICD-9-CM
7. ____ kinesic slip
8. ____ kinesics

9. ____ Medicaid
10. ____ Medicare
11. ____ phlebotomy
12. ____ polycythemia
13. ____ proxemics
14. ____ TAT
15. ____ tertiary care

a. advises the patient on healthcare needs and coordinates responses to those needs
b. biases or filters to communication
c. care by specialists who perform routine procedures
d. disorder characterized by excess iron deposits
e. disorder involving the overproduction of red blood cells
f. entitlement program that provides healthcare to people age 65 and older
g. evidence that an individual has mastered competencies in a particular area
h. federal and state program that provides medical care to the poor

i. group healthcare practices reimbursed on a prepaid basis
j. highly complex medical services
k. international coding system that groups similar diseases and operations together
l. involves nonverbal communication or body language
m. involves the concept and use of space
n. outpatient care
o. proof of continuing education
p. remove blood to a point at which life cannot be sustained
q. the process of removing blood from a vein
r. turnaround time from when a test is ordered until results are reported
s. verbal and nonverbal messages do not match

Choose the BEST answer.

16. Which of the following is an agency that certifies phlebotomists?
    a. American Society for Clinical Pathology (ASCP)
    b. Joint Commission on Accreditation of Healthcare Organizations (JCAHO)
    c. National Accrediting Agency for Clinical Laboratory Sciences (NAACLS)
    d. National Committee for Clinical Laboratory Standards (NCCLS)

17. The primary duty of a phlebotomist is to:
    a. access specimens.
    b. collect blood specimens.
    c. collect and document workload.
    d. perform skin tests.

18. Promoting good public relations is a part of the phlebotomist's role because:
    a. a phlebotomist is a representative of the laboratory.
    b. good public relations promotes a harmonious relationship with visitors, staff, and patients.
    c. patients often equate blood-drawing experiences with the caliber of overall care received while in the hospital.
    d. all of the above

19. *Primum non nocere* comes from the Hippocratic oath and means:
    a. first do no harm.
    b. first things first.
    c. quality is foremost.
    d. ready to serve.

20. All of the following are examples of good work ethics EXCEPT:
    a. accountability
    b. dependability
    c. liability
    d. reliability

21. Phlebotomy is used as a therapeutic treatment of:
    a. diabetes.
    b. hypothyroidism.
    c. phlebitis.
    d. polycythemia.

22. All of the following are reasons for a phlebotomist to participate in continuing education programs EXCEPT:
    a. to follow Centers for Disease Control (CDC) mandates
    b. to learn new techniques
    c. to remain current in phlebotomy technology
    d. to renew certification

23. The term "phlebotomy" is derived from Greek words that, literally translated, mean to:
    a. cut a vein.
    b. draw blood.
    c. stick a vein.
    d. suck blood.

24. All of the following are phlebotomist duties EXCEPT:
    a. collect blood specimens
    b. perform laboratory computer operations
    c. start intravenous lines (IVs)
    d. transport specimens to the laboratory

25. What are the credentials of an NCA-certified phlebotomist?
    a. RPT
    b. CLPlb
    c. CPT
    d. PBT

26. Which of the following ancient blood-letting instruments has a counterpart in a modern-day bleeding device?
    a. bleeding bowl
    b. cup
    c. fleam
    d. syringe

27. Proof of participation in a workshop to upgrade skills required by some agencies to renew certification is called:
  a. accreditation.
  b. continuing education units (CEUs).
  c. essentials.
  d. reciprocity.

28. All of the following are listed in the American Hospital Association (AHA) Patient's Bill of Rights EXCEPT the right to:
  a. a complete explanation of his or her bill.
  b. confidentiality of his or her records.
  c. refuse treatment.
  d. know the medical status of other patients.

29. Personal "zone of comfort" is a radius of:
  a. 1–18 inches
  b. 1.5–4 feet
  c. 4–12 feet
  d. more than 12 feet

30. Which of the following is an example of a barrier to effective communication with a patient? The patient:
  a. does not speak English.
  b. is a child.
  c. is emotionally upset.
  d. all of the above

31. Which of the following is an example of a confirming response to a patient?
  a. "I do not know what you mean."
  b. "I have no idea how long it will take."
  c. "I understand how you must be feeling."
  d. "I'm on a tight schedule right now."

32. Which of the following is an example of negative kinesics?
  a. eye contact
  b. frowning
  c. good grooming
  d. smiling

33. All of the following are part of a professional image EXCEPT:
  a. neat, clean appearance
  b. clean, pressed laboratory coat
  c. short clean fingernails and long hair pulled back
  d. wearing strong perfume or cologne

34. Which of the following examples is a good way to earn a patient's trust?
  a. act knowledgeably
  b. convey sincerity
  c. look professional
  d. all of the above

35. All of the following are proper telephone protocol EXCEPT:
  a. answer the phone promptly
  b. clarify and record information
  c. hang up on angry callers
  d. prioritize callers, if necessary

36. Which of the following is an example of proxemics?
  a. eye contact
  b. facial expression
  c. personal hygiene
  d. zone of comfort

37. All of the following are recognized elements of good communication in the healthcare setting EXCEPT:
  a. confirmation
  b. control
  c. distrust
  d. empathy

38. The best way to handle a "difficult" or "bad" patient is to:
  a. help the patient to feel in control of the situation.
  b. leave the room without collecting a specimen from the patient.
  c. speak firmly to the patient to show that you are in control of the situation.
  d. threaten to report the patient to his or her doctor.

39. Proxemics is the study of an individual's:
  a. body language.
  b. concept of space.
  c. facial expressions.
  d. verbal communication.

40. Which of the following situations allows the patient to feel in control?
  a. agreeing with the patient that it is his or her right to refuse to have a blood specimen drawn
  b. informing the patient that you are going to draw a blood sample
  c. insisting that the patient cooperate and let you draw blood
  d. telling the patient not to eat or drink anything during a test

41. What is the average speaking rate of a normal adult?
  a. 75–100 words per minute
  b. 125–150 words per minute
  c. 250–350 words per minute
  d. 500–600 words per minute

42. Another term for outpatient care is:
  a. ambulatory care.
  b. nonambulatory care.
  c. nursing home care.
  d. rehabilitation care.

43. Which laboratory department performs tests to identify abnormalities of the blood and blood-forming tissues?
  a. chemistry
  b. hematology
  c. microbiology
  d. urinalysis

44. What department is responsible for administering a patient's oxygen therapy?
  a. cardiodiagnostics
  b. electroencephalography
  c. physical therapy
  d. respiratory therapy

45. Which of the following tests would be performed in surgical pathology?
  a. compatibility testing
  b. enzyme immunoassay
  c. frozen section
  d. triglycerides

46. The phlebotomist is asked to collect a specimen from a patient in the nephrology department. A patient in this department is most likely being treated for a disorder of the:
  a. joints.
  b. kidneys.
  c. lungs.
  d. nose.

47. The phlebotomy supervisor asked a phlebotomist to collect a specimen in the otorhinolaryngology department. The phlebotomist proceeded to go to the department that provides treatment for:
  a. skin problems and diseases.
  b. eye problems or diseases.
  c. bone and joint disorders.
  d. ear, nose, and throat disorders.

48. Which of the following tests is performed in the coagulation department?
  a. blood urea nitrogen (BUN)
  b. complete blood count (CBC)
  c. glucose
  d. protime (PT)

49. Which medical specialty treats patients with tumors?
  a. geriatrics
  b. oncology
  c. ophthalmology
  d. orthopedics

50. The medical specialty that treats skeletal system disorders is:
  a. gastroenterology.
  b. neurology.
  c. orthopedics.
  d. pediatrics.

51. The specialty of this physician is the treatment of newborns.
    a. gerontologist
    b. neonatologist
    c. obstetrician/gynecologist
    d. pediatrician

52. Another name for blood bank is:
    a. immunohematology.
    b. immunology.
    c. microbiology.
    d. serology.

53. All of the following are hematology tests EXCEPT:
    a. glycosylated hemoglobin
    b. hematocrit
    c. platelet count
    d. reticulocyte count

54. Which department performs cerebrospinal fluid (CSF) analysis?
    a. chemistry
    b. hematology
    c. microbiology
    d. all of the above

55. With which other hospital department would the laboratory coordinate therapeutic drug monitoring?
    a. nuclear medicine
    b. pharmacy
    c. physical therapy
    d. radiology

56. Which department processes and stains tissue samples for microscopic analysis?
    a. chemistry
    b. coagulation
    c. histology
    d. microbiology

57. All of the following personnel are required to have a college degree or equivalent EXCEPT:
    a. clinical laboratory scientist
    b. medical technologist
    c. phlebotomist
    d. none of the above

58. An appendectomy performed in a free-standing ambulatory surgical center is an example of:
    a. managed care.
    b. primary care.
    c. secondary care.
    d. tertiary care.

59. What department would perform blood cultures?
    a. hematology
    b. microbiology
    c. serology
    d. urinalysis

60. Electrolyte testing includes:
    a. bilirubin and creatinine.
    b. blood urea nitrogen (BUN) and cholesterol.
    c. glucose and uric acid.
    d. sodium and potassium.

61. Which hospital department performs diagnostic tests and monitors therapy of heart patients?
    a. ECG
    b. EEG
    c. ER
    d. ICU

62. A basic metabolic panel (BMP) is performed in which department?
    a. chemistry
    b. hematology
    c. histology
    d. microbiology

63. Which laboratory department performs chromosome studies?
    a. chemistry
    b. coagulation
    c. cytogenetics
    d. hematology

64. A Pap smear is examined for the presence of cancer cells in this department.
    a. cytology
    b. hematology
    c. histology
    d. microbiology

65. Prepaid group healthcare organization in which members pay flat fees for defined services are called:
    a. DRGs
    b. HMOs
    c. PPOs
    d. None of the above

66. The term used to describe sophisticated and highly complex medical care is:
    a. managed care.
    b. primary care.
    c. secondary care.
    d. tertiary care.

67. A patient in labor would normally be admitted to which of the following medical specialty departments?
    a. cardiodiagnostics
    b. geriatrics
    c. obstetrics
    d. pediatrics

68. A function of the radiation therapy department is:
    a. administration of oxygen therapy.
    b. brain wave mapping and polysomnography.
    c. imaging by means of x-rays.
    d. treating cancer using high-energy x-rays.

69. Toxicology is often a part of which of the following laboratory departments?
    a. chemistry
    b. coagulation
    c. hematology
    d. urinalysis

70. A physician who is a specialist in diagnosing disease from laboratory findings is a(n):
    a. administrative technologist.
    b. laboratory director.
    c. medical technologist.
    d. pathologist.

71. Which of the following is a hematology test?
    a. BMP
    b. C&S
    c. CBC
    d. CSF

72. The department that injects patients with radioactive dyes that can interface with laboratory testing is:
    a. electroneurodiagnostics
    b. nuclear medicine
    c. pharmacy
    d. respiratory therapy

73. Which department performs carcinoembryonic antigen (CEA) testing?
    a. chemistry
    b. hematology
    c. microbiology
    d. urinalysis

74. Which department performs radiographic procedures and other imaging techniques to aid in diagnosis?
    a. occupational therapy
    b. pharmacy
    c. radiology
    d. respiratory therapy

75. Which of the following is an example of an inpatient care facility?
    a. day-surgery facility
    b. dentist's office
    c. hospital
    d. physician's office

76. Which of the following would most likely be performed in the serology department?
    a. blood urea nitrogen (BUN)
    b. complete blood cell count (CBC)
    c. prothrombin time (protime or PT)
    d. rapid plasma reagin (RPR)

77. Which of the following laboratory personnel has the same qualification as a medical technologist (MT)?
    a. clinical laboratory technician (CLT)
    b. clinical laboratory scientist (CLS)
    c. medical laboratory technician (MLT)
    d. pathologist

78. Which department would perform a hemogram?
    a. chemistry
    b. hematology
    c. immunohematology
    d. immunology

79. This department may examine specimens microscopically for the presence of crystals, casts, bacteria, and blood cells.
    a. chemistry
    b. hematology
    c. microbiology
    d. urinalysis

80. This hospital department provides therapy to restore patient mobility.
    a. cardiodiagnostics
    b. physical therapy
    c. radiology
    d. respiratory therapy

81. Brain wave mapping and evoked potential are performed by which department?
    a. ECG
    b. EEG
    c. OT
    d. RT

82. All of the following are primary objectives of managed care EXCEPT:
    a. enhance cost containment
    b. facilitate the management of patient care
    c. increase revenue from services offered
    d. maintain quality care

83. Which of the following describes a new category of multi-skilled personnel who work as part of the nursing team, performing nursing and phlebotomy duties along with ancillary testing?
    a. associate's degree nurse (ADN)
    b. certified nursing assistant (CNA)
    c. emergency medical technician (EMT)
    d. patient care technician (PCT)

84. Which laboratory worker has a bachelor's degree, or equivalent, in medical technology?
    a. clinical laboratory scientist (CLS)
    b. clinical laboratory technician (CLT)
    c. medical laboratory technician (MLT)
    d. phlebotomy technician (PBT)

85. Which of the following laboratory personnel has an associate's degree or equivalent?
    a. clinical laboratory scientist (CLS)
    b. clinical laboratory technician (CLT)
    c. medical technologist (MT)
    d. phlebotomist

86. A specimen for ova and parasite testing would be sent to:
    a. chemistry
    b. coagulation
    c. microbiology
    d. urinalysis

87. The process of identifying an organism and determining the appropriate antibiotic for treatment is called:
    a. antibody screening.
    b. culture and sensitivity testing.
    c. microscopic analysis.
    d. radioimmunoassay.

88. C&S tests on patient specimens are performed in which department?
    a. blood bank
    b. chemistry
    c. immunology
    d. microbiology

89. A glucose test would be performed in which department?
    a. chemistry
    b. hematology
    c. microbiology
    d. radioimmunoassay

90. Which medical specialty treats patients with blood disorders?
    a. dermatology
    b. hematology
    c. internal medicine
    d. urology

91. All of the following duties are performed by local public health agencies EXCEPT:
    a. diabetes screening
    b. insect control
    c. licensure of healthcare personnel
    d. sanitation inspections

92. Blood typing and compatibility testing are performed in which department?
    a. blood bank
    b. chemistry
    c. coagulation
    d. hematology

93. A sample for fibrin degradation products (FDP) testing would be sent to which department?
    a. blood bank
    b. chemistry
    c. coagulation
    d. microbiology

94. Which test performed in immunology detects streptococcus infection?
    a. ASO
    b. monospot
    c. RA
    d. RPR

95. A federal program that provides medical care for the indigent is:
    a. homecare services.
    b. Medicaid.
    c. Medicare.
    d. Workers' compensation.

96. Which department performs chemical screening tests on urine specimens?
    a. coagulation
    b. hematology
    c. microbiology
    d. urinalysis

97. Which department would perform an erythrocyte sedimentation rate?
    a. chemistry
    b. hematology
    c. immunology
    d. microbiology

98. Diagnosis and treatment of diseases characterized by joint inflammation is part of which medical specialty?
    a. dermatology
    b. gastroenterology
    c. internal medicine
    d. rheumatology

Match the test with the correct department.

99. _____ ABO type		**a.** blood bank
100. _____ antibody		**b.** chemistry
screen		
101. _____ potassium		**c.** coagulation
(K+)		
102. _____ bilirubin		**d.** hematology
103. _____ culture and		**e.** microbiology
sensitivity		**f.** serology
(C&S)		**g.** urinalysis
104. _____ cholesterol		
105. _____ glucose		
106. _____ hematocrit		
(HCT)		
107. _____ monospot		
108. _____ platelet count		
109. _____ partial throm-		
boplastin time		
(PTT)		
110. _____ retic		
111. _____ rapid plasma		
reagin (RPR)		
112. _____ U/A		
113. _____ white blood cell		
(WBC) count		

Match the condition with the medical specialty.

124. _____ anemia		**a.** dermatology
125. _____ arthritis		**b.** endocrinology
126. _____ diabetes		**c.** gerontology
127. _____ knee		**d.** gastroenterology
surgery		**e.** gynecology
128. _____ menopause		**f.** hematology
129. _____ senility		**g.** neurology
130. _____ skin		**h.** oncology
disorders		**i.** orthopedics
131. _____ spinal cord		**j.** rheumatology
injury		**k.** urology
132. _____ tumor		
133. _____ urinary tract		
disease		

Match the organ or body part with the medical specialty.

114. _____ brain		**a.** cardiology
115. _____ ear		**b.** dermatology
116. _____ eye		**c.** endocrinology
117. _____ heart		**d.** gastroenterology
118. _____ kidney		**e.** gerontology
119. _____ ovary		**f.** gynecology
120. _____ joint		**g.** neurology
121. _____ skin		**h.** ophthalmology
122. _____ stomach		**i.** orthopedics
123. _____ thyroid		**j.** otorhino-
		laryngology
		k. urology

ANSWERS AND EXPLANATIONS

1. **b.** Barriers are biases or filters to communication.

2. **g.** Certification is evidence that an individual has mastered competencies in a particular area.

3. **o.** Continuing education units (CEUs) are awarded as proof of continuing education.

4. **p.** Exsanguinate means to remove blood to a point where life cannot be sustained.

5. **d.** Hemochromatosis is an iron storage disorder characterized by excess iron deposits in organs and tissues.

6. **k.** International Classification of Diseases, Ninth Revision, Clinical Modification (ICD-9-CM) is an international coding system used for patient billing purposes that groups similar diseases and operations together.

7. **s.** When the verbal and nonverbal messages of an individual do not match, it is called a kinesic slip. In other words, a kinesic slip is when an individual says one thing but his or her body language conveys something else.

8. **l.** Kinesics involves nonverbal communication or body language.

9. **h.** Medicaid is a federal and state program that provides medical care to the poor.

10. **f.** Medicare is an entitlement program that provides healthcare to people age 65 and older.

11. **q.** Phlebotomy is the term used for the process of removing blood from a vein.

12. **e.** Polycythemia is a disorder involving the overproduction of red blood cells.

13. **m.** Proxemics involves the concept and use of space.

14. **r.** TAT stands for turnaround time and refers to the time from when a test is ordered until the results are reported to the physician.

15. **j.** Tertiary care refers to highly complex or specialized medical services.

16. **a.** ASCP is one of five national organizations that certifies phlebotomists. Certification is a process that indicates the completion of defined academic and training requirements and the attainment of a satisfactory score on a national examination.

17. **b.** A phlebotomist has many duties, but the primary one is to collect a quality blood specimen.

18. **d.** All of the above are correct because as a "public relations officer," everything the phlebotomist does reflects on the whole facility.

19. **a.** The primary objective in any healthcare professional's code of ethics must always be the patient's welfare: "first do no harm."

20. **c.** Good work ethics include accountability, dependability, and reliability. Liability, defined as an obligation to make good any loss or damage that occurs in a transaction, is invoked when malpractice occurs.

21. **d.** Polycythemia is a condition caused by overproduction of red blood cells, and therapy includes removing some of the blood to bring levels into the normal range.

22. **a.** Continuing education for a health professional should support the growth of knowledge in the increasingly complex field of health-

care. Proof of continuing education is necessary for a phlebotomist to be recertified by the National Credentialing Agency for Laboratory Personnel (NCA). The CDC is not involved in continuing education or recertification.

23. **a.** Literal translation of the word phlebotomy comes from the Greek words *phlebos,* meaning vein, and *tome,* meaning incision or to make an incision (cut) in a vein.

24. **c.** With the advent of multi-skilling in the healthcare field, phlebotomists' duties are expanding; however, starting IVs is not within phlebotomists' scope of practice at this time.

25. **b.** Each certifying agency awards a designated title and initials to phlebotomists who successfully pass the national examination. The National Certification Agency for Medical Laboratory Personnel (NCA) has chosen the initials CLPlb to designate the title of Clinical Laboratory Phlebotomist.

26. **c.** Today's lancet is the modern-day counterpart to the fleam. A typical fleam (Fig. 1-1) had a wide double-edged blade at a right angle to the handle. A fleam was used to slice a vein. The specimen was collected in a "bleeding bowl." A special suction device called a cup was placed on the skin to draw blood to the surface before making an incision with a lancet or fleam.

27. **b.** A number of organizations sponsor workshops and seminars to enable phlebotomists and other healthcare workers to earn credit required to renew their license or certification. Credits (in the form of certificates)

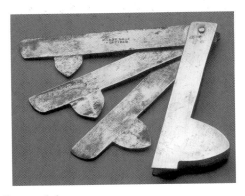

■ FIGURE 1-1 ■

Typical fleams. (Courtesy Robert Kravetz, MD, Chairman, Archives Committee, American College of Gastroenterology.)

awarded on completion of these events are called continuing education units (CEUs). Copies of these certificates can be sent to certifying agencies as "proof of continuing education."

28. **d.** According to the Patient's Bill of Rights, a medical institution has a responsibility to recognize certain established rights of a patient. These rights include the right to an explanation of the bill, confidentiality of records, and the ability to refuse treatment. A patient does not, however, have the right to know the medical status of another patient.

29. **b.** The "zone of comfort" varies with each individual, depending largely on how well the intruder is known and other circumstances surrounding the intrusion. For the average individual, intimate distance is a radius of 1–18 inches, personal distance is 1.5–4 feet, social distance is 4–12 feet, and public distance is a radius of more than 12 feet.

30. d. All of the examples can be barriers to communication and require special communication techniques for effective exchange of information to occur.

31. c. Confirming responses help a patient feel recognized as an individual and not a number. "I understand how you must be feeling" is a response that communicates an effort on your part to view the patient as an individual and empathize with his or her situation.

32. b. Kinesics is the study of nonverbal communication or body language. Frowning is an example of negative kinesics or body language. Eye contact, good grooming, and smiling are all examples of positive body language.

33. d. A neat, clean appearance plays a big part in presenting a professional image. A clean, pressed laboratory coat, short clean fingernails, and long hair pulled back also contribute to presenting a professional image. Wearing strong cologne is offensive to some people, especially those who are ill or allergic to perfume, and may interfere with their perceiving the individual who wears it as being professional.

34. d. Acting knowledgeably, conveying sincerity, and presenting a professional appearance are all part of portraying a professional image that earns a patient's confidence or trust.

35. c. Hanging up on an angry caller does nothing to diffuse the situation and may make it worse. Confirming responses are more apt to calm the caller and allow the problem or situation to be resolved.

36. d. "Zone of comfort" is an example of proxemics. It is a phrase used to describe the invisible "bubble" or range of personal territory that surrounds each of us. When another individual enters this personal territory, we may feel threatened.

37. c. Communication between the healthcare professional and the patient is complicated and involves the basic elements of empathy, control, and confirmation. Distrust can play a part in healthcare communication but is not a desirable element of communication.

38. a. A hospital is one of the few places where an individual gives up control over most of the personal tasks he or she normally performs. Because of this loss of control, the patient may respond by getting angry and is then characterized as a "difficult" or "bad" patient. The best approach is to help the patient feel in control of the situation.

39. b. Proxemics is the study of an individual's concept and use of space. To better relate to the patient in a healthcare setting, it is important to understand this subtle part of nonverbal communication.

40. a. Feeling in control is essential to a patient's well-being. Informing, insisting, and telling are all actions that may cause the patient to feel as if he or she has no control over the situation. Allowing the patient the right to either agree to or refuse a procedure allows the patient to exercise control over the situation and generally makes for a more agreeable patient.

41. b. The average speaking rate of an adult is 125–150 words per minute. Because the average person absorbs verbal messages at 500–600 words per minute (which is approximately 5 times the speaking rate), the listener must make an effort to stay actively involved in what the speaker is saying to communicate effectively.

42. a. The term "outpatient care" is synonymous with "ambulatory care." Ambulatory or outpatient care is offered to those who are able to come to the facility for care and go home the same day. Nonambulatory care is found in tertiary facilities where patients must stay over one or more nights. Nursing home or rehabilitation care is considered nonambulatory for the reasons stated above.

43. b. The hematology department identifies abnormalities of the blood by analyzing whole blood specimens in automated instruments (Fig. 1-2).

44. d. The respiratory therapy department is responsible for administering oxygen therapy.

45. c. A frozen section is a test performed by a pathologist in the surgical pathology department. Tissue re-

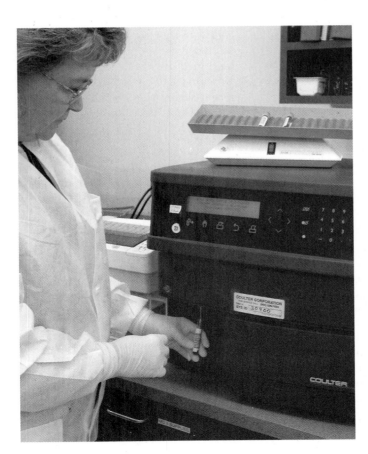

■ Figure 1-2 ■
Coulter MAXM automated hematology analyzer.

moved during surgery is quickly frozen, and a thin slice of the specimen is microscopically examined for abnormalities while the patient is still under anesthesia. Results of the frozen section analysis determine what further action is to be taken by the surgeon.

46. **b.** Nephrology means study of the kidneys. A patient being treated in the nephrology department is most likely being treated for a disorder associated with the kidneys.

47. **d.** "Oto" means *ear*, "rhino" means *nose*, and the "larynx" is a structure in the throat. The otorhinolaryngology department treats disorders of the ear, nose, and throat. Skin disorders are treated in the dermatology department. Eye problems are treated in the ophthalmology department, and bone and joint disorders are treated in the orthopedics department.

48. **d.** A prothrombin time (protime or PT) is performed in the coagulation department. It is most commonly performed to monitor the effects of anticoagulant drugs such as coumarin on the coagulation process. BUN and glucose tests are performed in the chemistry department. A CBC is performed in the hematology department.

49. **b.** The word "onco" means *tumor*, and the suffix "ology" denotes *the study of*. The term oncology is used to describe the medical specialty that treats patients with tumors. Geriatrics is the branch of medicine that deals with problems of aging. Ophthalmology deals with eye disorders, and orthopedics deals with musculoskeletal system disorders.

50. **c.** The term orthopedics is used to describe the medical specialty that treats disorders of the musculoskeletal system. Gastroenterology is the specialty that treats disorders of the digestive tract and related structures; neurology is the specialty that treats disorders of the brain, spinal cord, and nerves; and pediatrics is the specialty that treats children from birth to adolescence.

51. **b.** A neonate is a newborn up to the age of 1 month. A neonatologist is a physician who specializes in the study, treatment, and care of newborns. A gerontologist specializes in disorders related to ageing; an obstetrician/gynecologist specializes in pregnancy, childbirth, and treatment of disorders of the reproductive system; and a pediatrician treats children from birth to adolescence.

52. **a.** The blood bank department is sometimes called immunohematology. Immunology is another name for the serology department. An earlier name for the microbiology department was bacteriology.

53. **a.** Glycosylated hemoglobin is a chemistry test. Glycosylated hemoglobin is formed when glucose and hemoglobin combine. The most common glycosylated hemoglobin is hemoglobin A_{1c}.

54. **d.** A cerebrospinal fluid (CSF) analysis involves several different departments. Chemistry tests performed on CSF include glucose and protein analysis. Cell counts on CSF are performed in hematology, and culture and sensitivity testing on CSF is performed in microbiology. In addition, syphilis testing may be performed on CSF in the serology/immunology department.

55. b. Therapeutic drug monitoring is a team effort and requires cooperation between nursing, pharmacy, and the laboratory for quality results.

56. c. The histology department prepares tissue samples for microscopic examination by a pathologist.

57. c. A phlebotomist does not have to have a college degree and may not even be required to show any type of certification or proof of training to practice. A few states require licensing of phlebotomists, and many employers require their phlebotomists to be nationally certified. To become nationally certified, a phlebotomist must have a high school diploma or GED and have completed a formal, structured phlebotomy program or have a minimum of 1 year of full-time experience as a phlebotomist. A clinical laboratory scientist and a medical technologist are required to have a bachelor's degree either in medical technology or a chemical or biological science.

58. c. An appendectomy performed in an ambulatory surgical center is an example of secondary care. Managed care is a system of healthcare delivery and financing that involves primary, secondary, and tertiary care. Primary care involves initial consultation and treatment by a family physician or other caregiver. Tertiary care involves highly complex or specialized services delivered primarily in inpatient facilities to patients who stay overnight.

59. b. Blood cultures, performed in the microbiology department, are blood specimens collected in special nutrient substance or media designed to encourage the growth of microorganisms that might be present in a patient's blood stream. The process is often automated using a special system such as the BactALERT 3D system (Fig. 1-3).

60. d. Sodium and potassium are both electrolytes. They can be ordered as individual tests or as part of an electrolyte panel. A common electrolyte panel includes sodium, potassium, chloride, and bicarbonate (commonly measured as carbon dioxide [CO_2]).

61. a. ECG (formerly EKG) is used as an abbreviation for both the cardiodiagnostic department and the most common test performed by this department, an electrocardiogram. EEG is an abbreviation used for both the electroneurodiagnostic technology (ENT) department—also

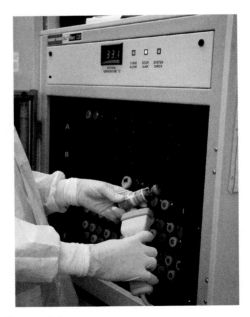

■ FIGURE 1-3 ■

Microbiologist reviews blood cultures processed by the BactALERT 3D.

called the electroencephalography (EEG) department—and its most common test, the electroencephalogram. The emergency room (ER or emergency department) initially deals with emergency situations involving all types of patients, not just heart patients. ICU stands for intensive care unit, which delivers specialized care for critically ill patients.

62. **a.** A BMP is a term used for one of the Health Care Financing Administration (HCFA)-approved disease and organ-specific panels that evaluate the functioning of various body systems. It includes glucose, blood urea nitrogen (BUN), creatinine, sodium, potassium, chloride, carbon dioxide (CO_2), and calcium. These tests are all performed in the chemistry department.

63. **c.** The cytogenetics department performs chromosome studies; however, not all laboratories have a cytogenetics department, in which case these studies are sent to a reference laboratory.

64. **a.** Cytology is the study of the formation, structure, and function of cells. The cells in body fluids and tissues are analyzed in the cytology department to detect signs of cancer. The Pap smear test is named after a cytology staining technique used to detect cancerous cells in specimens obtained from the cervix in the vagina.

65. **b.** An HMO charges members a flat fee for a complete package of healthcare services. The fee is normally paid by the member on a monthly basis and is paid regardless of whether the services are used. An additional fee, called a co-payment, is charged at the time services are used. The amount of the co-payment depends on the type of service chosen.

66. **d.** There are three basic levels of care offered in the United States: primary (basic) care through the physician, secondary (specialist) care offered on an outpatient basis, and tertiary (highly sophisticated and complex) care requiring a stay in an inpatient facility. The term managed care refers to efficient, cost-effective methods of care and applies to all three levels of care offered.

67. **c.** Obstetrics is the medical specialty that includes treating women throughout pregnancy and childbirth. This specialty also treats disorders of the female reproductive system and menopause.

68. **d.** The radiation therapy department uses ionizing radiation in the treatment of malignant tumors. The respiratory department administers oxygen therapy. Brain wave mapping and polysomnography are functions of the electroneurodiagnostic technology (ENT or EEG) department. X-ray imaging is performed in the x-ray department.

69. **a.** Toxicology is a subsection of the chemistry department. Toxicology tests determine the presence of poisons or toxic substances in blood or urine specimens.

70. **d.** A pathologist is a physician who specializes in diagnosing disease from abnormal changes detected in blood, body fluid, and tissue specimens.

71. **c.** A complete blood count (CBC) is the most common test performed in

the hematology department. Culture & sensitivity (C&S) is performed in the microbiology department. Cerebrospinal fluid (CSF) is analyzed in several different departments. A basic metabolic panel is a disease and organ-specific diagnostic test that is performed in the automated chemistry area of the laboratory.

72. b. Nuclear medicine uses radioactive substances such as dyes in procedures used to diagnose certain medical conditions. The radioactive substances are usually injected into the body and may interfere with tests on specimens collected while they are still in the body.

73. a. CEA is a substance released during malignant tumor growth and is classified as a "tumor marker." It was first associated with cancer of the colon. Because CEA levels increase in other types of cancer and some nonmalignant conditions, it is no longer considered specific for colon cancer. Monitoring CEA levels is, however, considered a useful tool in the treatment and management of certain cancers. CEA levels are performed in the chemistry department.

74. c. X-ray procedures and other imaging techniques are functions of the radiology department. Occupational therapy assists mentally, physically, or emotionally disabled patients in maintaining daily living skills. Pharmacy prepares and dispenses drugs, provides advice on selection and side effects of drugs, and helps coordinate therapeutic drug monitoring. Respiratory therapy aids in the diagnosis, treatment, and management of lung deficiencies.

75. c. There are two main types of healthcare facilities: inpatient and outpatient. An inpatient facility is designed for patients who stay overnight. A hospital is primarily an inpatient facility. Outpatient facilities are places where patients receive treatment and go home the same day. Physician's or dentist's offices and day-surgery centers are examples of outpatient facilities.

76. d. RPR is a common serology test used in the diagnosis of syphilis. BUN is a chemistry test. CBC is a hematology test. PT is a coagulation test.

77. b. Both the medical technologist (MT) and the clinical laboratory scientist (CLS) have the same qualifications, including a bachelor's degree in medical technology or a chemical or biological science. The title depends on which national certification examination was passed. A clinical laboratory technician (CLT) and medical laboratory technician (MLT) are both required to have a minimum of a 2-year associate's degree or equivalent. A pathologist is a physician with a specialty in laboratory diagnosis.

78. b. A hemogram is a hematology test. It is the name given to the graph or printed results of complete blood cell count (CBC) on an automated blood cell counter. It generally includes the major components of a CBC except a manual differential.

79. d. The urinalysis department performs urinalysis testing, a routine examination of urine that includes a microscopic examination of urine sediment for the presence of blood cells, bacteria, crystals, and other substances.

80. **b.** The physical therapy department provides many types of assistance to the patient who has physical handicaps, including therapy to restore mobility. The cardiodiagnostics department provides diagnosis, monitoring, and therapy for patients with cardiovascular problems. The radiology department diagnoses medical conditions using x-rays and other imaging techniques. The respiratory therapy department provides testing, therapy, and monitoring of patients with respiratory disease.

81. **b.** The electroencephalography (EEG) or electroneurodiagnostic technology (ENT) department performs evoked potentials testing to determine muscle function and brain wave mapping to diagnose and monitor neurologic disorders. ECG (formerly EKG) is the abbreviation used for an electrocardiogram and also the cardiodiagnostic department where electrocardiograms are performed. The occupational therapy (OT) department assists mentally, physically, or emotionally disabled patients in maintaining daily living skills. The respiratory therapy (RT) department provides testing, therapy, and monitoring of patients with respiratory disease.

82. **c.** The primary objectives of managed care are cost containment, more efficient management of patient care while maintaining quality care, and keeping costs down. Increasing revenue from services offered is not an objective.

83. **d.** A patient care technician (PCT) is a certified nursing assistant (CNA) with additional specialized patient care skills and phlebotomy skills.

An ADN is an associate's degree nurse. An EMT is also a multi-skilled person, but one who functions at an emergency level only.

84. **a.** A clinical laboratory scientist (CLS) and a medical technologist (MT) are required to have a bachelor's degree in medical technology or a chemical or biological science. A clinical laboratory technician (CLT) and a medical laboratory technician (MLT) normally have an associate's degree from a 2-year college or equivalent, or certification from a military or proprietary (private) college. A phlebotomist certified through the ASCP Board of Registry is called a phlebotomy technician (PBT) and has a high school diploma or GED as a minimum.

85. **b.** A clinical laboratory technician (CLT) and a medical laboratory technician (MLT) normally have an associate's degree from a 2-year college or equivalent, or certification from a military or proprietary (private) college. A clinical laboratory scientist (CLS) and a medical technologist (MT) are required to have a bachelor's degree in medical technology or a chemical or biological science. A phlebotomist may not be required to have any formal education or certification. However, to apply for certification a phlebotomist is typically required to have a high school diploma or GED as a minimum.

86. **c.** A subsection of the microbiology department is parasitology, where stool specimens are carefully examined for the presence of parasites or their eggs (ova).

87. **b.** The process used to identify microorganisms and determine the ap-

propriate antibiotic for treatment is called culture and sensitivity (C&S) testing.

88. d. Culture and sensitivity (C&S) testing is performed in the microbiology department.

89. a. The chemistry department performs tests to evaluate certain analytes such as glucose dissolved in the blood. Glucose levels are evaluated to diagnose or monitor diabetes.

90. b. The word root "hem" means *blood*, and the suffix "ology" denotes *the study of*. Hematology is the medical specialty that treats patients with blood disorders. Dermatology is the medical specialty that treats skin disorders. Internal medicine treats disorders of the internal organs and general medical conditions. Urology treats disorders of the urinary tract and male reproductive organs.

91. c. Public health agencies take care of large-scale healthcare problems at the federal, state, and local levels. Their designated services are to be used by the entire population of an area and include diabetes screening, insect control, and sanitation inspections. Licensure of personnel is not part of public health service responsibilities.

92. a. Blood typing and compatibility testing are performed in the blood bank department, which is sometimes called immunohematology.

93. c. FDP, also called fibrin split products (FSP), are the end-products of the breakdown of fibrin formed during the coagulation process. The test is performed in the coagulation department and is most commonly ordered to diagnose disseminated intravascular coagulation (DIC).

94. a. The antistreptolysin O (ASO) test is performed to demonstrate the presence of antibodies formed in response to an infection from streptococcus bacteria. A monospot test detects mononucleosis. RA is a rheumatoid arthritis test. Rapid plasma reagin (RPR) is a syphilis test.

95. b. Medicaid is a state-based, federal program that provides medical care for the poor. Homecare services provide medical care to patients in their homes. Medicare provides medical care to patients age 65 and older, and Workers' Compensation provides benefits to individuals who have been injured on the job.

96. d. The urinalysis department performs chemical screening tests on urine specimens as part of a urinalysis test. Chemical screening involves dipping a special strip (dipstick) into the urine. The dipstick contains special pads impregnated with chemical reagents that detect the presence of substances in the urine, such as blood cells, glucose, and protein.

97. b. An erythrocyte sedimentation rate is a whole blood test that is performed in the hematology department.

98. d. The medical specialty rheumatology is involved in the diagnosis and treatment of diseases characterized by joint inflammation. Dermatology involves the treatment of skin disorders. Gastroenterology involves the treatment of disorders of the digestive tract and related structures. Internal medicine involves the treatment of disorders of the internal organs and general medical conditions.

99. **a.** blood bank
100. **a.** blood bank
101. **b.** chemistry
102. **b.** chemistry
103. **e.** microbiology
104. **b.** chemistry
105. **b.** chemistry
106. **d.** hematology
107. **f.** serology
108. **d.** hematology
109. **c.** coagulation
110. **d.** hematology
111. **f.** serology
112. **g.** urinalysis
113. **d.** hematology
114. **g.** neurology
115. **j.** otolaryngology
116. **h.** ophthalmology

117. **a.** cardiology
118. **k.** urology
119. **f.** gynecology
120. **i.** orthopedics
121. **b.** dermatology
122. **d.** gastroenterology
123. **c.** endocrinology
124. **f.** hematology
125. **j.** rheumatology
126. **b.** endocrinology
127. **i.** orthopedics
128. **e.** gynecology
129. **c.** gerontology
130. **a.** dermatology
131. **g.** neurology
132. **h.** oncology
133. **k.** urology

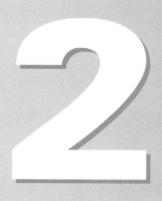

QUALITY ASSURANCE AND LEGAL ISSUES

A. Quality Assurance in Healthcare
1. National Standards and Regulatory Agencies
   a. Joint Commission on Accreditation of Healthcare Organizations
   b. College of American Pathologists
   c. Clinical Laboratory Improvement Amendments of 1988
   d. National Committee for Clinical Laboratory Standards
   e. National Accrediting Agency for Clinical Laboratory Sciences
2. Quality Improvement
3. Quality Assurance in Phlebotomy
   a. QA Defined
   b. QA Indicators
   c. Thresholds and Data
   d. Process and Outcomes
   e. QC Defined
4. Areas of Phlebotomy Subject to QC
   a Patient Preparation Procedures
   b. Specimen Collection Procedures
      1) Identification
      2) Equipment
         a) Puncture devices
         b) Evacuated tubes
      3) Labeling
      4) Technique
      5) Collection Priorities
      6) Delta Checks

5. Documentation
   a. Medical Record
   b. The User Manual
   c. Procedure Manual
   d. QA Forms
      1) Equipment Check Forms
      2) Internal Reports

B. Legal Issues
1. Divisions of the Law
   a. Criminal Law
   b. Civil Law
      1) Tort
         a) Assault
         b) Battery
         c) Fraud
         d) Invasion of privacy
         e) Breach of confidentiality
         f) Negligence
         g) Malpractice
      2) Standard of Care
      3) Respondeat Superior
      4) Vicarious Liability
      5) Malpractice Insurance
      6) Statute of Limitations
      7) Avoiding Lawsuits
2. Patient Consent
   a. Informed Consent
   b. Expressed Consent
   c. Implied Consent
   d. HIV Consent

e. Consent for Minors
f. Refusal of Consent
3. The Litigation Process
4. Risk Management
5. Patient Safety and Sentinel Events
6. Legal Cases Involving Phlebotomy Procedures
   a. A Negligence Case Settled Through Binding Arbitration

b. Jones Versus Rapids General Hospital
c. Congelton Versus Baton Rouge General Hospital
d. Montgomery Versus Opelousas General Hospital
e. Martin Versus Wentworth-Douglass Hospital

REVIEW QUESTIONS

Match the term with the BEST description.

1. ____ assault
2. ____ competencies
3. ____ civil action
4. ____ defendant
5. ____ delta check
6. ____ deposition
7. ____ implied consent
8. ____ malpractice
9. ____ negligence
10. ____ plaintiff
11. ____ proficiency testing
12. ____ QA indicator
13. ____ Respondeat superior
14. ____ threshold value
15. ____ tort
16. ____ vicarious liability

a. a civil wrong without just cause
b. actions indicate consent
c. compares current results with previous ones
d. concerned with actions between private parties
e. concerned with felonies and misdemeanors
f. educational standards for program accreditation
g. educational standards for program approval
h. employers are liable for actions of employees
i. employers are liable for actions of their subcontractors
j. failure to act in a reasonable and prudent manner
k. harmful or offensive touching without consent
l. injured party bringing a lawsuit
m. involves testing sample unknowns
n. involves the act or threat of harm
o. level of acceptable practice
p. monitors an important aspect of patient care
q. negligence by a professional
r. person against whom a lawsuit is filed
s. process in which an individual is questioned under oath
t. tests the efficiency of employees

Choose the BEST answer.

17. The abbreviation for an agency that has an approval process for phlebotomy programs is the:
    a. JCAHO.
    b. NAACLS.
    c. NCA.
    d. NCCLS.

18. Dr. W. Edwards Deming is famous for being a leader in:
    a. advancing the concept of total quality management (TQM).
    b. authoring the "Dimensions of Performance."
    c. describing the benefits of delta checks in patient testing.
    d. identifying the need for proficiency testing by laboratories.

19. The abbreviation for a national organization that established quality standards to ensure the accuracy, reliability, and timeliness of patient test results, regardless of the size, type, or location of the laboratory.
    a. BBP Standard
    b. CLIA
    c. CLIA '88
    d. OSHA

20. The abbreviation for an agency that sets standards for phlebotomy procedures.
    a. ASCP
    b. NAACLS
    c. NCA
    d. NCCLS

21. Areas of phlebotomy subject to quality control (QC) procedures include:
    a. patient identification.
    b. phlebotomy technique.
    c. specimen labeling.
    d. all of the above

22. A lab technician asked a phlebotomist to recollect a specimen on a patient. When the phlebotomist asked what was wrong with the specimen, the technician replied, "The specimen was OK, but the results were inconsistent." How would the laboratory technician have decided that the results were inconsistent?
    a. They did not compare with results of other patients tested at the same time.
    b. They did not compare with the results of control specimens.
    c. They did not compare with previous results when a delta check was conducted.
    d. All of the above

23. Which organization provides voluntary laboratory inspections and proficiency testing?
    a. College of American Pathologists (CAP)
    b. Joint Commission on Accreditation of Healthcare Organizations (JCAHO)
    c. National Certification Agency for Medical Laboratory Personnel (NCA)
    d. Occupational Safety and Health Administration (OSHA)

24. Quality control protocols prohibit use of outdated evacuated tubes because:
    a. additives that prevent clotting may no longer work.
    b. specimens collected in these tubes may yield erroneous results.
    c. the tubes may not fill completely.
    d. all of the above

25. All of the following are principles of total quality management EXCEPT:
    a. constant improvement
    b. customer satisfaction
    c. employee participation
    d. reduction in staff

26. All of the following are examples of quality control EXCEPT:
   a. check expiration dates of evacuated tubes.
   b. document maintenance on centrifuge.
   c. record refrigerator temperature daily.
   d. fill out your time sheet daily.

27. When the threshold value of a clinical indicator of quality assurance (QA) is exceeded and a problem is identified:
   a. a corrective action plan is implemented.
   b. an incident report must be filed.
   c. patient specimens must always be redrawn.
   d. the patient's physician must be notified.

28. All of the following represent a quality assurance (QA) procedure EXCEPT:
   a. checking needles for blunt tips and barbs
   b. following strict specimen labeling requirements
   c. recording results of refrigerator temperature checks
   d. keeping a record of employee sick leave

29. Which pre-analytical factor that can affect validity of test results is not always under the phlebotomist's control?
   a. patient preparation
   b. patient identification
   c. specimen collection
   d. specimen handling

30. Which of the following contains a chronologic record of a patient's care?
   a. delta check
   b. medical record
   c. specimen label
   d. user manual

31. The abbreviation for the agency that requires healthcare organizations to have a quality assurance (QA) program in place to be accredited is the:
   a. CAP.
   b. JCAHO.
   c. NCCLS.
   d. OSHA.

32. A specimen was mislabeled on the floor. You are required to fill out an incident report form. All of the following information would be included EXCEPT:
   a. description of the consequence
   b. details of the corrective action taken
   c. explanation of the problem
   d. suggestion for new guidelines

33. An example of a quality assurance (QA) indicator is:
   a. all phlebotomists will follow universal precautions.
   b. laboratory personnel will not wear laboratory coats when on break.
   c. no eating, drinking, or smoking are allowed in laboratory work areas.
   d. the contamination rate for blood cultures will not exceed the national contamination rate.

34. What laboratory document describes in detail the steps to follow for specimen collection?
   a. OSHA safety manual
   b. policy guidelines
   c. quality control procedures
   d. procedure manual/floor book

35. Drawing a patient's blood without his or her permission can result in a charge of:
   a. assault and battery.
   b. breach of confidentiality.
   c. malpractice.
   d. negligence.

36. What does the term "tort" mean?
    a. a criminal action
    b. a wrongful act for which damages may be awarded
    c. monetary awards for injustices
    d. personal injury or malpractice

37. All of the following are steps in the risk management process EXCEPT:
    a. breach of confidentiality
    b. education of employees and patients
    c. identification of risk
    d. treatment of risk using procedures already in place

38. All of the following would violate a patient's right to confidentiality EXCEPT:
    a. indicating the nature of a patient's disease on the door
    b. keeping a list of HIV-positive patients posted in the laboratory
    c. posting a patient's laboratory results on a bulletin board in his or her room
    d. sharing collection site information on a patient from whom it is difficult to draw blood

39. Unauthorized release of confidential patient information is called:
    a. assault.
    b. invasion of privacy.
    c. negligence.
    d. violation of informed consent.

40. Civil actions involve:
    a. actions between private parties.
    b. crimes against the state.
    c. laws established by governments.
    d. offenses for which a person may be imprisoned.

41. Malpractice is a claim of:
    a. battery.
    b. breach of confidentiality.
    c. improper treatment.
    d. invasion of privacy.

42. All of the following are examples of negligence EXCEPT:
    a. The phlebotomist does not return a bedrail to the upright position.
    b. The phlebotomist forgets to put a needle in the sharps container.
    c. The phlebotomist fails to report significant changes in a patient's condition.
    d. The phlebotomist fails to obtain a specimen from a combative patient.

43. A patient is told that she must remain still during blood collection or she will be restrained. Which tort is involved in this example?
    a. assault
    b. battery
    c. fraud
    d. malpractice

44. A patient agrees to undergo treatment after the method, risks, and consequences are explained to him. This is an example of:
    a. implied consent.
    b. informed consent.
    c. Respondeat superior.
    d. standard of care.

45. The period within which an injured party may file a lawsuit is know as:
    a. Respondeat superior.
    b. standard of care.
    c. statute of limitations.
    d. tort interval.

46. The definition of a minor is anyone:
    a. younger than 18 years of age.
    b. younger than 21 years of age.
    c. who has not reached the age of majority.
    d. who is not self-supporting.

47. Performing one's duties in the same manner as any other reasonable and prudent person with the same experience and training is referred to as:
    a. risk management.
    b. the statute of limitations.
    c. the standard of care.
    d. vicarious liability.

48. Doing something that a reasonable and prudent person would not do, or failing to do something that a reasonable and prudent person would do is:
    a. battery.
    b. breach of confidentiality.
    c. fraud.
    d. negligence.

49. A phlebotomist explains to an inpatient that he has come to collect a blood specimen. The patient extends his arm and pushes up his sleeve. This is an example of:
    a. expressed consent.
    b. refusal of consent.
    c. implied consent.
    d. informed consent.

50. A 12-year-old inpatient who refused to have his blood collected was restrained by a healthcare worker while the phlebotomist collected the specimen. This is an example of:
    a. assault and battery.
    b. malpractice.

    c. negligence.
    d. implied consent.

51. The standard of care used in phlebotomy malpractice cases is often based on guidelines from this organization.
    a. Joint Commission on Accreditation of Healthcare Organizations (JCAHO)
    b. College of American Pathologists (CAP)
    c. National Accrediting Agency for Clinical Laboratory Sciences (NAACLS)
    d. National Committee for Clinical Laboratory Standards (NCCLS)

52. Which of the following must be present to claim negligence?
    a. a breaking of a legal duty or obligation owed by one person to another
    b. a legal duty or obligation owed by one person to another
    c. harm done as a result of breach of duty
    d. all of the above

53. The process of gathering information by taking statements and interrogating parties involved in a lawsuit is called:
    a. collaboration.
    b. deposition.
    c. discovery.
    d. litigation.

ANSWERS AND EXPLANATIONS

1. **n.** involves the act or threat of harm
2. **g.** educational standards for program approval
3. **d.** concerned with actions between private parties
4. **r.** person against whom a lawsuit is filed
5. **c.** compares current results with previous ones
6. **s.** process in which an individual is questioned under oath
7. **b.** actions indicate consent
8. **q.** negligence by a professional
9. **j.** failure to act in a reasonable and prudent manner
10. **l.** injured party bringing a lawsuit
11. **m.** involves testing sample unknowns
12. **p.** monitors an important aspect of patient care
13. **h.** employers are liable for actions of employees
14. **o.** level of acceptable practice
15. **a.** a civil wrong without just cause
16. **i.** employers are liable for actions of their subcontractors
17. **b.** The National Accrediting Agency for Clinical Laboratory Sciences (NAACLS) is one of the agencies that approve phlebotomy programs. The Joint Commission on Accreditation of Healthcare Organizations (JCAHO) accredits healthcare organizations. The National Credentialing Agency for Laboratory Personnel (NCA) has a certification process for laboratory personnel. The National Committee for Clinical Laboratory Standards (NCCLS) develops guidelines for laboratory procedures.
18. **a.** Dr. W. Edwards Deming was a leader in advancing the concept of TQM. The "Dimensions of Performance" were developed by the JCAHO. Deming TQI concepts had to do with business management;

delta checks and proficiency testing are part of laboratory quality assurance.

19. **c.** The Clinical Laboratory Improvement Act (CLIA) was amended in 1988 (CLIA'88). CLIA '88 established quality standards to ensure accuracy, reliability, and timeliness of patient results, regardless of the size, type, or location of the laboratory. OSHA stands for the Occupational Safety and Health Act and also the Occupational Safety and Health Administration. The Bloodborne Pathogen (BBP) Standard was instituted to protect healthcare employees from bloodborne pathogens such as hepatitis B and human immunodeficiency virus.

20. **d.** The NCCLS develops guidelines and sets standards of performance for all areas of the clinical laboratory. These guidelines are often the basis of approval standards and certification examination questions. The ASCP Board of Registry (BOR) certifies laboratory personnel through examination. The NAACLS is one of the agencies that approve phlebotomy programs. The NCA is another organization that has a certification process for laboratory personnel.

21. **d.** Patient identification, phlebotomy technique, and specimen labeling are all areas of phlebotomy that are subject to QC procedures.

22. **c.** Delta checks compare current results of a test with previous results of the same test on the same patient. A patient's test results have no relationship to other patient's results or the results on control specimens.

23. **a.** CAP (College of American Pathologists) is a national organization of

board-certified pathologists that offers laboratory inspection and proficiency testing. JCAHO inspections are not voluntary, and the organization does not provide proficiency testing. The NCA certifies laboratory personnel. OSHA inspections involve safety violations.

24. d. Outdated tubes should never be used. The tube vacuum and the integrity of any additive that might be in the tube are guaranteed by the manufacturer, but only if the tube is used before the expiration date. After that date, the additive may break down and no longer function as intended. In addition, outdated tubes may lose some of the vacuum and no longer fill completely. In either situation, the results may be incorrect or erroneous.

25. d. Total quality management involves four principles: constant improvement, customer satisfaction, employee participation, and orientation to the process. Reduction in staff is not a part of total quality management, although it may be a result.

26. d. Quality control procedures involves checking all the operational procedures to make certain they are performed correctly, such as checking expiration dates, documenting centrifuge maintenance, and recording refrigerator temperature. Filling out your time sheet is important but is not considered a quality control procedure.

27. a. If the threshold of an indicator is exceeded, data are collected and organized to see if there is a problem. If a problem is identified, a corrective action plan is established and implemented.

28. d. QA procedures include checking for needle defects before use, following strict labeling requirements, and recording results of refrigerator temperature checks. Keeping a record of employee sick leave is an important personnel issue but is not a part of QA.

29. a. Preparing a patient for testing is not generally under the control of the phlebotomist. However, it is up to the phlebotomist to determine that preparation procedures have been followed. For example, if a test is ordered to be "fasting," the phlebotomist must check to see that the patient is indeed fasting. The phlebotomist is responsible for proper patient identification, collecting the specimen, and handling it properly after collection until turning it over to the laboratory for testing.

30. b. The medical record is a chronologic record of a patient's care. A delta check is a check to detect errors in testing. A specimen label contains patient information that often includes a medical record number. A user manual gives specimen requirements and collection information.

31. b. The JCAHO requires that healthcare facilities participate in a QA program. The CAP provides a voluntary inspection and proficiency testing program. The NCCLS develops standards and guidelines for laboratory procedures. OSHA regulates employee safety.

32. d. An incident report form (Fig. 2-1) must be filled out when a problem such as a mislabeled specimen occurs. Information on the form must identify the problem, state the consequence, and describe the corrective action. New guidelines are sometimes implemented as a result of an incident but are not included on the incident report form.

Quality Incident Report Form

Date: _____ Time: _____

Name of person filing the report: _____

Relationship to patient: Self _____ Family _____ Friend _____ Advocate _____

Attorney _____ Employee _____ Government _____

Telephone: (___) _____ E-mail: _____

Address: _____ Fax: _____

Provider Information (Where did problem occur?)

Name of organization: _____

Address: _____

_____

Telephone: (___) _____

Type of organization (Provider): Hospital _____ Ambulatory _____ Home Care _____

Laboratory _____ Long Term Care _____ Psychiatric/Behavioral Health _____

Network, PPO, HMO _____

Quality Incident: (Please state your concern) _____

_____

_____

(Attach additional pages, if required. Please keep to no more than two pages.)

Confidentiality required: _____ Yes

Were concerns made known to provider? _____ Yes _____ No

ACTIONS REQUIRED: (Office use only)

Referrals: _____

Quality Analyst: _____ Analyst

Signature: _____

■ FIGURE 2-1 ■

JCAHO incident report form. (Copyright Joint Commission on Accreditation of Healthcare Organizations, 2002. Reprinted with permission.)

QUALITY ASSESSMENT AND IMPROVEMENT TRACKING

CONFIDENTIAL A.R.S. 36-445

#: _____

STANDARD OF CARE/SERVICE: _____

DEPARTMENTS/POPULATION: LABORATORY-MICROBIOLOGY/ALL PATIENTS

IMPORTANT ASPECT OF CARE/SERVICE: LAB SVCS/BLOOD COLLECTION

DATA SOURCE(S): CULTURE WORKCARDS
DATA COLLECTOR: P. BABINA
FREQUENCY REVIEW: 3 MONTHS   100% SAMPLE
METHODOLOGY: RETROSPECTIVE
TYPE: OUTCOME
PERSON RESPONSIBLE FOR:
DATA ORGANIZATION: P. BABINA
ACTION PLAN: J. BENSON
FOLLOW-UP: J. BENSON
DATE MONITOR BEGAN: 1990
FOLLOW-UP: 3RD QTR.

SIGNATURES:
DIRECTOR:
MEDICAL DIRECTOR:
VICE PRESIDENT/ADMINISTRATOR:

INDICATORS	THRESHOLD			CRITICAL ANALYSIS/ EVALUATION	ACTION PLAN
	EXP.	ACT.	PREV.		
Blood culture contamination rate will not exceed 3% from three groups of drawing personnel.	3%			N= 1385 Patient Centered Care draws a Nursing line draws are out of compliance but show improvement from January to March.	A communication has gone out to Nursing reminding to follow established protocols for drawing. Microbiology has implemented new protocol disallowing a line draw unless two consecutive venipunctures have failed or protocol is over-ridden by physician order. PCC tecs have been reinserviced on proper technique.
LAB JAN	3%	1.1%			
FEB		1.8%			
MAR		1.7%			
PCC JAN	3%	5.6%			
FEB		4.8%			
MAR		3.2%			
LINE DRAWS JAN	3%	5.6%			
FEB		7.9%			
MAR		0.0%			

QICONFID

■ FIGURE 2-2 ■
Quality assessment form.

33. **d.** Answers a, b, and c are safety rules. QA indicators are not considered rules but are statements that serve as monitors of patient care. By setting a limit or threshold value, they serve as initiators of action plans (Fig. 2-2).

34. **d.** The laboratory procedure manual is a reference book that describes in detail the step-by-step processes for specimen collection and other procedures performed in the laboratory. A safety manual contains information on safety issues only. A policy manual details management issues, not test collection information. A quality control manual contains procedures and data for the quality control program.

35. **a.** Drawing a person's blood without permission can be perceived as assault, the act or threat of intentionally causing a person to be in fear of harm to his or her person, and battery, the intentional harmful or offensive touching of a person without consent or legal justification. Breach of confidentiality involves failure to keep medical information private or confidential. Malpractice is negligence by a professional. Negligence involves doing something that a reasonable person would not do, or not doing something a reasonable person would do.

36. **b.** A "tort" is a wrongful act resulting in injury for which a civil action can be brought.

37. **a.** Risk management is a process that focuses on identifying and minimizing situations that pose a risk to patients and employees through education and following procedures that are already in place. Breach of confidentiality caused by the unauthorized release of information concerning a patient can lead to the implementation of risk management techniques, but is not one of the designated step in the process.

38. **d.** As a professional, the phlebotomist should recognize that *all* patient information, including disease status and laboratory test results, is absolutely private or confidential. However, letting others know where the best site is to obtain a blood sample on a patient who is a "difficult stick" is part of proper patient care and not considered a violation of patient confidentiality.

39. **b.** Unauthorized release of confidential patient information is called invasion of privacy and can result in a civil lawsuit. Assault involves the act or threat of causing an individual to be in fear of harm. Negligence involves doing something that a reasonable person would not do, or not doing something a reasonable person would do. Failure to get informed consent before a procedure could lead to a claim of assault and battery.

40. **a.** Civil actions involve actions between private parties. The most common civil actions involve tort. For example, a claim of malpractice because of harm or injury to a patient by a phlebotomist is a civil wrong or tort. Crimes against the state or that violate laws established by governments are criminal actions for which a guilty individual may be imprisoned.

41. **c.** Malpractice can be described as improper or negligent treatment resulting in injury, loss, or damage. Battery is the intentional harmful touching of another person without consent or legal justification. Breach of confidentiality involves failure to keep medical information private or confidential. Invasion of

privacy can involve physical intrusion or the unauthorized publishing or releasing of private information.

42. d. Forgetting to return a bedrail to its upright position, failure to discard needles properly (such as dropping them in the trash instead of the sharps container), and not reporting an obvious problem with a patient's condition (such as severe breathing difficulties or inability to awaken) could all lead to serious consequences and are examples of negligence or failure to exercise reasonable care. Failing to obtain a specimen from a patient is not negligence. In addition, collecting a specimen from a combative patient against his or her will could be considered assault and battery.

43. a. Assault involves the act or threat of causing an individual to be in fear of harm. Threatening to restrain the patient can be considered assault. Restraining the patient and collecting a blood specimen can be considered assault and battery. Fraud is a type of deceitful practice or willful plan to produce unlawful gain. Malpractice is negligence by a professional.

44. b. Informed consent implies voluntary and competent permission for a medical procedure, test, or medication and requires that the patient be given adequate information as to the method, risks, and consequences involved before consent is given. In implied consent the patient's actions or condition (as in an emergency situation in which the patient is unconscious) indicate consent rather than a verbal or written statement. Respondeat superior is a term that means employers are responsible for actions of employees. Standard of care is a

level of care that protects clients from harm because it follows established standards of the profession and expectations of society.

45. c. Statute of limitations is the particular number of years within which one party can sue another. Respondeat superior is a term that means employers are responsible for actions of employees. Standard of care is a level of care that protects clients from harm because it follows established standards of the profession and expectations of society. Tort interval is a made up term, not a legal term.

46. c. The definition of a minor is anyone who has not reached the age of majority. The age of majority is determined by state law and normally ranges from 18–21 years of age regardless of whether the individual is self-supporting.

47. c. The standard of care is a level of care that protects clients from harm because it follows established standards of the profession and expectations of society. It requires that duties be performed the same way any other reasonable and prudent person with the same experience and training would perform those duties. Risk management is a process that focuses on identifying and minimizing risks. Statute of limitations is the particular number of years within which one party can sue another. Vicarious liability is a term that means organizations that hire subcontractors are liable for the actions of those subcontractors.

48. d. Negligence involves doing something that a reasonable and prudent person would not do, or not doing something that a reasonable and prudent person would do. Battery is the intentional harmful or offensive touching of another person without consent or legal justification. Breach of confidentiality involves failure to keep medical information private or confidential. Fraud is a type of deceitful practice or willful plan to produce unlawful gain.

49. c. In implied consent the patient's actions or condition (as in an emergency situation in which the patient is unconscious) indicate consent rather than a verbal or written statement. A patient who extends his arm and rolls up his sleeve after being told that the phlebotomist is there to collect a blood specimen is implying consent with his actions. The patient is obviously not refusing consent or he might have pulled his arm away and kept his sleeve down. To be expressed consent, the patient would have to give a written or verbal statement of consent. Implied consent can be informed consent; however, implied consent is the best choice because it is a more specific answer to the situation.

50. a. A 12 year old is not old enough to give consent for a medical procedure such as phlebotomy. A phlebotomist who collects a blood specimen from a minor without permission from a parent risks be-

ing charged with assault and battery. As long as no harm to the patient was involved, this would not be considered negligence or malpractice. The patient refused blood collection so this is in no way implied consent.

51. d. The NCCLS publishes standards for phlebotomy procedures. These national standards are recognized as the legal standard of care for phlebotomy procedures. The JCAHO and CAP set standards for healthcare organizations and laboratories, respectively, but not specifically for phlebotomy procedures. NAACLS approves phlebotomy programs.

52. d. To claim negligence, the following elements must be present: A legal obligation or duty owed by one person to another, a breaking of that duty or obligation, and harm done as a result of that breach of duty.

53. c. The process of gathering information by taking statements and interrogating parties involved in a lawsuit is called discovery. It involves taking depositions (questioning parties under oath). Some collaboration may be involved, but it is not the term used to describe the process. Litigation is the process used to settle disputes. Discovery is part of this process.

3 INFECTION CONTROL, SAFETY, FIRST AID, AND PERSONAL WELLNESS

A. Infection Control
 1. Infection
   a. Communicable Infections
   b. Nosocomial Infections
 2. The Chain of Infection
   a. Components of the Chain of Infection
    1) Source
    2) Modes of Transmission
      a) Contact transmission
      b) Droplet transmission
      c) Airborne transmission
      d) Vector transmission
      e) Vehicle transmission
    3) Susceptible Host
   b. Breaking the Chain of Infection
 3. Infection Control Programs
   a. Employee Screening and Immunization
   b. Evaluation and Treatment
   c. Surveillance
 4. Infection Control Methods
   a. Hand Washing
   b. Protective Attire
    1) Masks, Goggles, Face Shields, and Respirators
    2) Gowns
      a) Putting on/removing gowns
    3) Lab Coats
    4) Gloves
      a) Proper glove removal
    5) Order To Put On and Remove Protective Clothing
   c. Nursery and Neonatal Intensive Care Unit (ICU) Infection Control Technique
 5. Isolation Procedures
   a. Protective or Reverse Isolation
   b. Traditional Isolation Systems
   c. Universal Precautions
   d. Body Substance Isolation
   e. Revised Guideline for Isolation Precautions in Hospitals
    1) Standard Precautions
    2) Transmission-Based Precautions

B. Safety
 1. Biologic Hazards
   a. Biohazard Exposure Routes
    1) Airborne
    2) Ingestion
    3) Nonintact Skin
    4) Percutaneous
    5) Permucosal
   b. Bloodborne Pathogens
    1) HBV and Hepatitis D Virus
      a) Hepatitis B vaccination
      b) HBV exposure hazards
      c) Symptoms of HBV infection
    2) HCV
      a) HCV exposure hazards
      b) Symptoms of HCV infection

3) HIV
    a) HIV exposure hazards
    b) Symptoms of infection
  c. OSHA Bloodborne Pathogens
    Standard
  d. Exposure Control Plan
  e. Occupational Exposure to Bloodborne
    Pathogens
  f. Procedure for Needlesticks and Other
    Exposure Incidents
  g. Decontamination of Surfaces
  h. Blood Spill Clean-Up
  i. Biohazardous Waste Disposal
2. Electrical Safety
  a. Actions to Take if Electrical Shock
    Occurs
3. Fire Safety
  a. Components of Fire
  b. Classes of Fire
  c. Fire Extinguishers
4. Radiation Safety
5. Chemical Safety
  a. OSHA Hazardous Communication
    Standard
    1) HazCom Labeling Requirements

    2) Material Safety Data Sheets
  b. Department of Transportation Labeling
    System
  c. National Fire Protection Association
    Labeling System
  d. Safety Showers and Eye Wash
    Stations
  e. Chemical Spill Procedures
6. First Aid Procedures
  a. External Hemorrhage
  b. Shock
    1) Common Symptoms of Shock
    2) First Aid for Shock
  c. Cardiopulmonary Resuscitation and
    Emergency Cardiovascular Care
    1) International CPR and ECC
      Guidelines 2000
  d. American Heart Association Chain of
    Survival
7. Personal Wellness
  a. Introduction
  b. Personal Hygiene
  c. Proper Nutrition
  d. Rest and Exercise
  e. Back Protection
  f. Stress Management

REVIEW QUESTIONS

Match the term with the BEST description.

1. ____ avulsion
2. ____ biohazard
3. ____ engineering control
4. ____ fomite
5. ____ hepatitis
6. ____ microbe
7. ____ neutropenic
8. ____ nosocomial
9. ____ parenteral
10. ____ percutaneous
11. ____ permucosal
12. ____ systemic
13. ____ vector
14. ____ viability
15. ____ virulence

a. ability to live
b. able to neutralize disease
c. acquired from a parent
d. act of vomiting
e. affects the entire body
f. capable of creating an aerosol
g. degree of pathogenicity
h. device that isolates or removes a BBP
  hazard
i. forceful tearing away of a body part
j. hospital-acquired infection
k. insect, arthropod, or animal that transmits disease
l. liver inflammation
m. low neutrophil count
n. microorganism
o. object that harbors infectious material
p. other than the digestive tract
q. substance harmful to health
r. through mucous membranes
s. through the skin

Choose the BEST answer.

16. Which of the following is proper neonatal intensive care unit blood-drawing procedure?
    a. keep your blood drawing tray as close to the isolette as possible
    b. never awaken an infant to draw blood
    c. use povidone-iodine to clean a skin puncture site
    d. wear mask, gown, and gloves

17. What does the National Fire Protection Association (NFPA) codeword *RACE* mean?
    a. rescue, alarm, confine, extinguish
    b. rescue, activate, cover, extinguish
    c. run, alarm, counter, extinguish
    d. run, activate, confine, escape

18. All of the following statements concerning an employee bloodborne pathogen exposure incident are true EXCEPT:
    a. All exposure incidents should be reported to a supervisor.
    b. An exposed employee should have access to a free confidential medical evaluation.
    c. The exposure should be documented on an incident report form.
    d. The source patient must submit to HIV and HBV testing.

19. When the chain of infection is broken:
    a. an individual becomes immune.
    b. an individual becomes susceptible.
    c. infection is prevented.
    d. infection results.

20. The focus of infection control turned from preventing patient-to-patient transmission to preventing patient-to-personnel transmission with the introduction of this concept.
    a. category-specific isolation
    b. disease-specific isolation

    c. body substance isolation (BSI)
    d. universal precautions (UP)

21. The term used to describe an infection that infects the entire body is:
    a. communicable.
    b. local.
    c. nosocomial.
    d. systemic.

22. Which type of precautions would be used for a patient who has pulmonary tuberculosis?
    a. airborne
    b. droplet
    c. contact
    d. reverse

23. All of the following are recommended by the OSHA Bloodborne Pathogen Standard EXCEPT:
    a. dismissal of HIV-positive workers
    b. hand washing following glove removal
    c. HBV immunization
    d. use of barrier protection devices

24. The abbreviation for the virus that causes acquired immune deficiency syndrome (AIDS) is:
    a. HAV.
    b. HBV.
    c. HCV.
    d. HIV.

25. A person who has recovered from a particular virus and has developed antibodies against that virus is said to be:
    a. a carrier.
    b. immune.
    c. infectious.
    d. susceptible.

26. According to standard first aid procedures, severe external hemorrhage is *best* controlled by:
    a. applying direct pressure and elevation of the extremity.
    b. applying a tourniquet above the affected area.

c. keeping the injured extremity below the level of the heart.

d. raising the victim's head above the level of the injury.

27. The main purpose of an infection control program is to:
    a. determine the source of communicable infections.
    b. isolate infectious patients from other patients.
    c. prevent the spread of infection in the hospital.
    d. protect patients from outside contamination.

28. A pathogen is:
    a. a communicable virus.
    b. a microbe capable of causing disease.
    c. any microorganism anywhere.
    d. normal floral of the skin.

29. All of the following diseases involve a bloodborne pathogen EXCEPT:
    a. AIDS
    b. hepatitis B
    c. syphilis
    d. tuberculosis

30. Proper hand washing procedure involves all of the following EXCEPT:
    a. stand back so that clothing does not touch the sink
    b. wet hands with water before applying soap
    c. wash for at least 15 seconds
    d. turn the faucet off with the towel used to dry your hands

31. An example of a disease requiring droplet isolation is:
    a. pertussis.
    b. rubeola.
    c. respiratory syncytial virus (RSV).
    d. varicella.

32. A Class C fire involves:
    a. combustible metals.
    b. electrical equipment.
    c. flammable liquids.
    d. ordinary combustible materials.

33. Standard precautions should be followed:
    a. if a patient is in isolation.
    b. when a patient is known to be HIV positive.
    c. when a patient is known to have HBV.
    d. with all patients, at all times.

34. HBV vaccination involves:
    a. a dose of vaccine, another 1 month later, and a final dose 6 months later.
    b. a single dose of vaccine that confers lifetime immunity.
    c. three doses of vaccine, each 3 months apart, then yearly doses thereafter.
    d. there is no vaccine for HBV.

35. Objects capable of adhering to infectious material and transmitting disease are called:
    a. fomites.
    b. vectors.
    c. vehicles.
    d. none of the above

36. The "Right to Know" law primarily deals with:
    a. electrical safety.
    b. first aid procedures.
    c. hazardous materials information.
    d. universal precautions.

37. The body organ targeted by HBV is the:
    a. brain.
    b. heart.
    c. liver.
    d. lungs.

38. The two organizations responsible for the latest Guideline for Isolation Precautions in Hospitals are the:
    a. Centers for Disease Control and Prevention (CDC) and Hospital Infection Control Practices Advisory Committee (HICPAC).

b. Centers for Disease Control and Prevention (CDC) and Occupational Safety and Health Administration (OSHA).
c. Hospital Infection Control Practices Advisory Committee (HICPAC) and National Institute for Occupational Safety and Health (NIOSH).
d. National Institute for Occupational Safety and Health (NIOSH) and Joint Commission on Accreditation of Healthcare Organizations (JCAHO).

39. Gloves are worn to:
a. prevent contamination of hands when handling blood or body fluids.
b. reduce the chance of transmitting microorganisms on the hands of personnel to patients during invasive procedures.
c. minimize the possibility of transmitting infectious microorganisms from one patient to another.
d. all of the above

40. The three components of fire referred to as the fire triangle are:
a. combustible material, carbon dioxide, heat.
b. fuel, oxygen, heat.
c. fuel, oxygen, static electricity.
d. vapor, carbon dioxide, energy.

41. Which of the following are means of breaking the chain of infection?
a. hand washing and glove use
b. isolation procedures
c. stress reduction and proper nutrition
d. all of the above

42. Which of the following is a proper electrical safety procedure?
a. handling electrical equipment with wet hands
b. using frayed electrical cords
c. using extension cords when necessary
d. servicing electrical equipment when unplugged

43. Standard precautions apply to all body fluids except:
a. joint fluid.
b. saliva.
c. sweat.
d. urine.

44. The ability of a microorganism to survive on contaminated articles and equipment has to do with its:
a. susceptibility.
b. transmission.
c. viability.
d. virulence.

45. The component that turns the fire triangle into a fire tetrahedron is:
a. a chemical reaction.
b. an increase in temperature.
c. combustible material.
d. heat.

46. Airborne precautions require the phlebotomist to wear:
a. a mask.
b. a gown.
c. eye protection.
d. an N95 respirator.

47. The majority of exposures to HIV in healthcare settings occur:
a. during surgery.
b. from blood transfusion.
c. from needlesticks.
d. when touching patients with AIDS.

48. The most common type of nosocomial infection in the United States is:
a. hepatitis infection.
b. respiratory infection.
c. urinary tract infection.
d. wound infection.

49. Which of the following organizations instituted and enforces the Bloodborne Pathogen Standard?
a. College of American Pathologists (CAP)
b. Centers for Disease Control and Prevention (CDC)

c. Joint Commission on Accreditation of Healthcare Organizations (JCAHO)

d. Occupational Safety and Health Administration (OSHA)

50. All of the following are proper laboratory safety procedures EXCEPT:
    a. secure long hair away from the face
    b. never eat, drink, or apply makeup in the laboratory
    c. wear closed-toe shoes
    d. wear your laboratory coat at all times

51. You accidentally splash a bleach solution in your eyes while preparing it for cleaning purposes. What is the first thing to do?
    a. dry your eyes with a paper towel
    b. flush your eyes with water for a minimum of 15 minutes
    c. proceed to the emergency department as quickly as possible
    d. put 10 to 20 drops of saline in your eyes

52. What is the best way to clean up blood that has dripped on the arm of a phlebotomy chair?
    a. absorb it with a damp cloth and wash the area with soap and water
    b. absorb it with a paper towel or gauze pad and wipe the area with disinfectant
    c. wait for it to dry and then scrape it into a biohazard bag
    d. wipe it up with an alcohol pad using concentric circles

53. An example of employee screening for infection control is:
    a. purified protein derivative (PPD) testing.
    b. hepatitis B vaccination.
    c. measles vaccination.
    d. shot of immune globulin.

54. Which mode of infection transmission occurs from touching contaminated bed linens?

a. direct contact
b. droplet contact
c. indirect contact
d. vehicle contact

55. All of the following can be transmitted through blood transfusion EXCEPT:
    a. diabetes mellitus
    b. hepatitis B virus (HBV)
    c. human immunodeficiency virus (HIV)
    d. syphilis

56. Which of the following is required under the OSHA Bloodborne Pathogen (BBP) Standard?
    a. isolate HIV-positive patients
    b. special labeling for specimens from HIV-positive patients
    c. wear a mask when working with AIDS patients
    d. wear gloves when performing phlebotomy procedures

57. What is the meaning of the symbol W in Figure 3-1?
    a. biohazard
    b. flammable

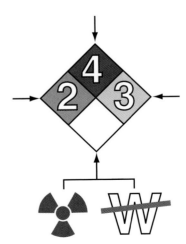

■ FIGURE 3-1 ■

National Fire Protection Association 704 marking system.

c. radiation hazard
d. water reactive

58. What type of isolation would be used for a patient who has a very low white cell count?
a. airborne
b. droplet
c. contact
d. neutropenic

59. What should the phlebotomist do if the outside of a patient specimen tube has blood on it?
a. discard it after pouring the contents into a clean tube
b. discard it in the patient's room and draw a new tube
c. place a biohazard label on it
d. wipe it with disinfectant

60. A laboratory or patient care activity that requires goggles to prevent exposure from sprays or splashes also requires this protective attire.
a. earplugs
b. mask
c. respirator
d. sterile gown

61. Which of the following conditions *would not necessarily* lead to work restrictions for a hospital employee?
a. a positive protein purified derivative (PPD) test
b. influenza
c. rubella
d. weeping dermatitis

62. How many classes of fire are identified by the National Fire Protection Association (NFPA)?
a. two
b. three
c. four
d. six

63. What is the *best* means of preventing nosocomial infection?

a. isolation procedures
b. proper hand washing
c. proper immunization
d. wearing gloves

64. The purpose of "protective" isolation is to:
a. prevent airborne transmission of disease.
b. protect others from patients with transmissible diseases.
c. protect susceptible patients from outside contamination.
d. provide a safe environment for psychiatric patients.

65. Which of the following involves possible exposure to bloodborne pathogens by a "percutaneous" exposure route?
a. getting struck with a contaminated needle
b. handling blood specimens with ungloved, badly chapped hands
c. ingesting infectious material
d. mucous membrane contact with infectious material

66. In which instance could an electrical shock to a patient most likely occur?
a. drawing a patient's blood during an electrical storm
b. drawing a patient's blood while standing in a puddle of water
c. drawing blood from a patient who is talking on the telephone
d. touching electrical equipment while drawing a patient's blood

67. The OSHA Hazardous Communication (HazCom) Standard is also commonly called the:
a. "Disclosure" Law.
b. Material Safety Data Sheets (MSDS) Act.
c. The "Right to Know" Law.
d. United Nations Placard Recognition System.

68. The *best* course of action when entering an isolation room is:
   a. follow the directions on the sign on the door.
   b. wear gown, mask, and gloves.
   c. wear only a gown.
   d. wear only a mask.

69. Which of the following diseases involve a bloodborne pathogen?
   a. influenza
   b. malaria
   c. rubella
   d. strep infection

70. The degree to which an organism is capable of causing disease is called:
   a. chain of infection.
   b. susceptibility.
   c. viability.
   d. virulence.

71. Any material or substance harmful to health is a(n):
   a. biohazard.
   b. chemical hazard.
   c. occupational exposure.
   d. pathogen.

72. What is the proper order for putting on protective clothing?
   a. gloves first, then gown, mask last
   b. gown first, then gloves, mask last
   c. gown first, then mask, gloves last
   d. mask first, then gown, gloves last

73. The blue quadrant of the National Fire Protection Association (NFPA) diamond-shaped symbol for hazardous materials (see Fig. 3-1) indicates:
   a. fire hazard.
   b. health hazard.
   c. reactivity hazard.
   d. specific hazard.

74. Which labeling system uses a diamond-shaped sign containing the United Nations hazard class number and a symbol representing the hazard?

   a. Centers for Disease Control and Prevention (CDC)
   b. Department of Transportation (DOT)
   c. National Fire Protection Association (NFPA)
   d. Occupational Safety and Health Administration (OSHA)

75. All of the following are unacceptable chemical safety procedures EXCEPT:
   a. adding acid to water
   b. familiarizing oneself with the material safety data sheets (MSDS) of a new reagent
   c. mixing bleach with other cleaners
   d. reporting a malfunctioning eye wash station to the proper authority

76. Federal law requires that hepatitis B vaccination be made available to employees assigned to duties with occupational exposure risk:
   a. immediately.
   b. once their probationary employment period has ended.
   c. within 1 month of employment.
   d. within 10 working days of initial assignment.

77. What is the *first* thing the phlebotomist should do in the event of an accidental needlestick?
   a. check the patient's medical records.
   b. decontaminate the site and fill out an incident report.
   c. go to employee health service and get a tetanus booster.
   d. leave the area so that the patient does not notice the injury.

78. All of the following are symptoms of shock EXCEPT:
   a. cold, clammy skin
   b. expressionless face and staring eyes
   c. increased shallow breathing
   d. strong, rapid pulse

79. The main principles involved in radiation exposure are:
   a. exposure time, amount of radiation, and glove thickness
   b. exposure time, distance, and shielding
   c. time of day, amount of radiation, and source
   d. time of day, distance, and eye protection

80. This organization requires healthcare facilities to have an infection control program.
   a. Centers for Disease Control and Prevention (CDC)
   b. Hospital Infection Control Practices Advisory Committee (HICPAC)
   c. Joint Commission on Accreditation of Healthcare Organizations (JCAHO)
   d. National Institute for Occupational Safety and Health (NIOSH)

81. Which of the following is an example of a nosocomial infection?
   a. catheter site of a patient in the intensive care unit becomes infected
   b. healthcare worker contracts hepatitis from a needlestick
   c. patient is admitted with Hantavirus
   d. pediatric patient breaks out with measles the day after admission for a tonsillectomy

82. This organization's regulations supersede those of all other organizations.
   a. College of American Pathologists (CAP)
   b. Centers for Disease Control and Prevention (CDC)
   c. Joint Commission on Accreditation of Healthcare Organizations (JCAHO)
   d. Occupational Safety and Health Administration (OSHA)

83. Which of the following contains regulations requiring the availability of personal protective equipment (PPE) in the medical laboratory?

   a. OSHA Bloodborne Pathogens (BBP) Standard
   b. Clinical Laboratory Improvement Amendments of 1988 (CLIA '88)
   c. Guideline for Isolation Precautions in Hospitals
   d. OSHA Hazardous Communication (HazCom) Standard

84. New American Heart Association recommendations for CPR on adults by laypersons include all the following recommendations EXCEPT:
   a. deletion of the pulse check.
   b. public access to and training in the use of automatic external defibrillators (AEDs).
   c. requiring a blind finger-sweep of the mouth before initiating CPR.
   d. standardizing the ratio of chest compressions to rescue breaths to 15:1 for both one- and two-rescuer CPR.

85. The most frequently occurring laboratory-acquired infection is:
   a. hepatitis A virus (HAV).
   b. hepatitis B virus (HBV).
   c. human immunodeficiency virus (HIV).
   d. tuberculosis (TB).

86. All of the following are requi͟ of an exposure control pla͟
   a. an exposure determ͟
   b. communication o͟
   c. isolation guide͟
   d. methods of ͟

87. Which clas͟ bustible
   a. A
   b. ͟

93. ͟

94. The sub͟ when det͟ firms.

88. Wi͟ patie͟
   a. airbo͟
   b. contact

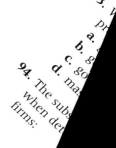

c. droplet
d. standard

89. All of the following are example of possible "parenteral" means of transmission EXCEPT:
   a. drinking contaminated water
   b. getting stuck by a needle used on a patient with AIDS
   c. rubbing the eye with a contaminated hand
   d. touching infectious material with chapped hands

90. All of the following affect a person's general susceptibility to infection EXCEPT:
   a. age
   b. gender
   c. health
   d. immune status

91. An example of vector infection transmission is:
   a. acquiring HIV infection from a blood transfusion.
   b. contracting hepatitis from a contaminated counter top.
   c. contracting plague from the bite of a rodent flea.
   d. contracting tuberculosis transmitted by droplet nuclei.

92. A patient might be placed in protective isolation if he or she has:
   a. chickenpox.
   b. hepatitis.
   c. severe burns.
   d. tuberculosis.

What is the correct order for removing protective clothing?
   gloves, mask, gown
   own, gloves, mask
   wn, mask, gloves
   k, gown, gloves

tance abbreviated as HBsAg
ected in a patient's serum con-

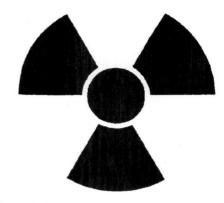

■ FIGURE 3-2 ■
Radiation hazard symbol.

   a. hepatitis A (HAV) infection.
   b. hepatitis B (HBV) immunity.
   c. hepatitis B (HBV) infection.
   d. human immunodeficiency virus (HIV) infection.

95. A radiation hazard symbol (Fig. 3-2) on a patient's door signifies a patient who:
   a. has gone to radiology.
   b. has had many radiographs.
   c. is being treated with radioactive isotopes.
   d. is scheduled to go to radiology.

96. Which of the following is an example of a work practice control that reduces risk of exposure to bloodborne pathogens?
   a. a biohazard symbol
   b. an exposure control plan
   c. hand washing after glove removal
   d. hepatitis B vaccination

97. Universal precautions, the precursor to standard precautions, were introduced by the:
   a. College of American Pathologists (CAP).
   b. Centers for Disease Control and Prevention (CDC).
   c. Joint Commission on Accreditation of Healthcare Organizations (JCAHO).
   d. Occupational Safety and Health Administration (OSHA).

98. Healthcare workers are considered immune to a disease if they have:
   a. a normal white blood cell count.
   b. had the disease.
   c. received gamma globulin within the past year.
   d. all of the above

99. What is the best thing to use to extinguish a flammable liquid fire?
   a. class A extinguisher
   b. class B extinguisher
   c. fire blanket
   d. water

100. Which federal agency instituted and enforces regulations requiring the labeling of hazardous materials?
   a. Centers for Disease Control and Prevention (CDC)
   b. Joint Commission on Accreditation of Healthcare Organizations (JCAHO)
   c. National Fire Protection Association (NFPA)
   d. Occupational Safety and Health Administration (OSHA)

101. Which mode of infection transmission involves transfer of an infective microbe to the mucous membranes of a susceptible individual by means of a cough or sneeze?
   a. contact
   b. droplet
   c. fomite
   d. vehicle

102. All of the following are links (component) in the chain of infection EXCEPT:
   a. means of transmission
   b. source
   c. surveillance
   d. susceptible host

103. The abbreviation for the organization specifically charged with the investigation and control of disease is the:
   a. CDC.
   b. JCAHO.

   c. HICPAC.
   d. OSHA.

104. What is the first action to take to help a victim in shock?
   a. call for help
   b. control bleeding
   c. keep victim lying down
   d. maintain an open airway

105. All of the following are healthy ways to deal with stress EXCEPT:
   a. exercising on a regular basis.
   b. learning how to relax.
   c. making several major life changes.
   d. taking time to plan your day.

106. A nosocomial infection is:
   a. a laboratory-acquired infection.
   b. acquired by a patient while in the hospital.
   c. always communicable.
   d. detected by pre-admission screening tests.

107. The mode of transmission that involves contaminated food, water, drugs, or a blood transfusion is:
   a. airborne.
   b. contact.
   c. vector.
   d. vehicle.

108. A phlebotomist who has b⌐ nosed with strep throat
   a. take antibiotics fo⌐ returning to w⌐
   b. be evaluate⌐ personne⌐
   c. have ⌐ are
   d. v⌐

109.
   ia⌐
   a. f⌐
   b. mos⌐
   c. isopro⌐
   d. isotonic s⌐

110. Which of the following is an example of an engineering control that helps eliminate hazards posed by bloodborne pathogens?
    a. gloves
    b. laboratory coat
    c. sharps container
    d. universal precautions statement

111. Manufacturers are required to supply material safety data sheets (MSDS) for their products by the:
    a. Bloodborne Pathogen Standard.
    b. Centers for Disease Control and Prevention (CDC) regulations.
    c. National Fire Protection Association (NFPA) guidelines.
    d. OSHA Hazardous Communication (HazCom) Standard.

112. What term is used to describe a type of infection that can be spread from person to person?
    a. communicable
    b. nonpathogenic
    c. nosocomial
    d. systemic

113. Which class of fire occurs with flammable liquids?
    a. A
    b. B
    c. C
    d. D

114. The first thing to do in the event of electrical shock to a co-worker or patient is:
    a. call for medical assistance.
    b. keep the victim warm.
    c. shut off the source of electricity.
    d. start CPR.

115. When a pathogen invades the body and causes disease, the result is called a(n):
    a. chain of infection.
    b. communicable disease.
    c. infection.
    d. systemic infection.

ANSWERS AND EXPLANATIONS

1. **i.** forceful tearing away of a body part

2. **q.** substance harmful to health

3. **h.** device that isolates or removes a BBP hazard

4. **o.** object that harbors infectious material

5. **l.** liver inflammation

6. **n.** microorganism

7. **m.** low neutrophil count

8. **j.** hospital-acquired infection

9. **p.** other than the digestive tract

10. **s.** through the skin

11. **r.** through mucous membranes

12. **e.** affects the entire body

13. **k.** insect, arthropod, or animal that transmits disease

14. **a.** ability to live

15. **g.** degree of pathogenicity

16. **d.** Typical proper nursery infection control techniques include wearing a mask, gown, and gloves because neonates in the intensive care unit are more susceptible to infections than older children or adults.

17. **a.** The code word or acronym *RACE* was established by the NFPA as a way to remember the order of action steps in the event of a fire. The "R" stands for *rescue* (step one is to rescue individuals in danger). The "A" stands for *alarm* (step two is to sound the alarm). The "C" stands for *confine* (step three is to confine the fire by closing doors and windows). The "E" stands for *extinguish* (step 4 is to extinguish the fire with the nearest fire extinguisher).

18. **d.** It is not mandatory for the source patient to submit to HIV or HBV testing. The source patient will be asked to submit to testing, and it is hoped that he or she will do so.

19. **c.** The process of infection requires the chain of infection to be complete. If the process is stopped or interrupted by such things as wearing gloves, immunization of susceptible individuals, or instituting isolation procedures, the chain is broken and infection will be prevented.

20. **d.** The concept that the blood and certain body fluids of all patients were potentially infectious for blood-borne pathogens originated with the introduction of universal precautions by the CDC. This concept changed the focus of infection control from prevention of patient-to-patient transmission to prevention of patient-to-personnel transmission. Category-specific and disease-specific precautions focused on patient-to-patient transmission. BSI focused on patient-to-personnel transmission, but came after UP.

21. **d.** Systemic means "pertaining to a whole body rather than one of its parts." A systemic infection infects the entire body. A communicable infection is one that is spread from person to person. A local infection is restricted to a small area of the body. A nosocomial infection is a hospital-acquired infection.

22. **a.** Under transmission-based precautions, airborne isolation is required in addition to standard precautions for a patient who has pulmonary tuberculosis. Under airborne precautions, anyone entering the pa-

tient's room is required to wear an N95 respirator.

23. **a.** Barrier protection devices (personal protective equipment or PPE), hand washing after glove removal, and HBV vaccination are all recommended by the OSHA Bloodborne Pathogen (BBP) Standard, but it is illegal to dismiss HIV-positive workers without just cause.

24. **d.** Human immunodeficiency virus (HIV) is the leading cause of AIDS. Hepatitis A virus (HAV), hepatitis B virus (HBV), and hepatitis C virus (HCV) cause hepatitis A, hepatitis B, and hepatitis C, respectively.

25. **b.** Immunity to a particular virus normally exists when a person's blood has antibodies directed against that virus. A person who does not display symptoms of the virus, but whose blood contains the virus and is therefore infectious (capable of transmitting the virus to others) is called a carrier. A person who is susceptible to a virus has no antibodies against that virus.

26. **a.** Control of hemorrhage or abnormal bleeding is most effectively accomplished by applying direct pressure to the wound and elevating the affected part above the level of the heart.

27. **c.** An infection control program is responsible for implementing procedures designed to break the chain of infection and prevent the spread of infection in the hospital.

28. **b.** Microorganisms (microbes) that are capable of causing disease are called pathogens. A communicable virus is a type of pathogen that can be spread from person to person. Most microbes (including the microbes that are normal flora of the skin)

are nonpathogenic, meaning they do not cause disease under normal conditions.

29. **d.** AIDS, hepatitis B, and syphilis are all bloodborne pathogens. Tuberculosis is an infectious disease caused by the *Mycobacterium tuberculosis* organism. This organism is not normally present in the blood, but is present in respiratory secretions and can be spread by droplets and airborne droplet nuclei.

30. **d.** A clean paper towel should be used to turn off the faucet after hand washing. Using the same paper towel that was used to dry the hands can contaminate the faucet handles.

31. **a.** Pertussis or whooping cough is a respiratory disease transmitted by droplets. Chickenpox and rubeola are highly contagious and require airborne precautions. RSV requires contact precautions.

32. **b.** Class C fires occur with electrical equipment. Class A fires involve ordinary combustible materials, Class B fires involve flammable liquids, and Class D fires involve combustible metals.

33. **d.** Standard precautions should be followed for all patients at all times with no exceptions.

34. **a.** HBV vaccination involves three separate injections: an initial dose, another dose 1 month later, and a final dose 6 months from the original dose.

35. **a.** Fomites are objects capable of adhering to infectious material and transmitting disease. Fomites can include telephones, computer terminals, and counter tops. A vector is an insect arthropod or animal involved in the

transmission of an infective microbe. A vehicle can be contaminated food, water, drugs, or a unit of blood involved in the transmission of an infective microbe.

36. c. The OSHA HazCom Standard is known as the "Right to Know Law" because it requires manufacturers of hazardous materials to provide material safety data sheets (MSDS) for their products. An MSDS contains general, precautionary, and emergency information about the product.

37. c. Hepatitis means inflammation of the liver. (The word root "hepat" means *liver*, and the suffix "itis" means *inflammation*.) Hepatitis B virus (HBV) and the other hepatitis viruses target the liver, causing liver inflammation.

38. a. The CDC and HICPAC together developed the latest Guideline for Isolation Precautions in Hospitals.

39. d. Reasons for wearing gloves include preventing contamination of hands when handling blood or body fluids, reducing the chance of transmitting microorganisms on the hands of personnel to patients during invasive procedures, and minimizing the possibility of transmitting infectious microorganisms from one patient to another.

40. b. The three components necessary for fire to occur are referred to as the fire triangle and include fuel, oxygen and heat.

41. d. The chain of infection can be broken or interrupted by such things as hand washing, wearing gloves, reducing stress, receiving proper nutrition, and instituting isolation procedures.

42. d. Electrical equipment should be unplugged before servicing to avoid electrical shock. Electrical equipment should never be handled with wet hands. Frayed electrical cords are dangerous and should be replaced rather than used. The use of extension cords should be avoided, if possible, because they lead to circuit overload, incomplete connections, and potential clutter in the path of workers.

43. c. Standard precautions apply to all body fluids, excretions, and secretions except sweat.

44. c. The definition of viability is the ability to live, grow, and develop. The ability of a microorganism to survive on a source depends upon its viability.

45. a. Fuel, oxygen, and heat make up the fire triangle. A fourth component, the chemical reaction that produces fire, creates a fire tetrahedron (Fig. 3-3), the latest way of looking at the chemistry of fire.

46. d. Anyone entering the room of a patient with airborne precautions must wear an N95 respirator, unless the precautions are for rubeola or varicella and the individual is immune.

47. c. Statistics compiled by the CDC have shown that needlesticks are the leading cause of HIV exposures that have occurred so far among health-care workers.

48. c. Approximately 5% of all hospitalized patients in the United States develop some type of nosocomial infection. The most common type of nosocomial infection developed is urinary tract infection.

Fire Tetrahedron

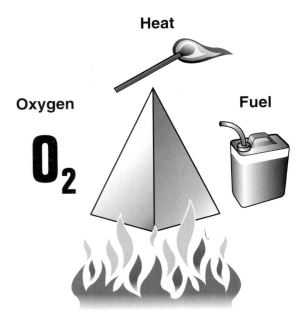

Heat

Oxygen

Fuel

O₂

Chemical Reaction

■ FIGURE 3-3 ■
Fire tetrahedron.

49. **d.** The Bloodborne Pathogen (BBP) Standard was instituted by OSHA when it was determined that healthcare employees face a serious health risk as a result of occupational exposure to bloodborne pathogens. Federal law mandates enforcement of the standard, and OSHA is responsible for enforcement.

50. **d.** Laboratory safety procedures include securing long hair away from the face; never eating, drinking, or applying makeup in the laboratory; and wearing closed-toe shoes. A laboratory coat is considered personal protective equipment and as such may become contaminated. It should be worn during procedures that require it, but it should not be worn on break, to lunch, or when leaving the lab to go home.

51. **b.** The immediate thing to do in the event of a chemical splash to the eyes is to flush them with water for 15 minutes.

52. **b.** The best way to clean up small amounts of blood is to absorb them with a paper towel or gauze pad and then clean the area with a disinfectant, being careful not to spread the blood over a wider area than the original spill. Dried spills should be moistened with disinfectant to avoid scraping, which could disperse infectious organisms into the air. Alcohol is not a disinfectant, nor is soap and water.

53. **a.** The PPD test is a screening test for tuberculosis. Hepatitis B and measles vaccination are examples of immunization measures to prevent the spread of infection. Immune globulin is sometimes given to employees who have had exposure incidents.

54. **c.** The indirect mode of infection transmission occurs when a susceptible individual touches contaminated inanimate objects such as bed linens. Direct transmission involves direct, physical transfer of an infective microbe through close or intimate contact such as touching or kissing. Droplet transmission involves the transfer of an infective microbe to the mucous membranes of a susceptible individual through sneezing, coughing, or talking. Vehicle transmission involves contaminated food, water, drugs, or blood for transfusion.

55. a. Diabetes mellitus is an endocrine disorder involving improper carbohydrate metabolism. It is not caused by a bloodborne pathogen and is not transmitted through blood transfusion. HBV, HIV, and syphilis are bloodborne pathogens that could be transmitted through blood transfusion if present in the transfused blood.

56. d. According to the OSHA Bloodborne Pathogens Standard, gloves are to be worn when performing vascular access procedures. This means that gloves are required for phlebotomy procedures. HIV-positive patients are not normally isolated unless they have AIDS and their immune systems are severely weakened, in which case they may be placed in protective isolation. It is against the law to label specimens from HIV-positive patients any differently than other specimens. A mask may be required in certain situations but is not normally required when working with AIDS patients.

57. d. Figure 3-1 represents the NFPA "water reactive" symbol used to label hazardous chemicals that should not come in contact with water.

58. d. Neutropenic means "a condition in which there is an abnormally low number of white blood cells (neutrophils)." A patient with a low white blood cell count has increased susceptibility to infection. For this reason, neutropenic patients are sometimes placed in a type of protective or reverse isolation called neutropenic isolation.

59. d. To prevent contamination of other articles in the phlebotomist's tray or other workers who may handle it, a tube that has blood on it should be wiped with disinfectant and placed in a biohazard bag before being placed in the tray.

60. b. If a laboratory or patient care activity requires a healthcare worker to wear goggles to prevent exposure from sprays or splashes, a mask must also be worn to prevent mucous membrane exposure of the nose and mouth.

61. a. A positive PPD test means that an individual has been exposed to tuberculosis (TB) and developed antibodies against it. It does not necessarily mean that the individual has TB. An employee with a positive PPD test would not have restrictions on working if the results of chest radiographs to detect signs of TB were negative. An employee with influenza, rubella, or weeping dermatitis, however, could spread the infection to others and would have work restrictions.

62. c. There are four classes of fire recognized by the NFPA. They are categorized by the fuel source of the fire.

63. b. Nosocomial infections can result from contact with infected personnel, other patients, visitors, or equipment. One of the best ways to prevent transmission of pathogenic microorganisms is proper hand washing.

64. c. Also called "reverse" isolation, protective isolation is a special kind of isolation that is used for patients who are highly susceptible to infections. Examples of patients requiring protective isolation are neutropenic patients (those with low white blood cell counts), severely burned patients, and patients with compromised immune systems.

65. a. Percutaneous means "through the skin." Percutaneous exposure routes involve direct inoculation of infectious material through previously intact skin, such as occurs with accidental needlesticks and injuries from other sharp objects. The exposure route involved when handling blood specimens with ungloved, badly chapped hands is non-intact skin contact. Mucous membrane contact with infectious material is a permucosal exposure route.

66. d. Touching electrical equipment while drawing a patient's blood could cause a short to travel through the needle and shock the patient. Drawing a patient's blood during an electrical storm, while standing in a puddle, or while the patient is talking on the telephone will not cause an electrical shock to the patient.

67. c. OSHA's HazCom Standard is known as the "Right to Know" Law because it requires all chemicals to be evaluated for health hazards, all chemicals found to be hazardous to be labeled as such, and the information communicated to employees.

68. a. Because different types of isolation require the use of different types of personal protective equipment, the *best* thing to do before entering an isolation room is to follow the directions on the precaution sign on the door. Precautions may be shown on the card on the door, or you may be directed to check with the patient's nurse first.

69. b. Bloodborne pathogen is a term applied to any infectious microorganism present in blood and other body fluids and tissues. It most commonly refers to HBV and HIV but also includes the organisms that cause syphilis, malaria, relapsing fever, and Creutzfeldt-Jakob disease. The microorganisms that cause influenza, rubella, and strep infections are not normally found in the blood.

70. d. The virulence of a microorganism is the degree to which the organism is capable of causing disease. The chain of infection refers to the three elements (source, means of transmission, and susceptible host) necessary for infection to result. Susceptibility has to do with the immune system of the host and is affected by such things as age and health. Viability is the ability of the microorganism to survive on a source.

71. a. Any material or substance harmful to health is a biological hazard or biohazard for short. Federal regulations require biohazardous material to be marked with a special symbol seen in Figure 3-4.

72. c. When putting on protective clothing, the healthcare worker puts on

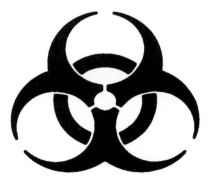

■ FIGURE 3-4 ■
Biohazard symbol.

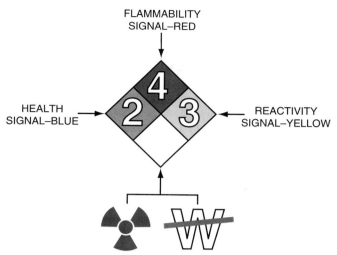

FLAMMABILITY
SIGNAL–RED

HEALTH
SIGNAL–BLUE

REACTIVITY
SIGNAL–YELLOW

RADIOACTIVE OR WATER REACTIVE

■ FIGURE 3-5 ■
National Fire Protection Association 704
marking system.

the gown first, being careful to touch only the inside surface. The mask is put on next. Gloves are applied last and pulled over the cuffs of the gown.

73. **b.** In the NFPA hazardous materials rating system (Fig. 3-5), health hazards are indicated in the blue quadrant on the left. The upper red quadrant indicates fire hazard. Stability or reactivity hazards are indicated in the yellow quadrant on the right, and the white quadrant on the bottom indicates other specific hazards.

74. **b.** The Department of Transportation (DOT) labeling system (Fig. 3-6) uses a diamond-shaped warning sign incorporating the United Nations hazard class number and symbol as well as a four-digit identification number. This symbol should not be confused with the NFPA's diamond-shaped sign divided into four quadrants used to signify specific hazards.

75. **c.** Mixing bleach with other cleaners can release dangerous gases.

76. **d.** OSHA regulations require employers to offer HBV vaccination free of charge to employees within 10 days of assignment to duties with risk of exposure.

77. **b.** If an accidental needlestick occurs, it is very important that the site be decontaminated immediately. The exposure should then be reported to the supervisor and an incident report filled out. The employee should also report to the employee health department for medical evaluation and possible treatment.

78. **d.** The symptoms of shock are pale, cold, clammy skin; expressionless face and staring eyes; increased shallow breathing; and a weak (not strong), rapid pulse.

79. **b.** Distance, time, and shielding are the principles involved in radiation exposure. This means that the amount of radiation you are exposed to depends on how far you are from the source of radioactivity, how long you are exposed to it, and what protection you have from it.

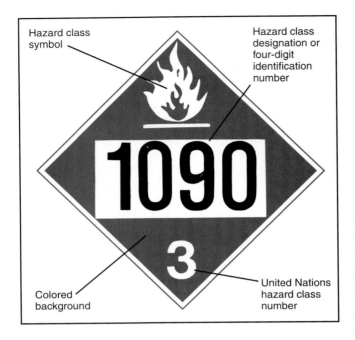

Hazard class symbol

Hazard class designation or four-digit identification number

1090

3

Colored background

United Nations hazard class number

■ FIGURE 3-6 ■

Example of Department of Transportation hazardous materials labels (flammable, poison, corrosive). (Used with permission from Jones SA, Weigel A, White RD, McSwain NE, Breiter M, eds. Advanced Emergency Care for Paramedics Practice (1992). Philadelphia: JB Lippincott.)

80. c. The JCAHO requires healthcare facilities to have an infection control program. The CDC and HICPAC develop guidelines for infection control. NIOSH is a federal agency that is responsible for conducting research and making recommendations for the prevention of work-related disease and injury and is part of the CDC.

81. a. A nosocomial infection is an infection that is acquired by a patient after admission to a healthcare facility. Therefore, a catheter site that becomes infected while a patient is in the intensive care unit is a nosocomial infection. Infection of a healthcare worker is not considered a nosocomial infection. The patient admitted with Hanta virus obviously acquired the virus before admission. Because the incubation period for measles is longer than 1 day, the patient with measles acquired the infectious organism before being admitted to the hospital. Although the others are not nosocomial infections in this case, they can be a source of nosocomial infections in other patients.

82. d. OSHA regulations, such as those concerning employee exposure to bloodborne pathogens, mandated by federal standard 1910.1030, are federal regulations or laws and therefore supersede all other organizations' requirements.

83. a. Availability of PPE in the laboratory is mandated by the OSHA Bloodborne Pathogens (BBP) Standard to minimize occupational exposure to HBV, HIV, and other bloodborne pathogens. CLIA '88 is concerned with laboratory testing. The CDC and HICPAC Guideline for Isolation Precautions in Hospitals describes what PPE to use for the different categories of precautions but has no authority to regulate availability of PPE. The OSHA HazCom standard deals with communicating hazards to employees.

84. c. The new American Heart Association (AHA) recommendations for CPR no longer require a blind finger-sweep of the mouth or a pulse check before initiating CPR. In addition, the ratio of chest compressions to rescue breaths has been standardized to 15:1 for both one- and two-rescuer CPR. AHA also advocates public access to AEDs.

85. b. According to OSHA, thousands of healthcare workers contract hepatitis B (HBV) every year and approximately 200 die as a result. This makes HBV the most frequently occurring laboratory-associated infection and a major infectious health hazard. HAV, HIV, and TB are also health hazards to healthcare workers but they do not occur as frequently as HBV.

86. c. To comply with OSHA standards, an exposure control plan must contain an exposure determination, communication of hazards, and methods of implementation. Isolation guidelines are not a required part of an exposure control plan.

87. d. Class D fires occur with combustible or reactive metals such as sodium, potassium, magnesium, and lithium. Class A fires occur with ordinary combustible materials. Class B fires occur with flammable liquids, and Class C fires occur with electrical equipment.

88. b. The word "enteric" is defined as pertaining to the small intestine. The route of exposure for enteric

pathogens is ingestion. HICPA isolation guidelines require contact isolation precautions in addition to standard precautions for enteric pathogens.

89. a. The word "parenteral" means *other than the digestive tract.* Therefore, something that is *not* parenteral involves the digestive tract. Drinking water involves the digestive tract and is therefore *not* parenteral. The other choices *are* examples of parenteral transmission.

90. b. Gender does not play a role in a person's general susceptibility to infection. Age, health, and immune status do. Gender may, however, play a role in the site of infection because of differences in male and female anatomy.

91. c. Vector transmission involves transfer of the microbe by an insect, arthropod, or animal, for example, the bite of a rodent flea. HIV acquired from a blood transfusion is vehicle transmission. Contracting hepatitis infection from a contaminated counter top is indirect contact transmission involving a fomite. Contracting tuberculosis from droplet nuclei is airborne transmission.

92. c. Protective or reverse isolation is used for patients who are highly susceptible to infections as in the case with a severely burned patient. Hepatitis requires standard precautions. Chickenpox and tuberculosis require airborne precautions in addition to standard precautions.

93. a. Protective clothing is removed in the opposite order that it is donned. For phlebotomy procedures, the gloves are considered the most con-

taminated article and are removed first. They are removed by grasping one glove at the wrist and pulling it inside-out off the hand and holding it in the gloved hand. Remove the second glove by slipping several fingers under it at the wrist and pulling it inside-out over the first glove so that the first glove ends up inside the second. Remove the mask next, being careful to touch only the strings. Remove the gown last by sliding the arms out of the sleeves. Then, while holding the gown away from the body, fold it with the outside (contaminated side) in.

94. **c.** HBV infection is indicated by the presence of HBsAg in the patient's serum. Eradication of HBV infection would be indicated by the absence of HBsAg in the patient's serum. HBV immunity is indicated by a certain titer (or level) of hepatitis B antibody (HBsAb) in the patient's serum.

95. **c.** A radiation hazard sign on a patient' door means the patient has been injected with radioactive dyes. Although in the patient, these radioactive isotopes can be hazardous to a fetus of a pregnant healthcare worker. In addition, a blood specimen collected at this time may be radioactive.

96. **c.** Work practice controls are routines that alter the manner in which a task is performed to reduce likelihood of exposure to bloodborne pathogens. Hand washing following glove removal is one example of a work practice control. A biohazard symbol, an exposure control plan, and HBV vaccination are all important in reducing the risk of exposure to bloodborne pathogens, but they are not considered work practices.

97. **b.** The CDC introduced the concept of universal precautions because it is not always possible to know if a patient is infected with a bloodborne pathogen.

98. **b.** Immunity to a particular disease is conferred by having had the disease and therefore developing antibodies against the disease-causing organism, or by vaccination against the particular organism. A shot of gamma globulin or immune globulin confers temporary immunity. A normal white blood cell count is necessary to fight infection but it is not an indication of immunity.

99. **b.** The Class B fire extinguisher was designed to put out flammable liquid fires. A flammable liquid or vapor fire requires blocking the source of oxygen or smothering the fuel to extinguish the fire. Class B and Class ABC (multipurpose) extinguishers use dry chemicals to smother the fire.

100. **d.** The Hazardous Communication (HazCom) Standard requires labeling of hazardous materials and the labeling must comply with the requirements set by the Manufacturers Chemical Association. OSHA instituted and enforces this standard.

101. **b.** Droplet contact transmission involves the transfer of infective organisms to the mucous membranes of the mouth, nose, or eyes of a susceptible individual by the sneezing, coughing, or talking of an infected person. The common cold is an example of infection that can be transmitted by droplets through coughing or sneezing.

102. **c.** A source of organisms, a means of transmission of the organism, and the presence of a susceptible host are all "links" in the chain of infection. Surveillance is a means of monitoring and preventing infection or breaking the chain of infection.

103. **a.** A division of the US Public Health Service called the Centers for Disease Control and Prevention (CDC) is charged with the investigation and control of various diseases, especially those that are communicable and have epidemic potential.

104. **d.** An immediate and proper first aid response to shock is important and includes the following in order: open the airway, call for assistance, keep the victim's head lower than the rest of the body, attempt to control bleeding or other cause if known, and keep the victim warm.

105. **c.** Healthy ways to deal with stress include exercising regularly, learning how to relax, and planning your day. Several major life changes at the same time can be a source of stress.

106. **b.** Approximately 5% of patients in the United States contract (acquire) some sort of infection after admission to a healthcare facility. Such infections are called nosocomial infections. A laboratory-acquired infection is an employee infection. A nosocomial infection can be, but is not normally, a communicable infection. Because a nosocomial infection is acquired *after* admission, it would not be detected by pre-admission screening tests.

107. **d.** Vehicle transmission involves the transmission of an infective microbe through contaminated food, water, drugs, or blood products. Shigella infection from contaminated water and hepatitis infection from blood products are examples of vehicle transmission. Airborne infection involves droplet nuclei. Contact transmission involves close or intimate contact with an infectious patient or articles contaminated by the patient. Vector transmission involves the transfer of an infectious microbe by an insect, arthropod, or animal.

108. **a.** A phlebotomist diagnosed with strep throat is not allowed to work until he or she has taken antibiotics for a minimum of 24 hours and is not exhibiting symptoms. Once allowed to return to work, a mask is not necessary and neither is an evaluation by infection control personnel.

109. **c.** Any product that has a hazardous warning on the label must have an MSDS supplied by the manufacturer. Isopropyl alcohol has a hazardous warning on the label and requires an MSDS. Laboratory coats, saline, and most patient medications do not have hazard warnings and do not require an MSDS.

110. **c.** An engineering control is an item or device, such as a sharps container, eye wash station, or shelf-sheathing needle, that isolates or removes the hazard from the work place. Gloves and laboratory coats are personal protective equipment or barrier protection. A universal precautions statement is required under the OSHA Bloodborne Pathogen (BBP) Standard but is not an engineering control.

111. **d.** The OSHA HazCom Standard requires chemical manufacturers to supply a material safety data sheet (MSDS) for any product with a hazardous warning on the label. An MSDS contains general information as well as precautionary and emergency information for the product.

112. a. An infection or disease that can spread from person to person is called a communicable infection. A nonpathogenic microorganism is not capable of causing disease or infection. A nosocomial infection is a hospital-acquired infection. Systemic is a term used to describe an infection that infects the entire body.

113. b. Class B fires occur with flammable liquids and vapors such as paint, oil, grease, or gasoline. Class A fires occur with ordinary combustible materials, Class C fires occur with electrical equipment, and Class D fires occur with combustible or reactive metals.

114. c. A person's first reaction during the event of an electrical shock is to try to remove the person from the source of the electricity, but this can result in shock to the rescuer if the source of electricity is still there. The first thing to do, therefore, is to shut off the source of electricity. Other actions to take after the source of electricity is shut off are to call for medical assistance, start CPR if indicated, and keep the victim warm.

115. c. If a pathogen invades the body and the conditions are favorable for it to multiply and cause injurious effects or disease, the resulting condition is called an infection. The chain of infection is the process of infection that involves three components or "links" that must be present for an infection to result. A communicable disease is a type of infection that can be spread from person to person. A systemic infection is a type of infection that affects the entire body.

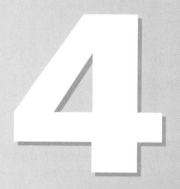

MEDICAL TERMINOLOGY

A. Introduction

B. Word Roots

C. Prefixes

D. Suffixes

E. Combining Vowels/Forms

F. Word Element Classification Discrepancies

G. Unique Plural Endings

H. Pronunciation

I. Abbreviations and Symbols

REVIEW QUESTIONS

Choose the BEST answer.

1. Hepatitis means:
   a. breakdown of blood cells.
   b. inflammation of the liver.
   c. kidney infection.
   d. muscle pain.

2. The abbreviation PT stands for:
   a. partial thromboplastin.
   b. patient temperature.
   c. prothrombin time.
   d. phenylketonuria.

3. What word is used to describe the breakdown of red blood cells?
   a. erythema
   b. erythrocytosis
   c. hemostasis
   d. hemolysis

4. The ability of the body to maintain equilibrium or "steady state" is called:
   a. hematology.
   b. homeostasis.
   c. hemochromatosis.
   d. hemostasis.

5. The combining form "erythro" means:
   a. cell.
   b. earth-like.
   c. oxygen.
   d. red.

6. The singular form of atria is:
   a. atris.
   b. atrium.
   c. atrion.
   d. atrius.

7. The pleural form of lumen is:
   a. lumena.
   b. lumina.
   c. lumeni.
   d. lumens.

8. What word means "large cell?"
   a. acromegaly
   b. cytoma
   c. macrocyte
   d. microcyte

9. What word means "controlling blood flow?"
   a. hemolysis
   b. hemostasis
   c. homeostasis
   d. venostasis

10. In which of the following pairs of letters is each letter pronounced separately?
    a. "ae" in chordae
    b. "es" as in nares
    c. "pn" as in dyspnea
    d. "ps" in psychology

11. The "e" is pronounced separately in:
    a. cavae.
    b. monocyte.
    c. supine.
    d. syncope.

12. Which of the following is a suffix?
    a. an
    b. neo
    c. oxia
    d. ren

13. In the term "bicuspid," bi- is a:
    a. combining form.
    b. prefix.
    c. suffix.
    d. word root.

14. The letter "c" has the sound of "s" in the term:
    a. brachial.
    b. glycolysis.
    c. hypoglycemia.
    d. pancreas.

Match the abbreviation with the word or phrase it identifies.

15. ___ RBC
16. ___ RPR
17. ___ diff
18. ___ EEG
19. ___ IM
20. ___ ASO
21. ___ CMV
22. ___ FUO
23. ___ DOB
24. ___ Rx
25. ___ ESR
26. ___ W
27. ___ LD
28. ___ O & P
29. ___ PKU
30. ___ RA
31. ___ NPO
32. ___ wt

a. gynecology
b. lactic dehydrogenase
c. phenylketonuria
d. erythrocyte sedimentation rate
e. rheumatoid arthritis
f. premature ventricular contraction
g. rapid plasma reagin
h. water reactive
i. weight
j. differential
k. central nervous system
l. antistreptolysin O
m. electroencephalogram
n. nothing by mouth
o. fever of unknown origin
p. intramuscular
q. electrocardiogram
r. date of birth
s. red blood cell
t. prescription
u. ova & parasites
v. cytomegalovirus

Match the word root with its meaning.

33. ___ arteri
34. ___ cardi
35. ___ cyte
36. ___ derm
37. ___ glyc
38. ___ hem
39. ___ hepat
40. ___ onco
41. ___ oste
42. ___ phleb
43. ___ pulmon
44. ___ scler
45. ___ thromb
46. ___ vas

a. vessel
b. skin
c. artery
d. chest
e. blood
f. heart
g. vein
h. brain
i. liver
j. hard
k. clot
l. cell
m. lung
n. bone
o. tumor
p. sugar

Match the prefix with its meaning.

47. ____ a/an-
48. ____ anti-
49. ____ brady-
50. ____ dys-
51. ____ homo-
52. ____ hypo-
53. ____ micro
54. ____ poly-

a. difficult
b. against
c. unequal
d. without
e. small
f. low, under
g. large
h. slow
i. many
j. same

Match the suffix with its meaning.

55. ____ -algia
56. ____ -cyte
57. ____ -emia

58. ____ -gram
59. ____ -itis
60. ____ -logist
61. ____ -lysis
62. ____ -oma
63. ____ -osis
64. ____ -pathy
65. ____ -penia
66. ____ -rrhage
67. ____ -stasis
68. ____ -tomy

a. tumor
b. inflammation
c. specialist in the study of
d. deficiency
e. disease
f. condition
g. cell
h. cutting, incision
i. blood condition
j. pain
k. bursting forth
l. breakdown, destruction
m. instrument that counts
n. recording, writing
o. enlargement
p. stopping, controlling

ANSWERS

1. **b.** inflammation of the liver
2. **c.** prothrombin time
3. **d.** hemolysis
4. **b.** homeostasis
5. **d.** red
6. **b.** atrium
7. **b.** lumina
8. **c.** macrocyte
9. **b.** hemostasis
10. **c.** "pn" as in dyspnea
11. **d.** syncope
12. **c.** oxia
13. **b.** prefix
14. **c.** hypoglycemia
15. **s.** red blood cell
16. **g.** rapid plasma reagin
17. **j.** differential
18. **m.** electroencephalogram
19. **p.** intramuscular
20. **l.** antistreptolysin O
21. **v.** cytomegalovirus
22. **o.** fever of unknown origin
23. **r.** date of birth
24. **t.** prescription
25. **d.** erythrocyte sedimentation rate
26. **h.** water reactive
27. **b.** lactic dehydrogenase
28. **u.** ova & parasites
29. **c.** phenylketonuria
30. **e.** rheumatoid arthritis
31. **n.** nothing by mouth
32. **i.** weight
33. **c.** artery
34. **f.** heart

35. **l.** cell
36. **b.** skin
37. **p.** sugar
38. **e.** blood
39. **i.** liver
40. **o.** tumor
41. **n.** bone
42. **g.** vein
43. **m.** lung
44. **j.** hard
45. **k.** clot
46. **a.** vessel
47. **d.** without
48. **b.** against
49. **h.** slow
50. **a.** difficult
51. **j.** same
52. **f.** low, under
53. **e.** small
54. **i.** many
55. **j.** pain
56. **g.** cell
57. **i.** blood condition
58. **n.** recording, writing
59. **b.** inflammation
60. **c.** specialist in the study of
61. **l.** breakdown, destruction
62. **a.** tumor
63. **f.** condition
64. **e.** disease
65. **d.** deficiency
66. **k.** bursting forth
67. **p.** stopping, controlling
68. **h.** cutting, incision

HUMAN ANATOMY AND PHYSIOLOGY REVIEW

8. Integumentary System
   a. Functions
   b. Structures
   c. Layers of the Skin
      1) Epidermis
      2) Dermis
      3) Subcutaneous
   d. Major Structures of the Skin
   e. Integumentary System Disorders
   f. Diagnostic Tests
9. Respiratory System
   a. Functions
   b. Structures
   c. Respiratory Tract
   d. Gas Exchange and Transport
   e. Respiratory System Disorders
   f. Diagnostic Tests

REVIEW QUESTIONS

Choose the BEST answer.

1. The gland that releases a hormone that follows diurnal rhythms.
   a. adrenal
   b. pineal
   c. thymus
   d. thyroid

2. All of the following are functions of the integumentary system EXCEPT:
   a. protection
   b. reception of environmental stimuli
   c. regulation of temperature
   d. manufacture of vitamin C

3. Which of the following is a test of a digestive system organ?
   a. bilirubin
   b. blood urea nitrogen (BUN)
   c. cortisol
   d. cerebral spinal fluid (CSF) analysis

4. The result of all chemical and physical reactions in the body that are necessary to sustain life is called:
   a. anabolism.
   b. cannibalism.
   c. catabolism.
   d. metabolism.

5. Which of the following structures in the skin give rise to fingerprints?
   a. arrector pili
   b. hair follicles
   c. papillae
   d. sebaceous glands

6. The fundamental unit of the nervous system is the:
   a. alveoli.
   b. meninges.
   c. neuron.
   d. pharynx.

7. Which body plane divides the body into equal portions?
   a. frontal
   b. midsagittal
   c. sagittal
   d. transverse

8. Which of the following is a nervous system disorder?
   a. hepatitis
   b. multiple sclerosis
   c. nephritis
   d. pruritus

9. An example of a dorsal cavity is the:
   a. abdominal cavity.
   b. pelvic cavity.
   c. spinal cavity.
   d. thoracic cavity.

10. Which of the following is a disorder associated with the skeletal system?
    a. atrophy
    b. cholecystitis

c. multiple sclerosis

d. osteochondritis

11. A major cause of respiratory distress in infants and young children is:
    a. cystic fibrosis.
    b. emphysema.
    c. *Mycobacterium tuberculosis.*
    d. respiratory syncytial virus.

12. Simple compounds are transformed by the body into complex compounds by a process called:
    a. anabolism.
    b. catabolism.
    c. digestion.
    d. hemoconcentration.

13. The ability of oxygen to combine with this substance in the red blood cells increases the amount of oxygen that can be carried in the blood by up to 70 times.
    a. carbon dioxide
    b. glucose
    c. hemoglobin
    d. potassium

14. This is the "master gland" of the endocrine system.
    a. pineal
    b. pituitary
    c. thymus
    d. thyroid

15. Elimination of waste products is a function of this body system.
    a. digestive
    b. endocrine
    c. nervous
    d. skeletal

16. Which of the following is a function of the urinary system?
    a. maintain electrolyte balance
    b. produce heat
    c. receive environmental stimuli
    d. remove carbon dioxide from the body

17. Which body system produces blood cells?
    a. muscular
    b. integumentary
    c. respiratory
    d. skeletal

18. Which of the following is a function of the reproductive system?
    a. produce gametes
    b. produce hormones
    c. produce sex cells
    d. all of the above

19. Female gametes are manufactured in the:
    a. cervix.
    b. fallopian tubes.
    c. ovaries.
    d. uterus.

20. Which of the following is a test of the urinary system?
    a. cortisol
    b. creatine kinase
    c. creatinine clearance
    d. pleuracentesis

21. This gland produces "fight or flight" hormones.
    a. adrenal
    b. pancreas
    c. pituitary
    d. thyroid

22. All of the following glands are part of the endocrine system EXCEPT:
    a. adrenal
    b. pituitary
    c. sebaceous
    d. thyroid

23. Glomeruli are structures found in which of the following systems?
    a. nervous
    b. reproductive
    c. respiratory
    d. urinary

24. The ability of the body to repair and maintain itself to achieve a "steady state" describes what term?
  a. anabolism
  b. catabolism
  c. hemostasis
  d. homeostasis

25. Prostate-specific antigen (PSA) is a test of which body system?
  a. endocrine
  b. nervous
  c. reproductive
  d. respiratory

26. Infant respiratory distress syndrome (IRDS) in premature infants is most often caused by a lack of:
  a. alveoli.
  b. carbon dioxide.
  c. hemoglobin.
  d. surfactant.

27. The gallbladder stores:
  a. bile.
  b. hormones.
  c. insulin.
  d. urine.

28. The rapid plasma reagin (RPR) test is a diagnostic test of which of the following body systems?
  a. endocrine
  b. reproductive
  c. respiratory
  d. urinary

29. Which of the following is (are) part of the peripheral nervous system (PNS)?
  a. afferent nerves
  b. brain
  c. cerebrospinal fluid (CSF)
  d. meninges

30. Which gland is most active before birth and during childhood?
  a. adrenal
  b. pituitary
  c. thymus
  d. thyroid

31. Renin is secreted by the:
  a. alveoli.
  b. kidneys.
  c. ovaries.
  d. sudoriferous glands.

32. Which of the following types of muscle is under voluntary control?
  a. cardiac
  b. skeletal
  c. smooth
  d. visceral

33. All of the following structures are part of the male reproductive system EXCEPT:
  a. epididymis
  b. fallopian tubes
  c. prostate
  d. vas deferens

34. Which of the following body cavities are separated by the diaphragm?
  a. abdominal and thoracic
  b. cranial and spinal
  c. pelvic and abdominal
  d. thoracic and cranial

35. Excessive growth hormone in adulthood can cause:
  a. acromegaly.
  b. Cushing's syndrome.
  c. encephalitis.
  d. goiter.

36. Which of the following is an abbreviation for a test of the respiratory system?
  a. ABGs
  b. CSF
  c. TSH
  d. UA

37. Which of the following tests is most likely a test of the integumentary system?
  a. ammonia
  b. occult blood
  c. fungal culture
  d. synovial fluid analysis

38. A hormone that increases metabolism is:
   a. cortisol.
   b. melatonin.
   c. renin.
   d. thyroxine.

39. The term distal means:
   a. farthest from the point of attachment.
   b. higher or above.
   c. nearest to the center of the body.
   d. toward the back.

40. When you are facing someone in normal anatomic position, at which body plane are you looking?
   a. frontal
   b. midsagittal
   c. sagittal
   d. transverse

41. Which of the following structures comprise the central nervous system?
   a. afferent and efferent nerves
   b. brain and spinal cord
   c. sensory and motor nerves
   d. voluntary and involuntary nerves

42. The layer of the epidermis where mitosis occurs is the:
   a. stratum corneum.
   b. stratum germinativum.
   c. subcutaneous.
   d. none of the above

43. Which of the following is a disorder of the urinary system?
   a. cystitis
   b. renal failure
   c. uremia
   d. all of the above

44. The medical term for elevated blood sugar is:
   a. diabetes.
   b. hyperglycemia.
   c. hypoglycemia.
   d. hypothyroidism.

45. Erythropoietin is a hormone secreted by the:
   a. islets of Langerhans.
   b. kidneys.
   c. pituitary gland.
   d. thyroid gland.

46. The layer(s) of the skin containing blood vessels is (are):
   a. epidermis only.
   b. epidermis and dermis.
   c. dermis and subcutaneous.
   d. subcutaneous only.

47. All of the following are functions of the muscular system EXCEPT:
   a. storing calcium.
   b. producing heat.
   c. maintaining posture.
   d. providing movement.

48. Hepatitis is inflammation of the:
   a. gallbladder.
   b. kidneys.
   c. liver.
   d. pancreas.

49. What infectious disease affecting the respiratory system is caused by a mycobacterium?
   a. asthma
   b. emphysema
   c. respiratory syncytial virus (RSV)
   d. tuberculosis (TB)

50. Which of the following terms describes the type of cells that make up the epidermis?
   a. epithelial
   b. keratinized
   c. stratified
   d. all of the above

51. T_4 and TSH are abbreviations for tests that measure the function of this gland:
   a. adrenal
   b. ovaries
   c. pancreas
   d. thyroid

52. The heart and lungs are located in this cavity.
    a. abdominal
    b. cranial
    c. spinal
    d. thoracic

53. Growth hormone (GH) levels test the functioning of which gland?
    a. adrenal
    b. ovary
    c. parathyroid
    d. pituitary

54. The exchange of O_2 and CO_2 in the lungs takes place in the:
    a. alveoli.
    b. bronchi.
    c. larynx.
    d. trachea.

55. Which of the following is true?
    a. the abdominal cavity is located superior to the diaphragm
    b. the elbow is on the ventral surface of the arm
    c. the head is located inferior to the neck
    d. the little toe is on the lateral surface of the foot

56. Which of the following substances is secreted by the islets of Langerhans of the pancreas?
    a. adrenaline
    b. estrogen
    c. glucose
    d. insulin

57. Which of the following structures is part of the digestive system?
    a. arrector pili
    b. gallbladder
    c. seminal vesicle
    d. ureter

58. Calcitonin levels test the functioning of which of the following glands?
    a. adrenal
    b. pituitary

c. thymus
d. thyroid

59. Which of the following laboratory tests is associated with the skeletal system?
    a. alkaline phosphatase
    b. bilirubin
    c. cortisol
    d. lactic acid

60. Antidiuretic hormone (ADH) is also called:
    a. adrenaline.
    b. cortisol.
    c. norepinephrine.
    d. vasopressin.

61. A person is having difficulty breathing. The term used to describe this condition is:
    a. asthma.
    b. dyspnea.
    c. emphysema.
    d. pneumonia.

62. This body system is responsible for releasing hormones directly into the blood stream.
    a. circulatory
    b. endocrine
    c. respiratory
    d. skeletal

63. Which of the following body planes divides the body into upper and lower portions?
    a. frontal
    b. midsagittal
    c. sagittal
    d. transverse

64. A disease in which the islets of Langerhans are unable to produce insulin is:
    a. diabetes insipidus.
    b. diabetes mellitus type I.
    c. diabetes mellitus type II.
    d. all of the above

65. Which of the following is a nervous system test?

    a. blood urea nitrogen (BUN)
    b. creatine kinase (CK)
    c. cerebrospinal fluid (CSF) analysis
    d. glucose

66. Which body system controls and coordinates the activities of all the other body systems?
    a. muscular
    b. nervous
    c. respiratory
    d. skeletal

67. Which of the following is a diagnostic test associated with the muscular system?
    a. BUN
    b. CK
    c. CSF analysis
    d. TSH

68. Which of the following is a disorder of the integumentary system?
    a. diabetes
    b. impetigo
    c. meningitis
    d. rhinitis

69. The avascular layer of the skin is the:
    a. dermis.
    b. epidermis.
    c. subcutaneous.
    d. none of the above

70. Pancreatitis is a disorder of this system.
    a. digestive
    b. reproductive
    c. respiratory
    d. skeletal

71. Which of the following is a true statement?
    a. a man who is supine is lying on his stomach
    b. the big toe is on the medial side of the foot
    c. the hand is at the proximal end of the arm
    d. the posterior curvature of the heel is a recommended heel puncture site

72. Which of the following organs has endocrine function?
    a. kidneys
    b. placenta
    c. stomach
    d. all of the above

73. Which of the following are male gametes?
    a. gonads
    b. ovum
    c. spermatozoa
    d. testes

74. Amylase and lipase are diagnostic tests associated with this system.
    a. circulatory
    b. digestive
    c. respiratory
    d. skeletal

75. Wasting or decrease in size of a muscle due to inactivity is called:
    a. atrophy.
    b. myalgia.
    c. osteomyelitis.
    d. tendonitis.

ANSWERS AND EXPLANATIONS

1. **b.** The pineal gland secretes the hormone melatonin. Melatonin secretion is inhibited by light and enhanced by darkness. Levels of melatonin in the blood, therefore, follow a diurnal rhythm with levels lowest around noon and highest at night.

2. **d.** Vitamin D, not vitamin C, is manufactured in the skin.

3. **a.** Bilirubin is a liver function test. The liver is an accessory organ of the digestive system. BUN is a kidney function test and therefore a urinary system test. Cortisol is an adrenal function test and therefore an endocrine system test. CSF is a nervous system test.

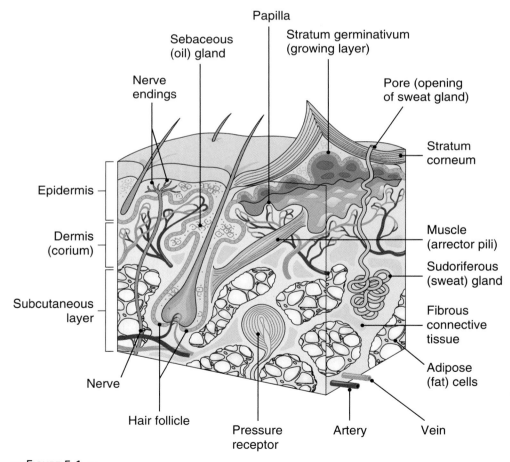

■ FIGURE 5-1 ■

Cross-section of the skin. (Used with permission from Cohen BJ, Wood DL. (2000). *Memmler's structure and function of the human body* (7th ed.). Philadelphia: Lippincott Williams & Wilkins, p. 56.)

4. **d.** Metabolism is defined as the sum of all chemical and physical reactions necessary to sustain life. Cannibalism is the eating of human flesh. Catabolism is the process by which complex substances are broken into simple ones. Anabolism is the name for the process in which simple compounds are transformed into complex compounds.

5. **c.** Papillae (Fig. 5-1), elevations and depressions in the dermis where it meets the epidermis, form the ridges and grooves of fingerprints.

6. **c.** The neuron is the fundamental unit of the nervous system. The meninges are the covering of the brain and spinal cord. Alveoli and pharynx are structures of the respiratory system.

7. **b.** A sagittal plane (Fig. 5-2) divides the body into right and left portions. If the portions are equal it is called a mid-sagittal plane. A frontal plane divides the body into front and back portions. A transverse plane divides the body into upper and lower portions.

8. **b.** Multiple sclerosis is a disorder involving the myelin sheath of the nerves. Hepatitis is liver inflammation. Nephritis is inflammation of the nephrons of the kidneys. Pruritus means itching.

9. **c.** Dorsal refers to the back. Dorsal cavities are to the back of the body. The spinal and cranial cavities are dorsal cavities. The abdominal, pelvic, and thoracic cavities are ventral cavities (Fig. 5-3).

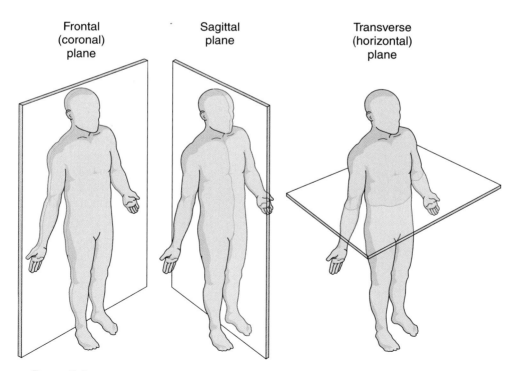

Frontal (coronal) plane

Sagittal plane

Transverse (horizontal) plane

■ FIGURE 5-2 ■

Body planes. (Used with permission from Cohen BJ, Wood DL. (2000). *Memmler's structure and function of the human body* (7th ed.). Philadelphia: Lippincott Williams & Wilkins, p. 7.)

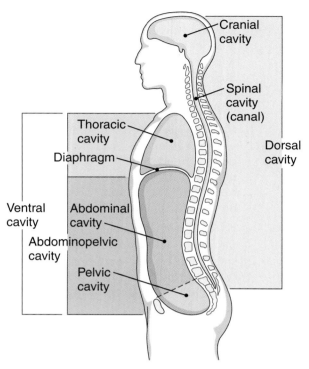

Cranial cavity

Spinal cavity (canal)

Thoracic cavity

Diaphragm

Dorsal cavity

Ventral cavity

Abdominal cavity

Abdominopelvic cavity

Pelvic cavity

■ FIGURE 5-3 ■

Body cavities. (Used with permission from Cohen BJ, Wood DL. (2000). *Memmler's structure and function of the human body* (7th ed.). Philadelphia: Lippincott Williams & Wilkins, p. 8.)

10. **d.** Osteochondritis means inflammation of the bone and cartilage. Atrophy means muscle wasting. Cholecystitis is gallbladder inflammation. Multiple sclerosis is an inflammatory disease of the nervous system that causes degeneration of the myelin sheath of the nerves.

11. **d.** Respiratory syncytial virus causes acute respiratory disease in children. Cystic fibrosis, emphysema, and *Mycobacterium tuberculosis* can cause respiratory distress in children but are not as common

12. **a.** Anabolism is the name for the process in which simple compounds are transformed into complex compounds. Catabolism is the process by which complex substances are broken into simple ones. Digestion is the process by which food is broken into simple usable components. Hemoconcentration is a term that means increased large molecules.

13. **c.** The ability of oxygen to combine with a protein in red blood cells called hemoglobin increases the oxygen-carrying capacity of the blood. Hemoglobin combined with oxygen is called oxyhemoglobin.

14. **b.** The pituitary gland (Fig. 5-4) releases hormones that stimulate other glands and is therefore referred to as the "master gland."

15. **a.** Elimination of waste products is a function of the digestive system (Fig. 5-5).

16. **a.** The primary function of the kidneys, which are a part of the urinary system (Fig. 5-6), is to maintain water and electrolyte balance. Electrolytes are sodium, potassium, chloride, and bicarbonate. Heat production is a function of the muscular system. The nervous system and the skin receive environmental stimuli, and the circulatory system removes carbon dioxide.

17. **d.** One function of the skeletal system is hematopoiesis or the production of blood cells.

18. **d.** Production of sex cells (gametes) and hormones are functions of the reproductive system.

19. **c.** Female gametes (ova) are manufactured by the ovaries. The uterus is another name for the womb. The fal-

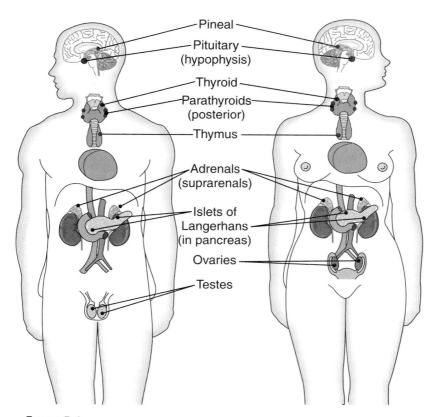

Pineal

Pituitary
(hypophysis)

Thyroid

Parathyroids
(posterior)

Thymus

Adrenals
(suprarenals)

Islets of
Langerhans
(in pancreas)

Ovaries

Testes

■ Figure 5-4 ■

Endocrine glands. (Used with permission from Cohen BJ, Wood DL. (2000). *Memmler's structure and function of the human body* (7th ed.). Philadelphia: Lippincott Williams & Wilkins, p. 166.)

lopian tubes are the pathway through which the ova reach the uterus. The cervix is the neck of the uterus.

20. **c.** Creatinine, a byproduct of muscle metabolism, is produced at a constant rate and is cleared from the blood by the kidneys. The creatinine clearance test measures the rate that creatinine is cleared from the blood by the kidneys and is a test of kidney function. Creatine kinase is a muscle enzyme and is a test of the muscular system. Cortisol is a test associated with endocrine function. Pleuracen-

tesis is a surgical puncture of the chest wall to remove fluid.

21. **a.** The adrenal glands (see Fig. 5-4) secrete the hormones epinephrine (adrenaline) and norepinephrine (noradrenaline), also referred to as the "fight or flight" hormones because of their effects when the body is under stress.

22. **c.** Sebaceous glands (see Fig. 5-1) are found in the skin and are part of the integumentary system. They secrete an oily substance called sebum that helps lubricate the skin.

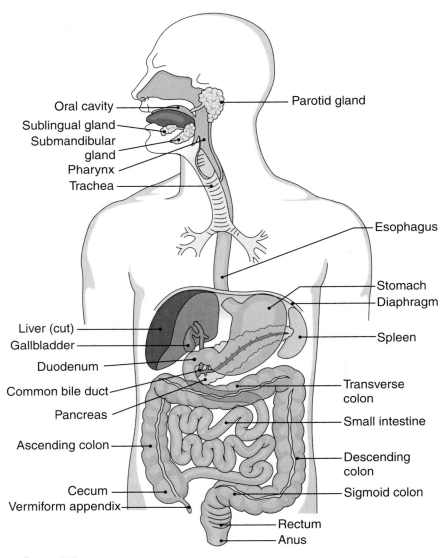

23. d. Glomeruli are structures of the kidney, which is part of the urinary system.

24. d. Homeostasis means "staying the same" and describes the balanced or "steady state" condition that the body strives to maintain. Anabolism is the part of the metabolism process in which the body converts simple substances into complex substances. Ca-

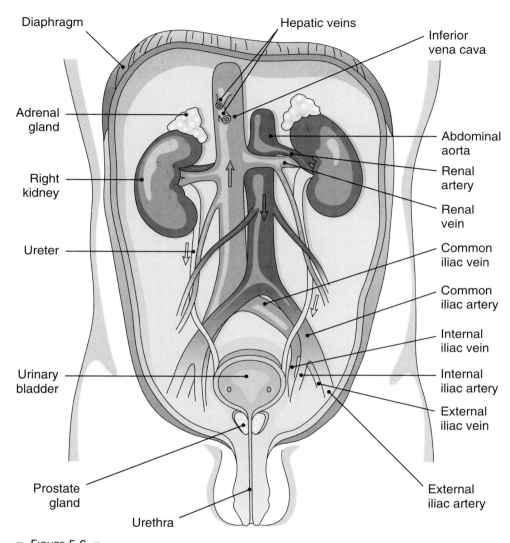

Diaphragm
Hepatic veins
Inferior vena cava
Adrenal gland
Abdominal aorta
Renal artery
Right kidney
Renal vein
Ureter
Common iliac vein
Common iliac artery
Internal iliac vein
Urinary bladder
Internal iliac artery
External iliac vein
Prostate gland
External iliac artery
Urethra

■ FIGURE 5-6 ■

Urinary system. (Used with permission from Cohen BJ, Wood DL. (2000). *Memmler's structure and function of the human body* (7th ed.). Philadelphia: Lippincott Williams & Wilkins, p. 294.)

tabolism is the process by which the body breaks complex substances into simple ones. Hemostasis refers to the stagnation of blood or stopping the flow of blood from the circulatory system.

25. c. The PSA test is a test associated with the prostate gland, which is part of the male reproductive system.

26. d. Surfactant is a fluid substance that coats the thin walls of the alveoli and keeps them from collapsing. Prema-

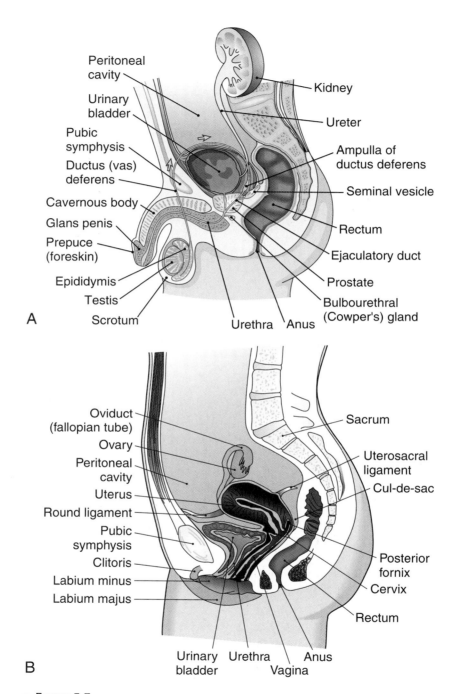

■ FIGURE 5-7 ■

Reproductive system. **A.** Male. **B.** Female. (Used with permission from Cohen BJ, Wood DL. (2000). *Memmler's structure and function of the human body* (7th ed.). Philadelphia: Lippincott Williams & Wilkins, pp. 314, 321.)

ture infants often lack sufficient surfactant to keep their lungs from collapsing.

27. **a.** The gallbladder (see Fig. 5-5) serves as a storage pouch for bile.

28. **b.** RPR is a test for syphilis, a sexually transmitted disease of the reproductive system.

29. **a.** Afferent nerves are part of the PNS (see answer to question 41). The brain, CSF, and meninges are part of the central nervous system.

30. **c.** The thymus gland (see Fig. 5-4), located in the chest behind the sternum, functions in the development of immunity and is most active before birth and during childhood.

31. **b.** Renin, a hormone secreted by the kidneys, increases blood pressure.

32. **b.** Skeletal muscle is under voluntary control. Cardiac and visceral (smooth) muscle are under involuntary control (Table 5-1).

33. **b.** The epididymis, prostate, and vas deferens are structures of the male reproductive system. The fallopian tubes are structures of the female reproductive system (Fig. 5-7).

34. **a.** The diaphragm is a muscular structure separating the thoracic cavity from the abdominal cavity.

35. **a.** Acromegaly is a condition characterized by the overgrowth of bones in the hands, feet, and face caused by excessive growth hormone in adulthood. Cushing's syndrome is caused by an excess of cortisone. Encephalitis means inflammation of the brain. Goiter is a term for an enlargement of the thyroid gland.

36. **a.** Arterial blood gases (ABGs) assess a patient's oxygenation and ventilation status, which are functions of the respiratory system. Cerebrospinal fluid (CSF) analysis is a nervous system test. Thyroid stimulating hormone (TSH) is a pituitary hormone that stimulates the thyroid and is a thyroid function test. Urinalysis (UA) is a urinary system test.

37. **c.** Fungal cultures are often performed on skin scrapings. The skin is part of the integumentary system. Ammonia, a liver function test, and occult blood, a test for hidden blood in feces, are digestive system tests. Synovial fluid comes from joint cavities, part of the skeletal system.

38. **d.** Thyroxine is a hormone released by the thyroid (see Fig. 5-4) that increases the metabolic rate. Cortisone is an adrenal hormone that suppresses inflammation. Melatonin is a hormone released by the pineal gland that plays a role in diurnal (daily) rhythms. Renin is secreted by the kidneys and stimulates vasoconstriction.

39. **a.** Distal means farthest from the center of the body, origin, or point of attachment. Superior means higher or above. Proximal means nearest to the center of the body. Dorsal refers to the back.

Table 5-1

Types of Muscles

Skeletal muscle is attached to bone, has **striated** (stri-a-ted) or banded muscle fibers, and is under **voluntary** (conscious) control

Visceral (vis-er-al) **muscle** lines the walls of blood vessels and most internal organs, is **nonstriated,** and is under **involuntary** or unconscious control; visceral muscle is often called **smooth** muscle

Cardiac muscle forms the wall of the heart, is a special kind of **striated** muscle, and is under **involuntary** control

40. a. The frontal plane divides the body vertically into front and back portions. When your are facing someone in normal anatomic position, he or she is also facing you, which means you are seeing the frontal plane. A midsagittal plane divides a body into equal right and left portions. A sagittal plane divides the body into right and left portions. A transverse plane divides the body into upper and lower portions (see Fig. 5-2).

41. b. The central nervous system (CNS) (Fig. 5-8) is composed of the brain and spinal cord. The afferent and efferent nerves, sensory and motor nerves, and voluntary and involuntary nerves are all part of the peripheral nervous system (PNS).

42. b. The layer of the epidermis where mitosis (cell division) occurs is the deepest layer, called the stratum germinativum. It is the only layer of living cells in the epidermis.

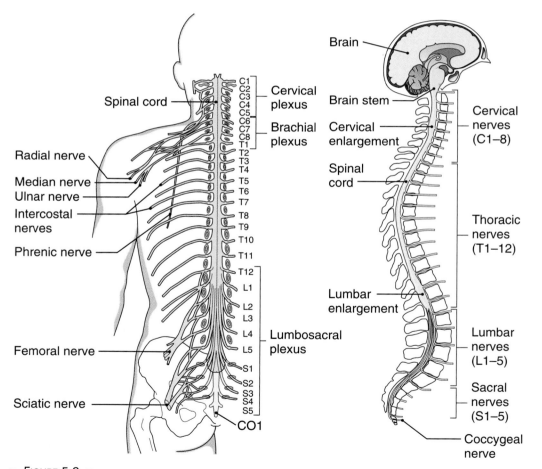

■ FIGURE 5-8 ■

Nervous system. (Used with permission from Cohen BJ, Wood DL. (2000). *Memmler's structure and function of the human body* (7th ed.). Philadelphia: Lippincott Williams & Wilkins, p. 114.)

43. **d.** Cystitis is inflammation of the bladder. Renal failure means kidney failure. Uremia is a build up a waste products in the body caused by impaired kidney function. The bladder and kidneys are part of the urinary system.

44. **b.** Hyperglycemia is the term for abnormally increased blood sugar. Hypoglycemia is a term for abnormally decreased blood sugar. Diabetes is a general term for diseases characterized by abnormally increased urination. Hypothyroidism is a disease caused by decreased thyroid secretion.

45. **b.** The kidneys release erythropoietin, a hormone that stimulates red blood cell production.

46. **c.** Blood vessels are found in the dermis and subcutaneous layers of the skin. The epidermis is avascular, which means it does not contain blood vessels.

47. **a.** Calcium storage is a function of the skeletal system.

48. **c.** Hepatitis comes from the Greek word *hepatos,* meaning "liver." The suffix "itis" means inflammation. The term for inflammation of the gallbladder is cholecystitis. Kidney inflammation is called nephritis. Inflammation of the pancreas is called pancreatitis.

49. **d.** TB is caused by *Mycobacterium tuberculosis.* This disease, once considered rare in the United States, is now in resurgence because of antibiotic resistance of the organism and an increase in world travel. As the name implies, RSV is caused by a virus, not a mycobacterium. Asthma and emphysema are conditions related to difficulty in breathing and are not infectious diseases.

50. **d.** Some cells of the epidermis can be described as stratified (layered), keratinized (hardened), epithelial cells.

51. **d.** Thyroxine (T_4), a hormone released by the thyroid gland (see Fig. 5-4), increases metabolic rate. Thyroid stimulating hormone (TSH) is released by the pituitary to stimulate the thyroid. Both T_4 and TSH are common tests of thyroid function.

52. **d.** The heart and lungs are located in the thoracic or chest cavity (see Fig. 5-3).

53. **d.** GH is secreted by the pituitary gland.

54. **a.** The larynx, trachea, bronchi, and alveoli are all part of the respiratory system (Fig. 5-9), but the exchange of oxygen and carbon dioxide occurs in the alveoli.

55. **d.** The little toe is on the outer or lateral side of the foot. The abdominal cavity is inferior or below the diaphragm. The elbow is on the back or dorsal surface of the arm. The head is above or superior to the neck.

56. **d.** The islets of Langerhans are part of the endocrine system. They secrete insulin, which is necessary for the cells to be able to utilize glucose. Adrenaline is secreted by the adrenal glands. Estrogen is secreted by the ovaries in the female reproductive system.

57. **b.** The gallbladder (see Fig. 5-5) is an accessory organ of the digestive system. Arrector pili are structures in the skin. Seminal vesicles are part of the male reproductive system. Ureters are structures of the urinary system.

58. **d.** Calcitonin is a hormone secreted by the thyroid that regulates the amount of calcium in the blood.

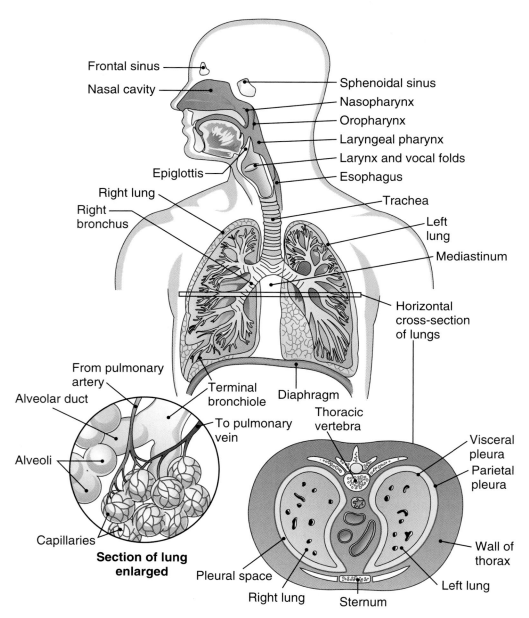

■ FIGURE 5-9 ■

Respiratory system. (Used with permission from Cohen BJ, Wood DL. (2000). *Memmler's structure and function of the human body* (7th ed.). Philadelphia: Lippincott Williams & Wilkins, p. 248.)

59. a. Alkaline phosphatase is an enzyme that functions in the mineralization of bone. Bilirubin is a liver function test. Cortisol is an endocrine system test. Lactic acid is a test associated with the muscular system.

60. d. Vasopressin is another name for ADH, which is secreted by the pituitary and decreases urine production.

61. b. The prefix "dys-" means difficult. "Pnea" comes from "pnoe," which means breathing. Asthma is a condition characterized by difficult breathing (dyspnea) accompanied by wheezing. Emphysema is a chronic obstructive pulmonary disease. Pneumonia is inflammation of the lungs most commonly caused by bacteria, viruses, or chemical irritation.

62. b. The endocrine system releases hormones directly into the blood stream.

63. d. The transverse plane divides the body into upper and lower portions (see Fig. 5-2).

64. b. In diabetes mellitus type I, also called insulin-dependent diabetes, the body is totally unable to produce insulin. In diabetes mellitus type II, also called non–insulin-dependent diabetes, the body is able to produce insulin, but either the amount produced is not sufficient or the insulin is not being properly used by the body. Diabetes insipidus, a condition characterized by increased thirst and increased urine production, is caused by inadequate secretion of antidiuretic hormone.

65. c. CSF is a clear, plasma-like fluid that fills the space between the meninges and the spinal cord and brain. BUN is a measure of the nitrogen portion of urine and is a kidney function test. Creatine kinase (CK) is a muscle enzyme. Glucose is a product of carbohydrate metabolism and a test of the digestive system.

66. b. The nervous system controls and coordinates the activities of all body systems. It does this by means of electrical impulses and chemical substances sent to and received from all parts of the body.

67. b. Creatine kinase (CK) is an enzyme present in skeletal and heart muscle. Blood urea nitrogen (BUN) is a urinary system test. Cerebrospinal fliud analysis (CSF) is a nervous system test. Thyroid stimulating hormone (TSH) is an endocrine system test.

68. b. The skin is part of the integumentary system. Impetigo is an inflammatory condition of the skin most often caused by staphylococcus or streptococcus infection. It is characterized by isolated blisters that rupture and crust over.

69. b. Avascular means "without blood vessels." The epidermis of the skin does not contain blood vessels. The blood vessels are in the dermis and subcutaneous layers of the skin.

70. a. Pancreatitis means inflammation of the pancreas. The pancreas is an accessory organ of the digestive system.

71. b. Medial means toward the midline of the body. The big toe is on the inner side of the foot, which is the side closest to the midline of the body. A man who is in a supine position is lying on his back. The hand is at the distal end ot the arm. The posterior curvature of the heel is not a recommended site for heel puncture.

72. d. The kidneys, placenta, and stomach all have endocrine function. The kidneys secrete erthropoietin, which stimulates red blood cell production.

The placenta secretes several hormones that function during pregnancy, including the human chorionic gonadotropin (HCG), which is detected in pregnancy tests. The lining of the stomach secretes the hormone gastrin, which stimulates digestion.

73. **c.** Male gametes or sex cells are called spermatozoa. An ovum is a female gamete. Gonads are the glands that manufacture the gametes. The male gonads are the testes.

74. **b.** Amylase and lipase are enzymes produced by the pancreas (an accessory organ of the digestive system) that aid the digestive process.

75. **a.** Atrophy means muscle wasting. Myalgia means muscle pain. Osteomyelitis means bone inflammation. Tendinitis means tendon inflammation.

THE CIRCULATORY SYSTEM

3. Types of Blood Specimens
  a. Serum
  b. Plasma
  c. Whole Blood
4. Blood Disorders
5. Diagnostic Tests

E. **Hemostasis**
  1. Primary Hemostasis
  2. Secondary Hemostasis

3. The Role of the Liver in Hemostasis
4. Hemostatic Disorders
5. Diagnostic Tests

F. **The Lymphatic System**
  1. Functions
  2. Structures
  3. Lymph Flow
  4. Lymphatic System Disorders
  5. Diagnostic Tests

REVIEW QUESTIONS

Using the choices on the right, identify the structures of the heart indicated by the arrows in Figure 6-1.

1. ____
2. ____
3. ____
4. ____
5. ____
6. ____
7. ____
8. ____

a. aortic arch
b. right atrium
c. left atrium
d. right ventricle
e. left ventricle
f. bicuspid valve
g. tricuspid valve
h. pulmonic valve
i. aortic valve
j. superior vena cava
k. inferior vena cava
l. right pulmonary artery (branches)
m. left pulmonary artery (branches)
n. right pulmonary veins
o. left pulmonary veins

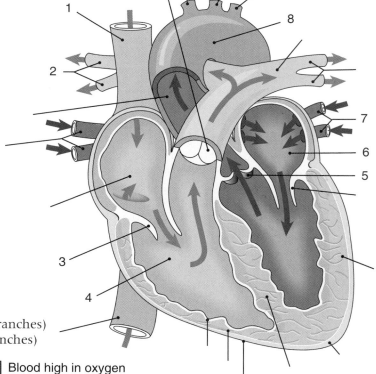

■ Blood high in oxygen
■ Blood low in oxygen

■ FIGURE 6-1 ■

Heart and great vessels. (Used with permission from Cohen, B.J. & Wood, D.L. (2000). Memmler's Structure and Function of the Human Body (7th ed.). Philadelphia: Lippincott Williams & Wilkins, p. 196.)

Choose the BEST answer.

9. The middle layer of heart muscle is called the:
   a. endocardium.
   b. epicardium.
   c. myocardium.
   d. pericardium.

10. The function of the left ventricle is to deliver:
    a. deoxygenated blood into the pulmonary artery.
    b. oxygenated blood into the aortic arch.
    c. oxygenated blood into the pulmonary vein.
    d. oxygenated blood to the left atrium.

11. How many chambers are in the human heart?
    a. 1
    b. 2
    c. 3
    d. 4

12. The medical term for a heart attack is:
    a. arrhythmia.
    b. ischemia.
    c. myocardial infarction.
    d. tachycardia.

13. The receiving chambers of the heart are the:
    a. atria.
    b. chordae tendineae.
    c. vena cavae.
    d. ventricles.

14. The heart is surrounded by a thin, fluid-filled sac called the:
    a. endocardium.
    b. epicardium.
    c. myocardium.
    d. pericardium.

15. The lower chambers of the heart are called:
    a. atria.
    b. septum.
    c. valves.
    d. ventricles.

16. The right atrioventricular valve is also called the:
    a. bicuspid valve.
    b. mitral valve.
    c. pulmonary valve.
    d. tricuspid valve.

17. The structure dividing the right and left halves of the heart is called:
    a. atrium.
    b. chordae tendineae.
    c. pericardium.
    d. septum.

18. The heart receives blood to supply its own needs via the:
    a. coronary arteries.
    b. pulmonary arteries.
    c. vena cavae.
    d. venules.

19. The relaxing phase of the cardiac cycle is called:
    a. bradycardia.
    b. diastole.
    c. infarction.
    d. systole.

20. The heart's "pacemaker" is the:
    a. atrioventricular node.
    b. bundle of His.
    c. semilunar valve.
    d. sinoatrial node.

21. A cardiac cycle lasts approximately:
    a. 0.5 seconds.
    b. 0.8 seconds.
    c. 1.5 seconds.
    d. 8 seconds.

22. The abbreviation for a test that monitors electrical impulses of the heart is:
    a. ABGs
    b. CK
    c. EEG
    d. ECG

23. On an electrocardiogram (ECG) tracing, atrial activity is represented by the:
    a. P wave.
    b. QRS complex.
    c. T wave.
    d. none of the above

24. On an electrocardiogram (ECG) tracing, which wave represents the activity of the ventricles?
    a. P and T
    b. P only
    c. QRS and P
    d. QRS and T

25. Abnormal heart sounds are called:
    a. arrhythmias.
    b. extrasystoles.
    c. fibrillations.
    d. murmurs.

26. Blood vessels that carry blood away from the heart are called:
    a. arteries.
    b. capillaries.
    c. veins.
    d. vena cavae.

27. A person's pulse is created by a wave of pressure caused by:
    a. atrial contraction.
    b. atrial relaxation.
    c. ventricular contraction.
    d. ventricular relaxation.

28. What keeps the blood moving through the venous system?
    a. expansion and contraction of the arteries
    b. movement of fluid through the lymph system veins
    c. pressure from the heart contractions
    d. skeletal muscle movement and the opening and closing of valves within the veins

29. An abnormally fast heart rate is called:
    a. bradycardia.
    b. extrasystole.
    c. fibrillation.
    d. tachycardia.

30. Which of the following is a normal blood pressure reading?
    a. 60/40 mm Hg
    b. 80/120 mm Hg
    c. 100/120 mm Hg
    d. 120/80 mm Hg

31. An infection of the lining of the heart is called:
    a. angina pectoris.
    b. aortic stenosis.
    c. endocarditis.
    d. pericarditis.

32. Which of the following are abbreviations for cardiac enzyme tests?
    a. ALP, ALT
    b. BUN, PT
    c. CK, LDH
    d. GTT, ESR

33. Systolic pressure measures pressure in the arteries during:
    a. atrial contraction.
    b. ventricular contraction.
    c. ventricular relaxation.
    d. none of the above

34. The pulmonary circulation:
    a. carries deoxygenated blood to the lungs and returns oxygenated blood to the heart.
    b. carries oxygenated blood from the heart to the tissues.
    c. delivers blood from the heart to the aorta.
    d. returns deoxygenated blood to the heart.

35. Which of the following represents the proper direction of blood flow in the circulatory system?
    a. arteries, veins, capillaries
    b. arterioles, capillaries, venules
    c. capillaries, arterioles, arteries
    d. veins, venules, capillaries

36. The right ventricle delivers blood to the:
    a. aorta.
    b. left atrium.
    c. pulmonary artery.
    d. pulmonary vein.

37. Normal systemic arterial blood is:
    a. blue.
    b. bright cherry red.
    c. dark red with a bluish tinge.
    d. dark blue with a reddish tinge.

38. The largest artery in the body is the:
    a. aorta.
    b. carotid.
    c. femoral.
    d. vena cava.

39. The pulmonary vein carries:
    a. arterial blood.
    b. lymph fluid.
    c. oxygen-rich blood.
    d. oxygen-poor blood.

40. A sphygmomanometer is a(n):
    a. blood pressure cuff.
    b. electrocardiogram.
    c. machine that records brain waves.
    d. pacemaker.

41. The smallest branches of veins are called:
    a. arterioles.
    b. capillaries.
    c. lumen.
    d. venules.

42. All of the following blood vessels are part of the systemic circulation EXCEPT:
    a. brachial artery
    b. cephalic vein
    c. pulmonary artery
    d. vena cava

43. Tiny one-cell-thick blood vessels are called:
    a. arterioles.
    b. capillaries.
    c. vena cavae.
    d. venules.

44. Which of the following blood vessels carries oxygenated blood?
    a. brachial vein
    b. pulmonary vein
    c. pulmonary artery
    d. superior vena cava

45. The outer layer of a blood vessel is called the tunica:
    a. adventitia.
    b. interna.
    c. intima.
    d. media.

46. The internal space of a blood vessel is called the:
    a. endothelium.
    b. lumen.
    c. tunica intima.
    d. tunica media.

47. The layers of arteries differ from the layers of veins in that the:
    a. inner lining is thicker in veins.
    b. outer layer is thinner in arteries.
    c. muscle layer is more elastic in veins.
    d. muscle layer is thicker in arteries.

48. The structure on the right in Figure 6-2 is a(n):
   a. artery.
   b. capillary.
   c. vein.
   d. none of the above

49. The inner layer of a blood vessel is called the:
   a. lumen.
   b. tunica adventitia.
   c. tunica intima.
   d. tunica media.

50. Which is the proper order of vein selection for venipuncture?
   a. basilic, cephalic, median cubital
   b. cephalic, median cubital, basilic
   c. median cubital, basilic, cephalic
   d. median cubital, cephalic, basilic

51. Oxygen and nutrients diffuse through the walls of the:
   a. alveoli.
   b. arterioles.
   c. capillaries.
   d. venules.

52. The antecubital fossa is located:
   a. anterior to and distal to the elbow.
   b. anterior to and distal to the ankle.
   c. posterior to and proximal to the elbow.
   d. proximal to the wrist.

53. A blood clot circulating in the blood stream is called a(n):
   a. aneurysm.
   b. embolism.
   c. embolus.
   d. thrombus.

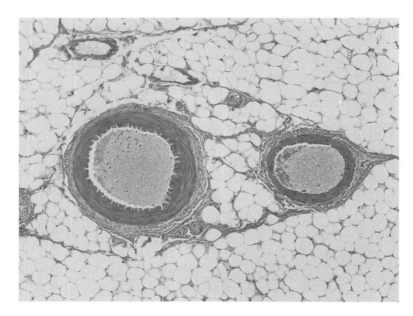

■ FIGURE 6-2 ■

Cross-section of an artery and a vein as seen through a microscope. (Used with permission from Cormac, D.H. (1993). Essential Histology. Philadelphia: JB Lippincott, Plate 11-1.)

Identify the veins in Figure 6-3 using the choices to the right.

54. ____   **a.** basilic

55. ____   **b.** brachial

56. ____   **c.** cephalic

                 d. median cubital

                 e. radial

Choose the BEST answer.

57. The basilic vein is the third choice for venipuncture because it is:
  a. more painful when punctured.
  b. near a major nerve.
  c. near the brachial artery.
  d. all of the above

58. A phlebotomist is allowed to perform a venipuncture on an ankle vein when:
  a. the patient has intravenous catheters in both arms.
  b. the patient's physician has given permission to do so.
  c. there are no acceptable antecubital or hand veins.
  d. there are no other accessible veins and the patient has no coagulation problems.

59. The longest vein in the body is the:
  a. aorta.
  b. femoral.
  c. great saphenous.
  d. vena cava.

60. A vein found on the lateral side of the ankle is the:
  a. femoral.
  b. lesser saphenous.
  c. popliteal.
  d. none of the above

61. Which of the following are normally found in the plasma portion of the blood?
  a. antibodies
  b. bacteria
  c. platelets
  d. red blood cells

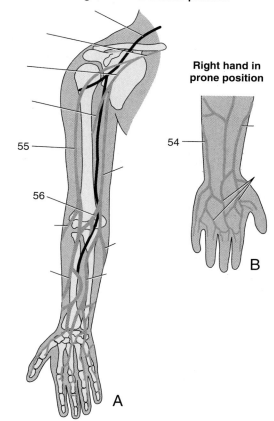

Right arm in anatomic position

Right hand in prone position

■ FIGURE 6-3 ■

A. Principal veins of the arm, including major antecubital veins subject to venipuncture. **B.** Forearm, wrist, and hand veins subject to venipuncture.

62. What is the medical term for vein inflammation?
  a. embolism
  b. hemostasis
  c. phlebitis
  d. thrombosis

63. Which of the following is the name or abbreviation for a vascular system test?
  a. bilirubin
  b. CSF
  c. DIC
  d. glucose

64. Lipid accumulation on the intima of an artery is called:
    a. atherosclerosis.
    b. cholesterol.
    c. endocarditis.
    d. phlebitis.

65. A localized dilation or bulging of an artery is called:
    a. an aneurysm.
    b. an embolism.
    c. arteriosclerosis.
    d. thrombophlebitis.

66. Inflammation of a vein in conjunction with formation of a blood clot is called:
    a. phlebitis.
    b. sclerosis.
    c. thrombophlebitis.
    d. vasculitis.

67. Normal adult blood volume is approximately:
    a. 2 L.
    b. 4 L.
    c. 5 L.
    d. 8 L.

68. The normal composition of blood is approximately:
    a. 10% plasma, 90% formed elements.
    b. 30% plasma, 70% formed elements.
    c. 55% plasma, 45% formed elements.
    d. 90% plasma, 10% formed elements.

69. Normal plasma is a:
    a. clear, colorless fluid that is 10% solutes.
    b. clear or slightly hazy, pale yellow fluid that is 90% water.
    c. cloudy, colorless fluid that is 45% solutes.
    d. hazy, pale yellow fluid that is 55% water.

70. When the hand is prone, the cephalic vein in the antecubital area is located in line with the:
    a. femoral artery.
    b. radial artery.

    c. little finger.
    d. thumb.

71. Which is the most numerous cell in the blood?
    a. platelet
    b. red blood cell
    c. reticulocyte
    d. white blood cell

72. Which blood cell contains a nucleus?
    a. erythrocyte
    b. leukocyte
    c. thrombocyte
    d. reticulocyte

73. A reticulocyte count measures immature:
    a. platelets.
    b. neutrophils.
    c. red blood cells.
    d. white blood cells.

74. Which blood cell increases in allergic reactions and pinworm infestations?
    a. eosinophil
    b. monocyte
    c. red blood cell
    d. segmented neutrophil

75. How large is a normal erythrocyte?
    a. 4–5 µm
    b. 7–8 µm
    c. 8–10 µm
    d. 10–12 µm

76. Where are leukocytes produced?
    a. blood stream
    b. bone marrow
    c. kidneys
    d. liver

77. What is the primary function of red blood cells?
    a. deliver nutrients to the cells of the body
    b. produce antibodies
    c. transport carbon dioxide from the tissues to the lungs
    d. transport oxygen from the lungs to the tissues

78. A leukocyte is a:
 a. lymph node.
 b. platelet.
 c. red blood cell.
 d. white blood cell.

79. Which blood cell has the ability to pass through the blood vessel walls?
 a. erythrocyte
 b. leukocyte
 c. reticulocyte
 d. thrombocyte

80. Which type of cell destroys pathogens by phagocytosis?
 a. erythrocyte
 b. neutrophil
 c. red blood cell
 d. thrombocyte

81. Which of the following is a another term for neutrophils?
 a. eos
 b. basos
 c. monos
 d. polys

82. Which formed element is first on the scene when an injury occurs?
 a. platelet
 b. red blood cell
 c. reticulocyte
 d. white blood cell

83. Which of the following is described as an anuclear, biconcave disc?
 a. erythrocyte
 b. granulocyte
 c. leukocyte
 d. thrombocyte

84. Which type of cell is sometimes called a macrophage?
 a. eosinophil
 b. basophil
 c. lymphocyte
 d. monocyte

85. Which type of cells give rise to plasma cells that produce antibodies?
 a. eosinophils
 b. lymphocytes
 c. monocytes
 d. neutrophils

86. Neutrophils are sometimes called segs because they have segmented:
 a. cytoplasm.
 b. granules.
 c. nuclei.
 d. none of the above

87. Platelets are also called:
 a. erythrocytes.
 b. leukocytes.
 c. segs.
 d. thrombocytes.

88. A platelet is actually a part of a cell called a:
 a. granulocyte.
 b. macrophage.
 c. megakaryocyte.
 d. T lymphocyte.

89. An individual's blood type is determined by the presence or absence of certain types of:
 a. antibodies on the surface of the white blood cells.
 b. antibodies on the surface of the red blood cells.
 c. antigens on the surface of the white blood cells.
 d. antigens on the surface of the red blood cells.

90. To prevent sensitization, Rh immunoglobulin is given to a(n):
 a. pregnant woman if there is bleeding during the pregnancy.
 b. Rh-negative mother on delivery of an Rh-positive baby.
 c. Rh-positive baby immediately after birth.
 d. Rh-positive mother on delivery of an Rh-negative baby.

91. A person who becomes "sensitized" to the Rh factor:
   a. has the Rh antigen.
   b. is Rh-positive.
   c. may produce antibodies to the Rh factor.
   d. should not have children.

92. A person who has A-negative blood has red blood cells that:
   a. have the A antigen and lack the Rh antigen.
   b. have the A antigen and the Rh antigen.
   c. lack the A antigen and have the Rh antigen.
   d. lack the A antigen and the Rh antigen.

93. Severe hemolytic disease of the newborn is most often caused by:
   a. ABO incompatibility between mother and baby.
   b. an incompatible blood transfusion.
   c. preformed Rh antibodies present shortly after birth.
   d. sensitization of an Rh-negative mother from a previous Rh-positive baby.

94. Incompatible blood given to a patient because of misidentification by a phlebotomist may result in the patient's:
   a. circulatory system constricting and shutting off blood supply.
   b. heart being overcome by hemoconcentration.
   c. immune system overacting to the antigen/antibody reaction.
   d. renal tubules being overcome by excess hemolysis and becoming totally dysfunctional.

95. Whole blood is made up of:
   a. aggregated platelets and water.
   b. formed elements suspended in plasma.
   c. serum and cells.
   d. serum and clotted red blood cells.

96. The liquid portion of a clotted specimen is called:
   a. fibrinogen.
   b. plasma.
   c. saline.
   d. serum.

97. The clear liquid portion of an anticoagulated specimen that has been centrifuged is called:
   a. buffy coat.
   b. plasma.
   c. saline.
   d. serum.

98. Figure 6-4 shows a centrifuged whole blood specimen. Identify the portion of the specimen indicated by arrow 1.
   a. buffy coat
   b. plasma
   c. serum
   d. red blood cells

99. Identify the portion of the specimen indicated by arrow 2 in Figure 6-4.

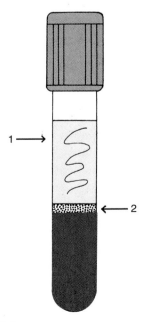

■ FIGURE 6-4 ■
Centrifuged plasma specimen

a. buffy coat
b. plasma
c. serum
d. red blood cells

100. How can you visually tell serum from plasma?
    a. serum is clear, plasma is cloudy
    b. serum is fluid, plasma is a gel
    c. serum is pale yellow, plasma is colorless
    d. you cannot visually tell serum from plasma

101. How soon should a blood smear be made from an ethylenediaminetetraacetate (EDTA) specimen? Within:
    a. 5 minutes.
    b. 30 minutes.
    c. 60 minutes.
    d. 12 hours.

102. The most common anticoagulants prevent clotting by:
    a. enhancing thrombin formation and releasing calcium.
    b. inhibiting glucose or binding fibrinogen.
    c. inhibiting thrombin or binding calcium.
    d. removing fibrinogen.

103. It is preferable to perform STAT chemistry tests on plasma rather than serum because plasma:
    a. is more stable than serum.
    b. is ready for testing sooner than serum.
    c. results are more accurate.
    d. tests require a smaller volume of specimen.

104. A test that assesses platelet plug formation is:
    a. bleeding time (BT).
    b. fibrin degradation products (FDP).
    c. prothrombin time (PT).
    d. partial thromboplastin time (PTT).

105. All of the following statements are true EXCEPT:
    a. serum is collected without an anticoagulant
    b. serum contains fibrinogen
    c. serum is normally clear, pale yellow in color
    d. serum is suitable for most chemistry determinations

106. A person with thrombocytosis has:
    a. abnormally decreased platelets.
    b. abnormally functioning platelets.
    c. abnormally increased platelets.
    d. normal platelets.

107. A disease characterized by an abnormally decreased red blood cell count is:
    a. anemia.
    b. leukopenia.
    c. polycythemia.
    d. thrombocytopenia.

108. The process of coagulation is also called:
    a. hemoconcentration.
    b. hemolysis.
    c. hemostasis.
    d. homeostasis.

109. Which of the following is a test of the formed elements?
    a. blood urea nitrogen (BUN)
    b. complete blood count (CBC)
    c. electrolytes
    d. glucose

110. Hemostasis refers to:
    a. broken red blood cells.
    b. increased large molecules in the blood stream.
    c. keeping the body in equilibrium.
    d. the coagulation process.

111. An abnormal increase in white blood cells is called:
    a. leukemia.
    b. leukocytosis.
    c. leukopenia.
    d. leukopoiesis.

112. The ion required in the coagulation process where prothrombin is converted to thrombin is:
    a. calcium.
    b. chloride.
    c. potassium.
    d. sodium.

113. The extrinsic pathway of coagulation is initiated by:
    a. events within the blood stream.
    b. factor VIII.
    c. platelet plug formation.
    d. tissue injury.

114. The first stage in the hemostatic process is:
    a. fibrin clot formation.
    b. fibrinolysis.
    c. platelet plug formation.
    d. vasoconstriction.

115. All of the following tests are used to diagnose blood cell disorders EXCEPT:
    a. complete blood count
    b. creatinine
    c. ferritin
    d. hemoglobin

116. Which stages of the coagulation process are called primary hemostasis?
    a. fibrin clot formation and fibrinolysis
    b. fibrin clot formation and vasoconstriction
    c. platelet plug formation and fibrin clot formation
    d. vasoconstriction and platelet plug formation

117. Lymph fluid is most like:
    a. serum.
    b. plasma.
    c. urine.
    d. whole blood.

118. A disease caused most often by the lack of factor VIII is:
    a. disseminated intravascular coagulation.
    b. hemophilia.

    c. leukemia.
    d. thrombocytopenia.

119. Coagulation problems may result from liver disease because the liver:
    a. filters blood improperly when diseased.
    b. manufactures coagulation factors.
    c. releases calcium.
    d. removes red blood cells.

120. Which stage of the coagulation process involves the action of the enzyme plasmin?
    a. fibrin clot formation
    b. fibrinolysis
    c. platelet plug formation
    d. vasoconstriction

121. Tests that measure the functioning of primary hemostasis are:
    a. fibrin degradation products and bleeding time.
    b. platelet count and bleeding time.
    c. platelet count and protime.
    d. protime and partial thromboplastin time.

122. Obstruction of a blood vessel by an embolus causes:
    a. a thrombus.
    b. an embolism.
    c. atherosclerosis.
    d. thrombophlebitis.

123. Which of the following is a coagulation test?
    a. electrolytes
    b. glycohemoglobin
    c. hemoglobin
    d. protime

124. When the arm is in the anatomic position, the basilic vein is:
    a. in line with the middle finger.
    b. in the center of the antecubital fossa.
    c. on the same side as the little finger.
    d. on the same side as the thumb.

125. Lymph fluid originates from:
    a. excess tissue fluid.
    b. lymph nodes.
    c. the liver.
    d. the kidneys.

126. A venipuncture site is normally healed by:
    a. fibrin clot formation.
    b. fibrinolysis.
    c. platelet plug formation.
    d. vasoconstriction only.

127. A malignant lymphoid tumor is called:
    a. lymphadenopathy.
    b. lymphangitis.
    c. lymphoma.
    d. lymphosarcoma.

128. A test associated with the lymph system is:
    a. arterial blood gases (ABGs).
    b. creatinine.
    c. disseminated intravascular coagulation (DIC).
    d. mononucleosis test.

129. Lymph fluid keeps moving in the right direction because of:
    a. functioning of the lymphatic ducts.
    b. lymphatic capillary structure.
    c. pressure created by the arterial system.
    d. valves in the lymph vessels.

130. All of the following are functions of the lymph nodes EXCEPT:
    a. process lymphocytes
    b. remove impurities
    c. synthesize coagulation factors
    d. trap and destroy bacteria

131. All of the following veins are antecubital veins EXCEPT:
    a. basilic
    b. cephalic
    c. median cubital
    d. femoral

132. The ability of platelets to stick to surfaces is called platelet:
    a. aggregation.
    b. adhesion.
    c. cohesion.
    d. inhibition.

133. Which test is performed on whole blood?
    a. blood urea nitrogen (BUN)
    b. complete blood count (CBC)
    c. creatine phosphokinase (CPK)
    d. protime

134. Which test is performed on plasma?
    a. complete blood count (CBC)
    b. erythrocyte sedimentation rate (ESR)
    c. hemoglobin (Hgb)
    d. protime

ANSWERS AND EXPLANATIONS

1. **j.** superior vena cava

2. **l.** right pulmonary artery (branches)

3. **g.** tricuspid valve

4. **d.** right ventricle

5. **i.** aortic valve

6. **c.** left atrium

7. **o.** left pulmonary veins

8. **a.** aortic arch

9. **c.** The heart (Fig. 6-5) has three layers: the epicardium is the thin outer layer; the myocardium is the thick muscular middle layer; and the endocardium is the thin membrane lining the heart. The pericardium is the double-layered sac enclosing the heart.

10. **b.** The left ventricle (see Fig. 6-5) pumps oxygenated blood into the systemic circulation via the aortic

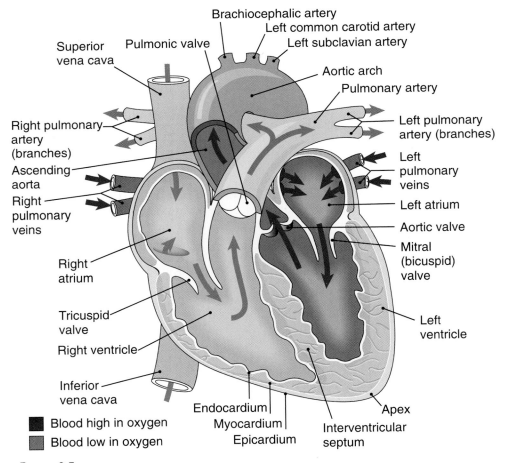

■ FIGURE 6-5 ■

Heart and great vessels. (Used with permission from Cohen, B.J. & Wood, D.L. (2000). Memmler's Structure and Function of the Human Body (7th ed.). Philadelphia: Lippincott Williams & Wilkins, p. 196.)

arch. The right ventricle pumps de-oxygenated blood into the pulmonary artery to be delivered to the lungs via the pulmonary circulation. The lungs deliver oxygenated blood to the pulmonary veins, which deliver it to the left atrium.

11. **d.** The human heart has four chambers: the right and left atria and the right and left ventricles (see Fig. 6-5).

12. **c.** Myocardial infarction or heart attack is a condition caused by occlusion of one or more of the coronary arteries which leads to ischemia or insufficient blood supply to the heart muscle. The term arrhythmia or dysrhythmia means irregularity or loss of heart rhythm. Tachycardia signifies a fast heart rate (greater than 100 beats per minute).

13. **a.** Atria is the plural form of atrium. The atria are the upper chambers of the heart and are called receiving chambers because they receive blood as it returns to the heart. The chordae tendineae are thin tissues that attach the atrioventricular valves to the walls of the ventricles to keep the valves from flipping back into the atria. The vena cavae are two large veins that deliver blood to the right atrium. The ventricles are the lower chambers of the heart that deliver blood to vessels exiting the heart.

14. **d.** The pericardium is a thin, double-layered sac enclosing the heart. The root word "cardi" means *heart* and the following prefixes indicate position of the layers: peri = *around;* epi = *upon, over;* myo = *muscle;* and endo = *within.*

15. **d.** Ventricles, from the Latin word "ventriculus" meaning *little belly,* are

the lower chambers of the heart. The atria are the upper chambers that are connected to the ventricles by valves. The septum is the partition that divides the heart into two sides, right and left.

16. **d.** The right atrioventricular (AV) valve found between the right atrium and ventricle is also called the tricuspid valve because it has three flaps or cusps. The bicuspid valve or left AV valve has two cusps and is also called the mitral valve. The pulmonary valve (right semilunar valve) is so named because it allows blood to pass into the pulmonary artery from the right ventricle (see Fig. 6-5).

17. **d.** The septum (see Fig. 6-5) is the partition that divides the heart into two sides, each side containing two chambers: an atrium and a ventricle. The pericardium is the membranous sac covering the heart. The chordae tendineae are thin threads of tissue that attach the valves to the walls of the ventricles to keep them from flipping back into the atria as the ventricle contracts.

18. **a.** The coronary or cardiac arteries, which are the first branches off the aorta, furnish the blood supply to the heart. The pulmonary arteries carry blood from the right atrium to the lungs. The vena cavae deliver blood to the heart from the systemic system. Venules are the smallest branches of veins.

19. **b.** One complete contraction and subsequent relaxation of the heart is called a cardiac cycle. The relaxing phase is called diastole, and the contracting phase is called systole. A heart attack is called a myocardial infarction. Bradycardia is the term used to de-

scribe an irregular slow heart rate of less than 60 beats per minute.

20. **d.** The sinoatrial (SA) node (Fig. 6-6) is called the heart's "pacemaker" It generates an electrical impulse that initiates the contraction of both atria pushing the blood into the ventricles. The impulse is picked up by the atrioventricular (AV) node and relayed through the bundle of His and along the Purkinje fibers throughout the ventricles, causing them to contract. The semilunar or crescent-shaped valves open as the ventricles contract to allow the blood to flow into the exit arteries.

21. **b.** The complete cardiac cycle involving the simultaneous contraction of both atria pushing the blood into the ventricles followed by the simultaneous contraction of the ventricles pushing the blood into the exit arteries and then the relaxation of both takes approximately 0.8 seconds.

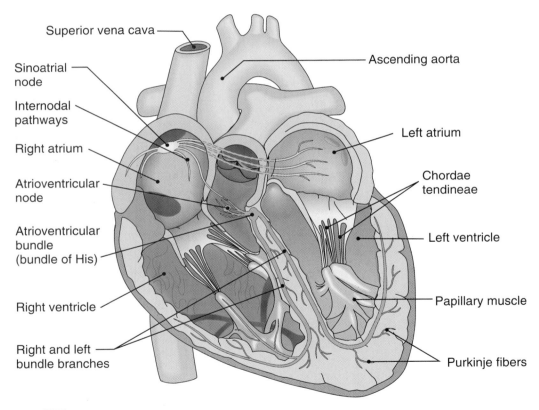

Sinoatrial node and internodal pathways

Atrioventricular node and the bundle of His with its branches

■ FIGURE 6-6 ■

Electrical conduction system of the heart. (Used with permission from Cohen, B.J. & Wood, D.L. (2000). Memmler's Structure and Function of the Human Body (7th ed.). Philadelphia: Lippincott Williams & Wilkins, p. 201.)

22. **d.** An electrocardiogram (ECG) is the actual record of electrical currents that correspond to each event in the heart muscle contraction. An electroencephalogram (EEG) measures electrical currents from the brain. Creatine kinase (CK) and arterial blood gases (ABGs) are diagnostic blood tests used to measure heart muscle damage and changes in the acid-base balance of blood, respectively

23. **a.** The P wave represents the activity of the atria and is usually the first wave seen. The QRS complex along with the T wave represents the activity of ventricles (Fig. 6-7).

24. **d.** The QRS complex (collection of three waves) along with the T wave represents the electrical activity of the ventricles, while the P wave represents the activity of the atria (see Fig. 6-7).

25. **d.** Murmurs are abnormal heart sounds, usually caused by faulty valve action. Extrasystoles, fibrillations, and arrhythmias are abnormal contractions, not sounds.

26. **a.** An artery is a vessel that carries blood away from the heart. Veins, such as the vena cava, carry blood to the heart. Capillaries are vessels that connect the ends of the smallest arteries (arterioles) to the smallest veins (venules).

27. **c.** The wave of increased pressure created as the ventricles contract and blood is forced out of the heart through the arteries creates the throbbing beat known as the pulse.

28. **d.** Unlike the arterial system, veins do not have sufficient pressure from the heart's contractions to keep the blood moving through them. Veins rely on skeletal muscle movement around them and the opening and closing of the valves to keep the blood moving toward the heart.

29. **d.** All of the choices deal with heart rates or rhythm. Tachycardia is an

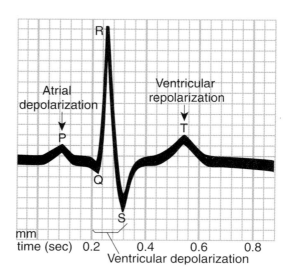

■ FIGURE 6-7 ■

Normal ECG tracing showing one cardiac cycle. (Used with permission from Cohen, B.J. & Wood, D.L. (2000). *Memmler's structure and function of the human body* (7th ed.). Philadelphia: Lippincott Williams & Wilkins, p. 205.)

abnormally fast rate. Bradycardia is a slow rate. Extrasystole is the term for an extra beat before the normal beat. Fibrillation is the term for rapid, uncoordinated contractions.

30. d. Blood pressure is a measure of the pressure exerted on the walls of a blood vessel. It is commonly measured in a large artery, such as the brachial. Blood pressure is expressed in millimeters of mercury and has two components: the systolic pressure, which is the highest pressure reached during ventricular contraction, and the diastolic pressure, which occurs during relaxation of the ventricles. Systolic pressure for the normal, relaxed, sitting adult averages 120 mm Hg, whereas diastolic averages 80 mm Hg.

31. c. Endocarditis means inflammation of the endocardium. The endocardium is the thin membrane lining the inner surface of the heart. Pericarditis is inflammation of the pericardium which is the thin, fluid-filled sac that surrounds the heart. Angina pectoris refers to pain in the area of the heart caused by decreased blood flow to the muscle layer of the heart. Aortic stenosis is the term used to describe a narrowing of the aorta or its opening.

32. c. Creatine kinase (CK) and lactate dehydrogenase (LDH) are enzymes present in cardiac muscle. They are released during myocardial infarction. Alkaline phosphatase (ALP) and alanine aminotransferase (SGPT) are enzymes measured most commonly to determine liver function. Blood urea nitrogen (BUN) is a kidney function test, and prothrombin time (PT) is a coagulation test used to monitor anticoagulant

therapy. A glucose tolerance test (GTT) measures glucose metabolism, and erythrocyte sedimentation rate (ESR) is a nonspecific indicator of disease, especially inflammatory conditions such as arthritis.

33. b. Systolic pressure is the pressure in the arteries during contraction of the ventricles. Diastolic pressure is the arterial pressure when the ventricles are relaxed. Because the atrial contraction is so very close to the ventricle contraction, blood pressure for atrial contraction cannot easily be detected and is not normally measured.

34. a. Pulmonary circulation carries deoxygenated blood from the right ventricle of the heart to the lungs via the pulmonary artery. It also returns oxygenated blood from the lungs to the left atrium of the heart via the pulmonary vein. The left ventricle pumps the oxygenated blood into the arterial systemic circulation via the aorta. The arterial systemic circulation delivers the blood to the tissues. The venous systemic circulation returns deoxygenated blood to the heart (Fig. 6-8).

35. b. Blood flows from the heart into arteries, which branch into smaller and smaller arteries, the smallest of which are called arterioles. Arterioles connect with capillaries, which in turn are connected to the smallest veins, which are called venules. Blood from the arterioles passes through the capillaries where the exchange of gases, nutrients, and waste products takes place. From the capillaries the blood flows into the venules, which merge with larger and larger veins until the blood returns to the heart. Choices

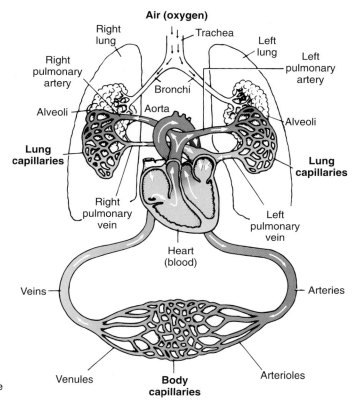

■ FIGURE 6-8 ■

Representation of the vascular flow. (National Tuberculosis and Respiratory Disease Association, New York, NY.)

"a" and "c" are obviously incorrect. In choice "d" the blood would be traveling in the wrong direction (see Fig. 6-8).

36. **c.** The right ventricle delivers blood to the pulmonary artery. The left ventricle delivers blood to the aorta by way of the aortic arch. The lungs deliver oxygenated blood to the pulmonary veins, which deliver it to the left atrium (see Fig. 6.8).

37. **b.** Because it is full of oxygen, normal systemic arterial blood is bright cherry red. Normal systemic venous blood is dark red with a bluish tinge. Regardless of what some people think, no one has blue blood.

38. **a.** The aorta, at the start of the systemic arterial circulation, is the largest artery in the body. The largest vein in the body is the vena cava. The femoral artery is a large artery in the leg. The carotid artery is a large artery in the neck.

39. **c.** The pulmonary vein carries oxygenated (oxygen-rich) blood from the lungs to the heart. All vessels that return blood to the heart are called veins. All vessels that carry blood away from the heart are called arteries. The general rule of

thumb that arteries carry oxygenated blood is only true for the
systemic circulation. In the pulmonary circulation, the vessel that
carries oxygenated (oxygen-poor)
blood from the lungs is called a vein
because it is returning the blood to
the heart. The vessel that carries deoxygenated (oxygen-poor) blood to
the lungs is called the pulmonary
artery because it is carrying the
blood away from the heart.

40. **a.** Sphygmomanometer is the technical name for a blood pressure cuff.
An electrocardiogram (ECG) is a
record (tracing) of the electrical activity of the heart. A machine that
records brain waves is used in electroencephalography (EEG). A pacemaker is an electrical device that
automatically generates electrical
impulses to initiate the heart beat.

41. **d.** The smallest veins are called
venules. Arterioles are the smallest
arteries. Capillaries connect the arterioles (which are the end of the
arterial system) to the venules
(which are the beginning of venous
system). Lumen is the term for the
internal space of any vessel.

42. **c.** The pulmonary artery, as its name
infers, is part of the pulmonary circulation. The brachial artery,
cephalic vein, and vena cava are all
part of the systemic circulation.

43. **b.** Capillaries are tiny one-cell-thick
vessels that form the fine network
that delivers oxygen and nutrients
to the tissues and carries carbon
dioxide and other waste products
away. Arterioles and venules, on
the other hand, have multiple layers like arteries and veins. The vena
cava, the larges vein in the body,
also has multiple layers.

44. **b.** The pulmonary vein is part of the
pulmonary circulation and carries
oxygenated blood from the lungs to
the heart so that it can be pumped
to the body. The superior vena cava
and the brachial vein are part of the
systemic venous circulation and
carry deoxygenated blood back to
the heart. The pulmonary artery
carries deoxygenated blood from
the heart to the lungs.

45. **a.** The tunica adventitia is the term
applied to the outer layer of an
artery or vein. It is made up of connective tissue and is thicker in arteries than veins. The tunica media
is the middle layer, composed of
smooth muscle and some elastic
fibers. The tunica media is much
thicker in arteries than in veins.
The tunica intima, sometimes also
called tunica interna, is the inner
layer or lining of a blood vessel and
is composed of a single layer of en-
dothelial cells with an underlying
basement membrane, connective
tissue layer, and elastic membrane.

46. **b.** The space within a blood vessel is
called the lumen. The tunica intima
and tunica media are blood vessel
layers. The endothelium is the inner lining of a blood vessel.

47. **d.** The smooth muscle of the tunica
media is much thicker in arteries
than in veins. The tunica adventitia
or outer layer is also thicker in arteries. Both veins and arteries are
lined with a single layer of en-
dothelial cells (Fig. 6-9). Arteries
typically have more elastic tissue
than veins.

48. **c.** You can tell the structure on the
right in Figure 6-2 is a vein because
it has a valve. Arteries do not have
valves. See Figure 6-9 for a compar-

ison diagram of artery, vein, and capillary structure.

49. c. The inner layer of a blood vessel is called the tunica intima. The lumen is the internal space within a blood vessel. The tunica adventitia and media are the outside layer and middle layer, respectively (see Fig. 6-9).

50. d. In choosing the best vein, the first selection is the median cubital because it is large, bruises less easily, and is well anchored. The cephalic vein is the next choice because it is better anchored and less painful to puncture than the basilic. The basilic vein is the last choice because it rolls easily and there is the possibility of accidentally puncturing the brachial artery and a major nerve when this vein is used (Fig. 6-10).

51. c. Capillaries are the smallest blood vessels. They are one-cell-thick which allows for the exchange of oxygen and nutrients between the cells and the blood. Alveoli are thin-walled saclike chambers within the lungs where oxygen and carbon dioxide are exchanged between the air and blood. Arterioles are tiny arteries that connect with and deliver blood to the capillaries. Venules are tiny veins at the junction where the capillaries merge with the venous circulation.

52. a. The antecubital fossa is located in front of (anterior) and below (distal to) the elbow.

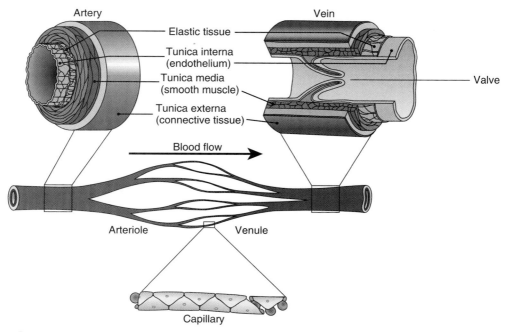

■ FIGURE 6-9 ■

Artery, vein, and capillary structure. (Used with permission from Cohen, B.J. & Wood, D.L. (2000). Memmler's Structure and Function of the Human Body (7th ed.). Philadelphia: Lippincott Williams & Wilkins, p. 211.)

53. c. A blood clot or other undissolved matter circulating in the bloodstream is called an embolus. An aneurysm is a bulging or dilation of a blood vessel. An embolism is the obstruction of a blood vessel by an embolus. A thrombus is a stationary blood clot that obstructs or partially obstructs a blood vessel.

54. a. basilic

55. c. median cubital

56. d. median cubital

57. d. The basilic vein is the third choice of veins in the antecubital fossa area for all of the reasons listed.

58. b. Ankle and foot veins should *never* be punctured routinely. They are used only when no other suitable sites are available *and* the patient's physician has given permission to do so. Coagulation problems and poor circulation may cause serious problems as well as erroneous results when ankle or foot veins are used.

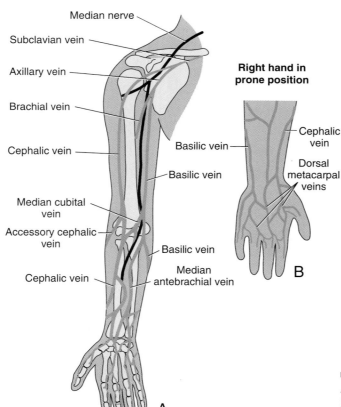

Right arm in anatomic position

Median nerve

Subclavian vein

Axillary vein

Brachial vein

Cephalic vein

Median cubital vein

Accessory cephalic vein

Cephalic vein

Basilic vein

Basilic vein

Basilic vein

Median antebrachial vein

A

Right hand in prone position

Cephalic vein

Dorsal metacarpal veins

B

■ Figure 6-10 ■

A. Principal veins of the arm, including major antecubital veins subject to venipuncture. **B.** Forearm, wrist, and hand veins subject to venipuncture.

59. **c.** The great saphenous vein runs the entire length of the leg and is considered the longest vein in the body. The largest vein and artery in the body are, respectively, the vena cava and the aorta. There is a femoral vein and a femoral artery. Both are located in the leg (Fig. 6-11).

60. **b.** The lesser or small saphenous vein is found on the lateral side of the ankle. It goes up the back of the leg and then goes deeper behind the knee. The femoral vein is found deep in the upper part of the leg. The popliteal vein is found deep in the area of the knee.

61. **a.** Blood is a mixture of fluid and cells. The fluid portion is called *plasma*. Plasma is approximately 90% water and 10% dissolved substances such as antibodies, nutrients, minerals, and gases. Red blood cells (erythrocytes) and platelets are part of the cellular portion of blood referred to as the *formed elements*. Bacteria are not normally found in the blood.

62. **c.** Phlebitis is the medical term for vein inflammation. An embolism is the obstruction of a blood vessel by a blood clot or other undissolved foreign matter. Hemostasis is the process by which bleeding is stopped. Thrombosis means the formation or existence of a blood clot in the vascular system.

63. **c.** A disseminated intravascular coagulation (DIC) screen is a series of tests to detect diffuse uncontrolled coagulation throughout the vascular system. In DIC situations, continuous generation of thrombin causes depletion of several clotting factors to such an extent that generalized bleeding may occur. Bilirubin is a liver function test. Glucose is a test of carbohydrate metabolism. A cerebrospinal fluid (CSF) test is considered a nervous system test.

64. **a.** Atherosclerosis is a form of arteriosclerosis involving changes in the intima of the artery caused by the accumulation of lipid material. Increased blood cholesterol levels constitute an increased risk of developing coronary heart disease. Endocarditis means inflammation of the lining membrane of the heart and may be caused by invasion of microorganisms. Phlebitis means inflammation of a vein.

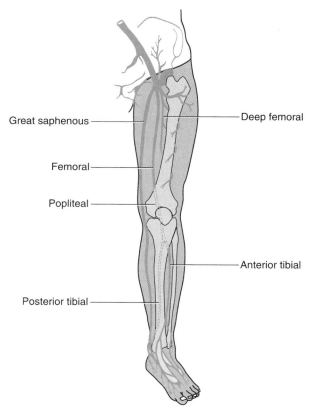

Great saphenous

Femoral

Popliteal

Posterior tibial

Deep femoral

Anterior tibial

■ Figure 6-11 ■
Major leg and foot veins.

65. a. An aneurysm is a localized dilation or bulging of a blood vessel, usually an artery. An embolism is the obstruction of a blood vessel by a blood clot or other undissolved foreign matter. Arteriosclerosis is a hardening or thickening and loss of elasticity of the wall of the artery. Thrombophlebitis is defined as inflammation of the vein in conjunction with the formation of a blood clot.

66. c. Thrombophlebitis is defined as inflammation of a vein in conjunction with the formation of a blood clot. Vasculitis is a general term meaning inflammation of a blood vessel. Phlebitis is more specific and means vein inflammation. Phlebitis can lead to thrombophlebitis. Sclerosis, when pertaining to the vascular system, refers to a thickening or hardening of the wall of a blood vessel.

67. c. The average 154-lb adult has approximately 5 L or 5.2 qt of blood. More exact blood volume can be calculated based on the fact that the average adult has 70 mL of blood per each kilogram of weight.

68. c. The normal ratio of plasma to formed elements is approximately 55% plasma and 45% cells. That means approximately half of a normal blood specimen will be serum or plasma. This is important when determining how much blood to collect for testing purposes.

69. b. Normal plasma is a clear to slightly hazy, pale yellow fluid that is 90% water.

70. c. When the hand is prone (in pronation), the palm faces downward, causing the cephalic vein in the an-

tecubital area to be in line with the little finger. When the arm is in the normal anatomic position, the palm is up and the cephalic vein is on the same side as the thumb.

71. b. The type of cell that is most numerous in the blood is the erythrocyte or red blood cell, averaging 4.5–5.0 million per cubic millimeter of blood.

72. b. All mature leukocytes or white blood cells contain nuclei. Thrombocytes (platelets) and mature erythrocytes (red blood cells) do not have nuclei. A reticulocyte is an immature red blood cell that contains remnants of nuclear material but not a complete nucleus (Fig. 6-12).

73. c. Reticulocytes are immature red blood cells in the blood stream that contain nuclear remnants.

74. a. The granulocytes called eosinophils (eos) are increased in allergic reactions and parasitic infestations such as a case of pinworms. Eos ingest and detoxify foreign protein and help turn off immune reactions.

75. b. Normal erythrocytes are anuclear, biconcave disks approximately 7–8 μm in diameter.

76. b. Leukocytes (white blood cells) are produced in the bone marrow and lymphatic tissue.

77. d. The primary function of red blood cells is to transport oxygen from the lungs to the tissues. A secondary function of red blood cells is to transport carbon dioxide from the tissues to the lungs. Nutrients and antibodies are not transported by red blood cells but are carried dissolved in the plasma.

78. d. Leukocyte is the medical term for a white blood cell.

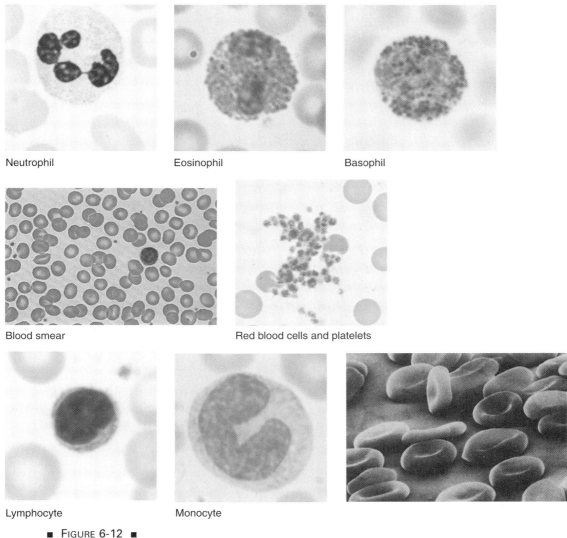

Neutrophil   Eosinophil   Basophil

Blood smear   Red blood cells and platelets

Lymphocyte   Monocyte

■ FIGURE 6-12 ■

A. Normal blood smear and close-up view of individual blood cells. **B.** Red blood cells as seen by scanning electron microscopy. (Used with permission from Cohen, B.J. & Wood, D.L. (2000). Memmler's Structure and Function of the Human Body (7th ed.). Philadelphia: Lippincott Williams & Wilkins, p. 184.)

79. b. Leukocytes have extravascular function, which means they do their job outside the blood stream. They have the ability to pass through the walls of blood vessels by a process called diapedesis. Ery-throcytes, reticulocytes, and thrombocytes have intravascular function and cannot pass through intact blood vessel walls.

80. b. Neutrophils are a type of leukocyte that are able to destroy bacteria and small particles by a process called phagocytosis.

81. **d.** The term "polys" comes from the word polymorphonuclear. Neutrophils are sometimes called polys because they have a nucleus with several lobes.

82. **a.** The first cell on the scene when an injury occurs is the platelet. The role of the platelet is to aggregate with other platelets and adhere to the injured area, forming a platelet plug to help stop the flow of blood from the injured blood vessel.

83. **a.** Erythrocytes (red blood cells) are anuclear (non-nucleated), biconcave disks approximately 7–8 μm in diameter (see Fig. 6-12).

84. **d.** Monocytes that have left the blood stream are sometimes referred to as macrophages because they are found in the loose connective tissue where they phagocytize particles much like cells of the reticuloendothlial (RE) system.

85. **b.** A type of lymphocyte called a B-lymphocyte differentiates into a plasma cell.

86. **c.** A typical neutrophil is polymorphonuclear, meaning its nucleus has several lobes or segments. Thus, the natural tendency is to call this cell a "seg" (see Fig. 6-12).

87. **d.** "Thrombo" and "cyte" mean *clotting* and *cell*, respectively. Thrombocyte is a medical term for platelets that function in the clotting process.

88. **c.** A platelet is not a true cell but a cytoplasmic fragment of a large bone marrow cell called a megakaryocyte. When separated into parts (mega-karyo-cyte), this term means large-nucleated-cell.

89. **d.** An individual's blood type is inherited and is determined by the presence or absence of certain types of antigens on the surface of the red blood cells. The ABO blood group system recognizes four blood types based on two antigens called A and B. A type A individual has the A antigen; type B has the B antigen; type AB has both antigens; and type O has neither A nor B. The Rh system is based on the presence or absence of the Rh antigen. An Rh-positive individual has the Rh antigen, and an Rh-negative individual lacks the Rh antigen.

90. **b.** To prevent sensitization from an Rh-positive fetus, an Rh-negative woman may be given Rh immunoglobulin at certain times during her pregnancy as well as immediately after the baby's birth. Rh immunoglobulin will destroy any Rh-positive fetal cells that may have entered her blood stream, thus preventing sensitization. Only an Rh-negative person can become sensitized to the Rh factor.

91. **c.** Becoming sensitized means that the individual may produce antibodies against the Rh factor. Rh antibodies produced by the mother can cross the placenta into the fetal circulation and cause the destruction of red blood cells of a subsequent Rh-positive fetus.

92. **a.** An individual whose blood type is A-negative has red blood cells that have the A antigen but lack the Rh antigen. (See explanation of question 89.)

93. **d.** Hemolytic disease of the newborn is most often the result of an Rh-negative mother being sensitized by a previous Rh-positive fetus, caus-

ing her to form Rh antibodies. During a subsequent pregnancy, these antibodies can cross the placenta into the fetal circulation and attack the red blood cells of the fetus and cause hemolysis.

94. **d.** If a person is given an incompatible type of blood, antibodies in the blood may agglutinate and hemolyze the red blood cells. The excess hemoglobin puts physical stress on the renal tubules and may damage them permanently.

95. **b.** Whole blood, like the blood found in the body, is made up of a liquid portion called plasma which contains formed elements (red blood cells, white blood cells, and platelets) suspended in it.

96. **d.** Clotted blood is made up of two parts, a clotted portion containing cells enmeshed in fibrin and a liquid portion called serum.

97. **b.** After centrifugation of whole blood, the clear liquid portion called plasma is at the top of the tube and the cellular portion is at the bottom.

98. **b.** Arrow 1 in Figure 6-4 points to the plasma portion of the specimen. A whole blood specimen is collected in an anticoagulant such as EDTA to keep it from clotting. If the specimen is centrifuged or allowed to settle, the clear liquid portion at the top of the specimen is called plasma.

99. **a.** Arrow 2 in Figure 6-4 points to the thin layer of white blood cells and platelets on top of the red blood cells that is commonly called the buffy coat.

100. **d.** You cannot visually tell serum from plasma because both serum and plasma are mostly clear, pale yellow fluids. Plasma is sometimes slightly hazy because of the fibrinogen in it, but serum may also be slightly hazy when fats are present, a condition called lipemia.

101. **c.** EDTA is the anticoagulant of choice for hematology studies. However, if a blood smear is to be made from an EDTA specimen, it should be made within 1 hour of collection because prolonged contact with EDTA may change the staining characteristics of the formed elements.

102. **c.** The most common anticoagulants are EDTA, sodium citrate, and heparin. EDTA and sodium citrate prevent coagulation by binding calcium into a calcium salt. Without calcium ions, the coagulation process cannot take place. Heparin inhibits thrombin. Without thrombin, the blood cannot form a fibrin clot.

103. **b.** Most chemistry tests are ideally performed on serum because nothing has to be added to the blood during collection. Unfortunately, to obtain serum, a normal blood specimen must be allowed to clot for at least 20–30 minutes before being centrifuged. With the exception of fibrinogen, plasma contains the same analytes as serum; however, because a plasma specimen does not clot, it can be spun immediately after collection and tested 20–30 minutes sooner. A fast turnaround time is vitally important for STAT requests.

104. **a.** A bleeding time (BT) test assesses the ability of the platelet to aggregate (degranulate and stick to one another) and form a platelet plug. FDP, PT, and PTT test other parts of the coagulation process.

105. b. To obtain serum, blood must be allowed to clot. During the clotting process, fibrinogen is split into fibrin, which enmeshes the cells to form the clot. Once the clotting is complete, the specimen is centrifuged and the clear liquid obtained is called serum. Serum does not contain fibrinogen because it was used up in the clotting process.

106. c. "Thrombo," "cyt," and "osis" mean *clotting, cell,* and *condition,* respectively. The term is used to describe a condition in which the clotting cells (platelets) are abnormally increased.

107. a. Anemia is a blood disorder usually characterized by an abnormal reduction in the number of red blood cells in the circulating blood. Leukopenia is characterized by abnormally decreased white blood cells. Polycythemia is overproduction of red blood cells. Thrombocytopenia is abnormally decreased platelets.

108. c. The process of coagulation, which means stopping or controlling the flow of blood, is also called hemostasis. Hemoconcentration means increased nonfilterable elements. Hemolysis is destruction of red blood cells. Homeostasis is the state of equilibrium or balance the body strives to maintain.

109 b. Assessing the formed elements (red blood cells, white blood cells, and platelets) is part of a CBC. It is performed on whole blood. BUN, electrolytes, and glucose are chemistry tests performed on serum or plasma.

110. d. "Hemostasis" means *blood-stopping or controlling* and refers to the process of coagulation.

111. b. When broken into parts, "leukocyt-osis" means *white-cells-condition.* The term is used to describe an abnormal increase of white blood cells.

112. a. The ion (particle carrying an electrical charge) necessary to convert prothrombin to thrombin in the coagulation cascade is calcium (Ca+).

113. d. The word "extrinsic" means *from or coming from, without.* The extrinsic pathway is initiated by tissue injury, causing the release of thromboplastin (factor III) and the activation of factor VII. The intrinsic pathway of coagulation is initiated by events within the blood stream. Factor VIII (antihemophilic factor) is part of the intrinsic pathway. Platelet plug formation is the second stage in the coagulation process and occurs before the initiation of either pathway.

114. d. There are four stages to the hemostasis process, the initial stage is the constriction of vessels (vasoconstriction) to slow down blood loss. The second stage is platelet plug formation, which involves platelet aggregation and adhesion. These first two stages are called primary hemostasis. Stage three is fibrin clot formation, which involves activation of the intrinsic and extrinsic pathways of the coagulation cascade. Stage four is fibrinolysis, the process by which the fibrin clot is dissolved.

115. b. Both complete blood count and hemoglobin are hematology tests used to assess blood disorders. Ferritin, the form in which iron is stored in the tissues, is a whole blood chemistry test that is also used in the diagnosis of blood disorders. Creatinine is a kidney function test performed in the chemistry department.

116. **d.** The word "primary" means *first*. The first two stages of the hemostasis/coagulation process are vasoconstriction and platelet plug formation. These first two stages combined are called primary hemostasis and are sometimes all that is needed to stop blood loss, and the process goes no further.

117. **b.** Lymph fluid is similar to plasma but is 95% water instead of 90%. Unlike serum, lymph does contain fibrinogen. It is unlike urine or whole blood.

118. **b.** Hemophilia is a hereditary blood disorder characterized by very long bleeding times. The most common type of hemophilia is caused by the lack of clotting factor VIII.

119. **b.** The liver plays a major role in coagulation. It synthesizes the clotting factors fibrinogen and prothrombin and is the source of heparin, a naturally formed anticoagulant found in the blood stream.

120. **b.** The last stage of the coagulation process is called fibrinolysis. In this stage the protein plasminogen is converted to the enzyme, plasmin. Plasmin splits fibrin into small fragments called fibrin degradation products (FDP), which are removed by phagocytic cells of the reticuloendothelial system.

121. **b.** Tests used to evaluate primary hemostasis or platelet plug formation are platelet count and bleeding time. The other choices are tests that measure the functioning of secondary hemostasis.

122. **b.** Obstruction of a blood vessel by an embolus causes an embolism.

123. **d.** A prothrombin test (PT), or protime, is a coagulation test. Electrolytes are chemistry tests. Glycohemoglobin is a chemistry test that measures glucose bound to hemoglobin. Hemoglobin is a hematology test.

124. **c.** The anatomic position refers to the body as if the patient is standing erect, arms at the side with palms facing forward. In this position, the basilic vein is on the same side as the little finger.

125. **a.** Body cells are nourished from the tissue fluid acquired from the blood stream. Much of the fluid diffuses back into the capillaries along with waste products of metabolism. Excess tissue fluid filters into lymphatic capillaries, where it is called lymph.

126. **c.** Stage 1, vasoconstriction, and stage 2, platelet plug formation, are referred to as primary hemostasis. Normally a needle puncture of a vein can be healed through primary hemostasis alone.

127. **d.** The word parts, "lympho-sarc-oma" combine to mean *lymphoid-fleshy-malignant tumor.*

128. **d.** The test most often associated with the lymph system is the mononucleosis test. Mononucleosis is an acute infectious disease that primarily affects lymphoid tissue.

129. **d.** The lymph fluid moves through the lymph vessels primarily by skeletal muscle contraction, much like blood moves through the veins. Like veins, the lymph vessels have

valves to keep the lymph flowing in the right direction.

130. **c.** The lymph nodes function to remove impurities, process lymphocytes, and trap and destroy impurities. Lymph nodes *do not* synthesize coagulation factors.

131. **d.** The femoral vein is found in the upper portion of the leg and is a continuation of the popliteal vein. The basilic, cephalic, and median cubital are antecubital veins.

132. **b.** The word "adhesion" means *the uniting of two surfaces or parts,* as in platelet adhesion to the injured area. The ability of platelets to stick to one another is called platelet aggregation.

133. **b.** To perform hematology tests, such as a CBC, the specimen must be whole blood. This allows the laboratory technologist to look at and count the cells in suspension as they are in the body.

134. **d.** CBC, ESR, and Hgb are all hematology tests that require whole blood specimens. A protime is a coagulation test that is performed on plasma.

7 BLOOD COLLECTION EQUIPMENT, ADDITIVES, AND ORDER OF DRAW

REVIEW QUESTIONS

Match the term with the BEST description.

1. ____ additive
2. ____ anticoagulant
3. ____ antiglycolytic agent
4. ____ antiseptics
5. ____ bevel
6. ____ butterfly needle
7. ____ clot activator
8. ____ citrate phosphate dextrose (CPD)
9. ____ disinfectants
10. ____ evacuated tube
11. ____ gauge
12. ____ glycolysis
13. ____ hub
14. ____ hypodermic needle
15. ____ lumen
16. ____ multisample needle
17. ____ order of draw
18. ____ plasma separator tube (PST)
19. ____ shaft
20. ____ sharps container
21. ____ serum separator tube (SST)

a. additive used for donor collections
b. blood collection tube with a pre-measured vacuum
c. breakdown or metabolism of glucose
d. double-pointed needle used with the evacuated tube system
e. end of a needle that attaches to a blood collection device
f. forms a barrier between cells and serum or plasma
g. heparinized tube containing a gel separator
h. inhibits calcium metabolism
i. inhibit the growth of bacteria
j. internal space of a needle or vein
k. kill bacteria
l. long cylindrical portion of a needle
m. number related to the diameter of a needle
n. prevents blood from clotting
o. prevents the metabolism of glucose
p. sequence of tube collection in a multi-tube draw
q. slanted end of a needle
r. special container used to dispose of needles and other sharp objects
s. specimen collection priority
t. substance added to a blood collection tube other than a tube coating or stopper
u. substance that enhances clotting of blood
v. tube containing a gel separator and silica to activate clotting
w. type of needle that is used with a syringe
x. winged infusion set

Match the additive with the tube stopper color.
(Some stopper choices may be used more than once.)

22. _____ ACD
23. _____ EDTA
24. _____ heparin
25. _____ no additive
26. _____ potassium oxalate
27. _____ silica
28. _____ sodium citrate
29. _____ sodium fluoride
30. _____ SPS
31. _____ thixotropic gel

a. gold or mottled red and gray
b. gray
c. dark green
d. lavender
e. light blue
f. red (glass tube)
g. yellow

Choose the BEST answer.

32. Disinfectants are all of the following EXCEPT:
    a. corrosive chemical compounds
    b. safe to use on human skin
    c. used on surfaces and instruments
    d. used to kill pathogenic microorganisms

33. A solution used to clean the site before routine venipuncture is:
    a. 5.25% sodium hypochlorite.
    b. 70% isopropyl alcohol.
    c. 70% methanol.
    d. povidone iodine.

34. Which of the following is typically used to clean the site when collecting blood culture specimens?
    a. benzalkonium chloride
    b. isopropanol
    c. povidone iodine
    d. sodium hypochlorite

35. Which of the following is the *best* solution to use to clean up blood spills?
    a. 1:10 sodium hypochlorite
    b. 70% alcohol
    c. povidone iodine
    d. soap and water

36. Why are gauze pads a better choice than cotton balls for covering the site and holding pressure following venipuncture?

a. cotton balls are not as absorbent
b. cotton ball fibers tend to stick to the site
c. gauze pads are more sterile
d. gauze pads create more pressure

37. All of the following can be used on infants younger than 2 years of age EXCEPT:
    a. adhesive bandages
    b. evacuated tubes
    c. isopropyl alcohol
    d. tourniquet

38. Which of the following is a required characteristic of a sharps container?
    a. leak-proof and puncture-resistant
    b. locking lid
    c. marked with a biohazard symbol
    d. all of the above

39. When a disposable latex tourniquet becomes soiled with blood, it is best to:
    a. autoclave it before reuse.
    b. throw it away.
    c. wash it with a bleach solution.
    d. wipe it with alcohol.

40. Wearing gloves during phlebotomy procedures is mandated by the:
    a. Centers for Disease Control and Prevention (CDC).
    b. Food and Drug Administration (FDA).

c. Hospital Infection Control Practices Advisory Committee (HICPAC).
d. Occupational Safety and Health Administration (OSHA).

41. What criterion do you use to decide which needle gauge to use for venipuncture?
a. depth of the vein
b. personal preference
c. size and condition of the vein
d. type of test being collected

42. To what does the "gauge" of a needle relate?
a. diameter
b. length
c. strength
d. volume

43. Which needle gauge has the largest bore?
a. 18
b. 20
c. 21
d. 22

44. Multisample needles are typically available in these gauges.
a. 16–18
b. 18–20
c. 20–22
d. 22–24

45. The slanted tip of a needle is called the:
a. bevel.
b. hub.
c. lumen.
d. shaft.

46. The purpose of the rubber sleeve that covers the tube end of a multiple-sample needle is to:
a. enable smooth tube placement and removal.
b. maintain sterility of the sample.
c. prevent leakage of blood during tube changes.
d. protect the needle and keep it sharp.

47. A phlebotomy needle that does not have a safety feature:
a. cannot be used for venipuncture.
b. must be used with a tube holder that has a safety feature.
c. requires immediate recapping after use.
d. should be removed from the holder before disposal.

48. What criterion do you use to decide what size tubes to use for ETS blood collection?
a. age of the patient
b. amount of blood needed for the test
c. size and condition of the patient's vein
d. all of the above

49. Evacuated tubes are coated with silicon to:
a. allow tubes to fill more quickly.
b. keep blood from clinging to the sides of the tube.
c. prevent glycolysis.
d. prevent reflux of tube contents.

50. Which of the following stopper colors designates a tube used for coagulation testing?
a. green
b. lavender
c. light blue
d. red

51. Which of the following tubes will yield a serum specimen?
a. green top
b. lavender top
c. light blue top
d. red top

52. This test requires preparation of a blood film on a glass slide.
a. blood culture
b. glucose
c. manual differential
d. prothrombin time

53. All of the following tube stopper colors indicate the presence (or absence) and type of additive in the tube EXCEPT:
  a. green
  b. lavender
  c. light blue
  d. royal blue

54. Heparin prevents blood from clotting by:
  a. activating calcium.
  b. activating thrombin.
  c. binding calcium.
  d. inhibiting thrombin.

55. Which department would most likely perform the test on a specimen collected in a sodium polyanethol sulfonate (SPS) tube?
  a. chemistry
  b. coagulation
  c. hematology
  d. microbiology

56. A royal blue top with green color-coding on the label contains:
  a. EDTA.
  b. heparin.
  c. sodium citrate.
  d. no additive.

57. All of the following substances interfere with the action of calcium in the clotting process EXCEPT:
  a. EDTA.
  b. heparin.
  c. potassium oxalate.
  d. sodium citrate.

58. It is important to fill oxalate tubes to the stated fill capacity because excess oxalate:
  a. causes hemolysis.
  b. changes the staining characteristics of WBCs.
  c. increases potassium levels.
  d. leads to microclot formation.

59. Which of the following substances is contained in a serum separator tube?

  a. EDTA
  b. heparin
  c. sodium citrate
  d. thixotropic gel

60. What is the purpose of an antiglycolytic agent?
  a. enhance clotting
  b. inhibit electrolyte breakdown
  c. preserve glucose
  d. prevent clotting

61. Glass particles present in serum separator tubes:
  a. accelerate clotting.
  b. deter clotting.
  c. inhibit glycolysis.
  d. prevent hemolysis.

62. Which is the *best* tube for collecting an ethanol (ETOH) specimen?
  a. gray top
  b. green top
  c. lavender top
  d. light blue

63. Identify the tubes needed to collect a complete blood count (CBC), partial thromboplastin time (PTT), and STAT potassium by color and in the proper order of collection for a multi-tube draw.
  a. lavender top, SST, royal blue top
  b. gold top, yellow top, light blue top
  c. light blue top, green top, lavender top
  d. red top, gray top, light blue top

64. During venipuncture the tourniquet should not be left on longer than:
  a. 30 seconds.
  b. 1 minute.
  c. 2 minutes.
  d. 5 minutes.

65. Which of the following tubes is filled first when multiple tubes are filled from a syringe?
  a. blood culture tube
  b. CBC tube
  c. STAT potassium
  d. nonadditive tube

66. This test is collected in a light blue top tube.
    a. glucose
    b. platelet count
    c. prothrombin time
    d. red blood count

67. Which of the following STAT tests is typically collected in a lithium heparin tube?
    a. blood type and screen
    b. complete blood cell (CBC) count
    c. electrolytes
    d. partial thromboplastin time (PTT)

68. This tube stopper indicates that the tube contains EDTA.
    a. green
    b. lavender
    c. light blue
    d. royal blue

69. Which anticoagulant is contained in a serum separator tube?
    a. EDTA
    b. heparin
    c. sodium citrate
    d. none of the above

70. The purpose of sodium citrate in specimen collection is to:
    a. accelerate clotting.
    b. inhibit glycolysis.
    c. preserve glucose.
    d. protect coagulation factors.

71. The part of a syringe that shows measurements in cc or mL is called the:
    a. adapter.
    b. barrel.
    c. hub.
    d. plunger.

72. The part of the evacuated tube holder that is meant to aid in smooth tube removal.
    a. barrel
    b. flange
    c. hub
    d. sleeve

73. The *best* choice of equipment for drawing difficult veins is:
    a. butterfly and evacuated tube holder.
    b. lancet and microtainer.
    c. needle and evacuated tube holder.
    d. needle and syringe.

74. Mixing equipment from different manufacturers can result in:
    a. improper needle fit.
    b. needle coming unscrewed.
    c. tubes popping off.
    d. all of the above

75. You are *most* likely to increase the chance of hemolyzing a specimen if you use a:
    a. 21-gauge needle and evacuated tube system to collect a specimen from the median cubital vein.
    b. 22-gauge needle and syringe to collect a specimen from a difficult vein.
    c. 23-gauge butterfly needle to collect a specimen from a hand vein.
    d. 25-gauge butterfly needle to collect a specimen from a child.

76. The purpose of a tourniquet in the venipuncture procedure is to:
    a. block arterial blood flow to the area.
    b. enlarge veins so they are easier to find and enter.
    c. obstruct blood flow to concentrate analytes.
    d. all of the above

77. If a blood pressure cuff is used for venipuncture in place of a tourniquet, the pressure used must be:
    a. below the patient's diastolic pressure.
    b. between the patient's diastolic and systolic pressure.
    c. equal to the patient's systolic pressure.
    d. equal to the patient's venous pressure.

78. An anticoagulant:
    a. binds calcium or inhibits thrombin.
    b. keeps the blood from clotting.

c. prevents coagulation.
d. all of the above

79. Needle safety devices are required to have all of the following qualities EXCEPT:
   a. allow the user's hand to remain behind the needle at all times.
   b. create a barrier between the hands of the user and the needle after use.
   c. one-handed activation.
   d. provide temporary containment of the needle.

80. An EDTA tube that contains gel separator is called a(n):
   a. EST.
   b. PST.
   c. PPT.
   d. SST.

81. Which additive contains a substance that inhibits phagocytosis of bacteria by white blood cells?
   a. heparin
   b. silica
   c. SPS
   d. thixotropic gel

82. Which type of test is most affected by tissue thromboplastin contamination?
   a. chemistry
   b. coagulation
   c. microbiology
   d. serology

83. Which of the following tests would be most affected by carryover of K_2EDTA?
   a. blood urea nitrogen (BUN)
   b. glucose

c. potassium
d. sodium

84. Which of the following microcollection containers should be filled first if collected by skin puncture?
   a. gray stopper
   b. green stopper
   c. lavender stopper
   d. red stopper

85. The intent of the alternate syringe order of draw is to:
   a. minimize microclot formation in anticoagulant tubes.
   b. prevent additive carryover.
   c. reduce microbial contamination.
   d. none of the above

86. A pink top tube containing EDTA is primarily used for:
   a. blood bank tests.
   b. chemistry tests.
   c. coagulation tests.
   d. microbiology tests.

87. A blood smear made from blood collected in a container with a lavender stopper should be prepared within:
   a. 1 hour of specimen collection.
   b. 4 hours of specimen collection.
   c. 6 hours of specimen collection.
   d. 24 hours of specimen collection.

88. Which Becton Dickinson (BD) tube contains a clot activator?
   a. glass red top
   b. glass royal blue top
   c. plastic gray top
   d. plastic red top

ANSWERS AND EXPLANATIONS

1. **t.** substance added to a blood collection tube other than a tube coating or stopper

2. **n.** prevents blood from clotting

3. **o.** prevents the metabolism of glucose

4. **i.** inhibit the growth of bacteria

5. **q.** slanted end of a needle

6. **x.** winged infusion set

7. **u.** substance that enhances clotting of blood

8. **a.** additive used for donor collections

9. **k.** kill bacteria

10. **b.** blood collection tube with a pre-measured vacuum

11. **m.** number related to the diameter of a needle

12. **c.** breakdown or metabolism of glucose

13. **e.** end of a needle that attaches to a blood collection device

14. **w.** type of needle that is used with a syringe

15. **j.** internal space of a needle or vein

16. **d.** double-pointed needle used with the evacuated tube system

17. **p.** sequence of tube collection in a multi-tube draw

18. **g.** heparinized tube containing a gel separator

19. **l.** long cylindrical portion of a needle

20. **r.** special container used to dispose of needles and other sharp objects

21. **v.** tube containing a gel separator and silica to activate clotting

22. **g.** yellow

23. **d.** lavender

24. **c.** dark green

25. **f.** red (glass tube)

26. **b.** gray

27. **a.** gold or mottled red and gray

28. **e.** light blue

29. **b.** gray

30. **g.** yellow

31. **a.** gold or mottled red and gray

32. **b.** Disinfectants are corrosive chemical compounds that are bactericidal (kill bacteria). Some also kill viruses, such as human immunodeficiency virus and hepatitis. Disinfectants are used on surfaces and instruments to kill potential pathogens. They are *not* safe for use on human skin.

33. **b.** The most common antiseptic used for routine blood collection is 70% isopropyl alcohol (isopropanol). Bleach (5.25% sodium hypochlorite) is a disinfectant and is not safe to use on human skin. Methanol can be toxic when absorbed through the skin and is not used as a skin antiseptic. Povidone iodine is used for collection of sterile specimens such as blood cultures.

34. **c.** Povidone iodine, often referred to by the trade name Betadine, is the recommended antiseptic for cleaning blood culture collection sites (Fig. 7-1).

35. **a.** A 1:10 dilution of household bleach (5.25% sodium hypochlorite) in water is recommended for cleaning

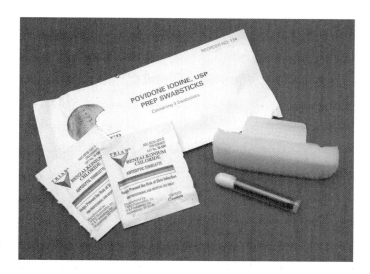

■ FIGURE 7-1 ■

Three types of blood culture cleaning supplies. *Left,* Povidone-iodine swabsticks. (The Purdue Frederick Co., Norwalk, CT.) *Center,* Benzalkonium chloride. (Triad Disposables Inc., Brookfield, WI.) *Right,* Frepp/Sepp povidone-iodine cleaning kit components. (Medi-Flex Inc., Overland Park, KS.)

blood spills because it has been shown to be effective in killing hepatitis B virus and human immunodeficiency virus. Benzalkonium chloride is an alternate antiseptic for routine venipuncture. Isopropanol (isopropyl alcohol) is the most common antiseptic used for routine venipuncture. Diluted 5.25% sodium hypochlorite (bleach) is a disinfectant used to clean surfaces and instruments but is not safe for use on human skin.

36. b. Gauze or gauze-like pads are preferred for holding pressure over a venipuncture site because the fibers from cotton, Dacron, or rayon balls tend to stick to the site and reinitiate bleeding when removed.

37. a. Adhesive bandages should not be used on infants younger than 2 years of age because of the danger of aspiration and suffocation.

38. d. The Occupational Safety and Health Administration (OSHA) requires that sharps containers (Fig. 7-2) be rigid, leak-proof, puncture-resistant, disposable, and have locking lids that can be easily sealed when the container is full. OSHA also requires that they be marked with a biohazard symbol.

39. b. Because latex tourniquets are relatively inexpensive, they are usually discarded if soiled with blood. Autoclaving a latex tourniquet would destroy it. Bleach disintegrates latex

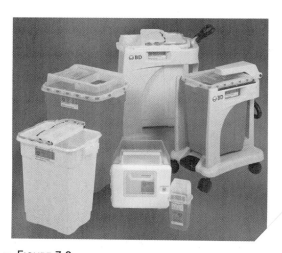

■ FIGURE 7-2 ■

Several styles of sharps containers. (Courte Dickinson, Franklin Lakes, NJ.)

and makes it gummy. Alcohol is an antiseptic and would not necessarily destroy bloodborne pathogens.

40. **d.** OSHA's Bloodborne Pathogen Standard is a federal law that mandates wearing of gloves during most phlebotomy procedures. The CDC and HICPAC provide guidelines for wearing gloves but the guidelines are not federal laws. The FDA regulates glove quality.

41. **c.** The needle gauge for venipuncture is selected according to the size and condition of the patient's vein, the type of procedure, and the equipment being used. Personal preference and the depth of the vein influence the length of needle used, rather than the gauge. The type of test being collected does not normally influence selection of the needle gauge or length.

42. **a.** The gauge of a needle is a number that is inversely related to the diameter of the lumen or internal space of the needle. It is an indication of the size of the needle; the larger the number, the smaller its diameter, and vice-versa. Most needles are color-coded according to

gauge; however, color-coding varies by manufacturer. Multisample needles typically have color-coded caps (Fig. 7-3).

43. **a.** Bore is a term used to describe the diameter of a needle and the size of the hole it makes. There is an inverse relationship between the gauge number and the bore or diameter of the lumen of a needle.. Therefore, the needle gauge with the largest bore or lumen is the one with the smallest number.

44. **c.** ETS multisample needles (see Fig. 7-3) are generally available in 20-, 21-, and 22-gauge. A 21-gauge needle is considered the standard needle for routine venipuncture. Syringe needles and butterfly needles are available in smaller diameter gauges for difficult draw situations.

45. **a.** The end of the needle that is inserted into the vein is called the bevel (Fig. 7-4) because it is cut on a slant or "beveled" to allow the needle to penetrate the vein easily and prevent coring (removal of a portion of the skin or vein). The hub of a needle is the end that attaches to a syringe or tube holder. The lumen of

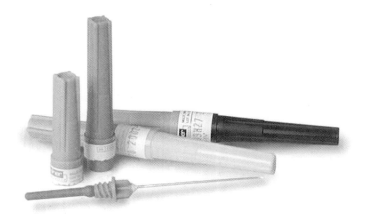

■ FIGURE 7-3 ■

Multisample needles with color-coded caps; yellow 20g, green 21g, and black 22g. (Greiner Bio-One, Kremsmünster, Austria.)

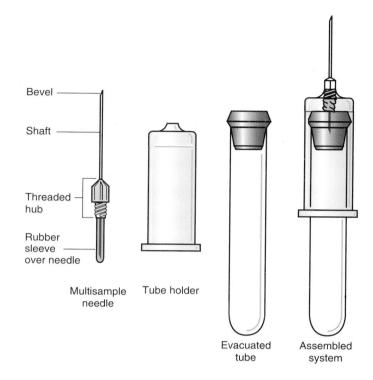

Bevel

Shaft

Threaded hub

Rubber sleeve over needle

Multisample needle   Tube holder

Evacuated tube

Assembled system

■ FIGURE 7-4 ■

Traditional components of the evacuated tube system (ETS).

a needle is the internal space of the needle. The shaft is the long cylindrical part of the needle.

46. **c.** The rubber sleeve (see Fig. 7-4) of a multiple sample needle retracts as the needle is inserted into the tube, allowing the tube to fill with blood, and recovers the needle as the tube is removed, preventing leakage of blood into the tube holder.

47. **b.** A needle without a safety feature can be used for blood collection. However, according to OSHA regulations, it must be used with a tube holder that has a safety feature (Fig. 7-5). In addition, needles must never be recapped or removed from holders after use unless it has been demonstrated that it is specifically required by a medical procedure or there is no feasible alternative. In

such instances, a mechanical device or some method other than a two-handed procedure must be used.

48. **d.** The age of the patient, the amount of blood needed for the test, and the size and condition of the patient's vein all play a role in selecting the appropriate size tubes to use to collect a venipuncture specimen.

49. **b.** Glass evacuated tubes are often coated on the inside with silicon to fill tiny cracks and other imperfections in the glass and create a smooth surface. The smooth surface prevents destruction of red blood cells and helps keep blood from sticking to the sides of the tube. The silicon coating also prevents activation of the clotting factors in tubes used for coagulation studies. In contrast, plastic tubes are so

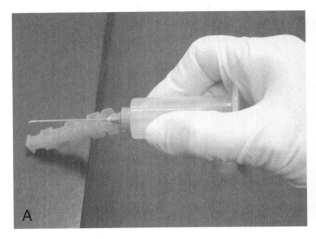
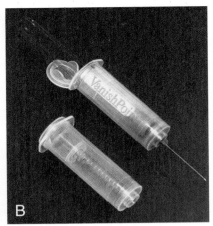

■ FIGURE 7-5 ■

Safety tube holders. **A.** Venipuncture Needle-Pro with needle resheathing device. (SIMS, Inc., Keene, NH.) **B.** Vanishpoint tube holder with needle retracting device.

that platelet aggregation and adhesion is inhibited, and a clot activator must be added to the ones that are used to collect serum specimens.

50. c. A light blue top tube typically contains the anticoagulant sodium citrate as the additive. Sodium citrate prevents coagulation by binding calcium. It is used for coagulation specimens because it does the best job of preserving the coagulation factors, and adding calcium back to the specimen during testing easily reverses its binding effects. The most common use of green tops is to collect plasma for chemistry tests. Lavender tops are most commonly used to collect whole blood for hematology tests Red tops are most often used for chemistry, serology, and blood bank tests.

51. d. Glass red top tubes are additive free. Plastic red top tubes contain a clot activator. Blood collected in either of these tubes will eventually clot. When centrifuged, clear fluid

called serum separates from the clotted cells. Green, lavender, and light blue top tubes contain anticoagulants. Specimens that are collected in anticoagulant tubes are prevented from clotting and yield whole blood specimens. Some tests, such as hematology tests, collected in tubes with lavender tops are performed on whole blood specimens. When blood in anticoagulant tubes is centrifuged, clear fluid separates from the cells and is called plasma. Green top tubes are typically centrifuged to yield plasma for certain chemistry tests. The most common use of light blue tops is to provide plasma for coagulation tests.

52. c. A manual differential is a hematology test performed using a microscope to count white blood cells and evaluate cell morphology in a specially stained blood film prepared on a glass slide.

53. d. Most tube stopper colors indicate the presence (or absence) and type of additive in a tube. A green stopper indicates heparin, a lavender stopper indicates EDTA, and light blue normally indicates sodium citrate. A royal blue stopper, however, indicates that the tube and stopper are virtually trace-element–free. A royal blue top can contain no additive, EDTA, or heparin. Additive color-coding of a royal blue top tube is typically indicated on the label.

54. d. Heparin prevents coagulation by inhibiting thrombin during the coagulation process. Thrombin is necessary for the formation of fibrin from fibrinogen. Without thrombin, a fibrin clot cannot form.

55. d. SPS tubes are used to collect blood cultures, which are performed in the microbiology department. SPS is an anticoagulant with special properties that inhibit proteins that destroy bacteria, prevent phagocytosis of bacteria by white blood cells, and reduce the activity of some antibiotics.

56. b. A royal blue stopper signifies that the tube and stopper contain the lowest levels of trace elements available (i.e., they are virtually trace-element–free). Royal blue top tubes are available with EDTA, heparin, or no additive. Color-coding on the label indicates what additive, if any, is in the tube. Green color-coding on the label of a royal blue top indicates that it contains heparin.

57. b. Calcium is essential to the coagulation process. EDTA, potassium oxalate, and sodium citrate bind or precipitate calcium, making it unavailable to the coagulation process. Heparin prevents coagulation by inhibiting the clotting component thrombin.

58. a. Excess oxalate causes hemolysis, the destruction of red blood cells and the liberation of hemoglobin into the plasma. White blood cells are evaluated in hematology. Hematology tests are collected in EDTA, not oxalate. Hemolysis increases potassium levels, but oxalate is not used to collect potassium specimens. Microclot formation can result from too little anticoagulant, rather than too much.

59. d. Thixotropic gel is an inert (nonreacting) synthetic substance that forms a physical barrier between the cellular portion of a specimen and the serum or plasma portion after the specimen has been centrifuged. When used in a serum collection tube, it is called serum separator and the tube is referred to as a serum separator tube (SST). When used in a tube that contains heparin, it is called plasma separator and the tube is referred to as a plasma separator tube (PST). If it is used in a tube that contains EDTA, the tube is called a plasma preparation tube (PPT). So far there is no gel tube that contains sodium citrate.

60. c. An antiglycolytic agent is a substance that inhibits or prevents glycolysis (metabolism of glucose) by the cells of the blood. The most common antiglycolytic agents are sodium fluoride and lithium iodoacetate.

61. a. Glass (silica) particles are called clot activators and are present in serum separator tubes to make the blood clot faster. Glass particles enhance or accelerate clotting by providing increased surface for platelet activtion, aggregation, and adhesion. Other substances that function as clot activators in other types of tubes include inert clays, such as siliceous earth, kaolin, and Celite, and the clotting components thromboplastin and thrombin.

62. **a.** A gray top tube typically contains sodium fluoride, which prevents glycolysis. It is used for alcohol determinations and glucose tests. Alcohol values are stable because glycolysis (the metabolism of glucose or sugar is prevented). Sodium fluoride also inhibits growth of bacteria and protects the specimen from an increase in alcohol due to fermentation by bacteria.

63. **c.** A CBC is a hematology test collected in a lavender top. A PTT is a coagulation test collected in a light blue top. A STAT potassium is a chemistry test collected in a green top. The proper order of draw for these tubes is light blue first, green next, and lavender last.

64. **b.** Proper tourniquet application allows arterial blood flow into the area below the tourniquet but obstructs venous flow away from the area. This causes the veins to enlarge and makes them easier to find and pierce with a needle. However, the obstruction of blood flow can change blood components if the tourniquet is left in place for more than 1 minute.

65. **a.** Tubes or containers for specimens such as blood cultures that must be collected in a sterile manner are always collected first in both the syringe and ETS system of venipuncture.

66. **c.** A prothrombin time (PT) is a coagulation test and is collected in a light blue top containing sodium citrate. The best tube for collecting a glucose specimen is a gray top containing an antiglycolytic agent such as sodium fluoride. A platelet count is sometimes ordered to assess coagulation, but is a hematology test collected in a lavender top. A red blood count is a hematology test and is collected in a lavender top.

67. **c.** Most chemistry tests have been traditionally performed on serum, but to save the time it takes for a serum specimen to clot before it can be tested, STAT electrolytes and other STAT chemistry tests are often performed on plasma specimens collected in lithium heparin tubes. Sodium heparin tubes must not be used for STAT electrolytes because sodium is one of the electrolytes measured. In addition, new studies show that heparinized plasma may be the best specimen for potassium tests regardless of whether they are STAT.

68. **b.** A lavender stopper indicates that the tube contains EDTA. A green stopper indicates a heparin-containing tube, and a light blue stopper indicates the presence of sodium citrate unless it has a special yellow label. A royal blue stopper indicates that the tube and stopper are as free of trace elements as possible. A royal blue stopper sometimes contains EDTA, but only if it has lavender color-coding on the label.

69. **d.** There is no anticoagulant in a serum separator tube (SST). An SST typically contains silica to enhance coagulation and an inert gel that forms a physical barrier between the serum and the cells after centrifugation. Anticoagulants are used to obtain either whole blood or

plasma specimens. A plasma separator tube (PST) contains heparin. A plasma preparation tube (PPT) contains EDTA.

70. d. Sodium citrate is the anticoagulant contained in light blue top tubes used to collect plasma for coagulation tests. It is used for coagulation tests because it does the best job of protecting the coagulation factors. The ratio of blood to anticoagulant is critical in coagulation testing, so it is important for sodium citrate tubes to be filled to their stated capacity.

71. b. The barrel of a syringe holds the fluid being aspirated or administered and is measured in cc or mL.

The hub is where the needle attaches to the syringe. The plunger fits within the barrel. Pulling on the plunger creates the vacuum that allows the syringe to fill with the fluid being aspirated (Fig. 7-6). An adapter is not part of a syringe.

72. b. The flanges or extensions on the sides of the tube end of the holder are there to aid in tube placement and removal.

73. a. The butterfly needle (Fig. 7-7) is an indispensable tool for collecting blood from small or difficult veins, because it allows much more flexibility and precision than either a regular needle and evacuated tube holder or needle and syringe. A

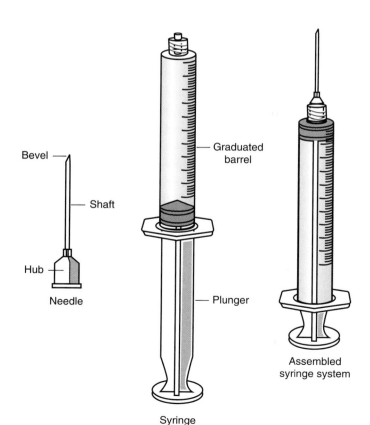

Bevel

Shaft

Hub

Needle

Graduated barrel

Plunger

Assembled syringe system

Syringe

■ FIGURE 7-6 ■

Traditional syringe system components.

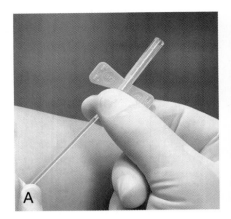
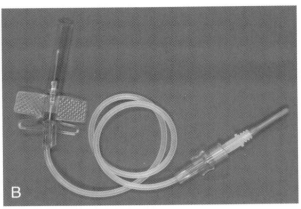

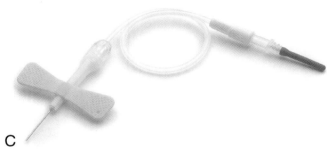

■ FIGURE 7-7 ■

Examples of winged infusion sets. **A.** SAFETY-LOK Blood Collection Set for use with the evacuated tube system. (Becton Dickinson Vacutainer Systems, Franklin Lakes, NJ.) **B.** Monoject Angel Wing blood collection set. (Kendall CO, LP, Mansfield, MA.) **C.** Vacuette safety blood collection systems. (Greiner Bio-One, Kremsmünster, Austria.)

lancet and microtainer can be used for some specimens, but there are a number of tests that cannot be collected by skin puncture.

74. d. Although evacuated tube collection system components from different manufacturers are similar, they are not necessarily interchangeable. Mixing components from different manufacturers can lead to problems such as improper needle fit and needles coming unscrewed, or tubes popping off during venipuncture procedures.

75. d. The 25-gauge butterfly needles are sometimes successfully used to collect blood specimens from infants and others with difficult veins. However, any time a needle smaller than 23g is used to collect blood,

the chance of trauma to the red blood cells and resulting hemolysis is increased.

76. b. The purpose of a tourniquet in the venipuncture procedure is to block the venous flow, not the arterial flow, so that blood flows freely into the area but not out. This causes the veins to enlarge, making them easier to find and penetrate with a needle. The tourniquet must not be left on for longer than 1 minute because obstruction of blood flow changes the concentration of some analytes, leading to erroneous test results.

77. a. A blood pressure cuff may be used in place of a tourniquet by those familiar with its operation. The patient's blood pressure is taken, and the pressure is then maintained below the patient's diastolic pressure.

78. d. An anticoagulant prevents coagulation or clotting of the blood either by binding calcium and making it unavailable to the coagulation process, or by inhibiting thrombin.

79. d. A needle safety device (Fig. 7-8) should allow the user's hand to remain behind the needle at all times, create a barrier between the hands of the user and the needle after use, be activated using a one-handed technique, and provide permanent (not temporary) containment of the needle. A needle safety feature should never be a temporary measure.

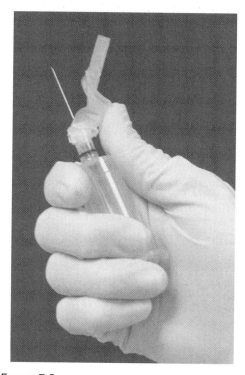

■ Figure 7-8 ■

BD Eclipse multisample safety needle attached to traditional tube holder. (Courtesy Becton Dickinson, Franklin Lakes, NJ.)

80. c. An EDTA tube that contains a separator gel is called a plasma preparation tube (PPT). There is no separator gel tube called an EPT. A plasma separator tube (PST) contains heparin and gel. A serum separator tube (SST) contains silica particles or clot activator and gel.

81. c. Sodium polyanethol sulfonate (SPS) is used in tubes for microbiology tests and is formulated to inhibit phagocytosis of bacteria by white blood cells. Heparin inhibits thrombin. Silica activates or enhances clotting. When a specimen is centrifuged, thixotropic gel becomes a physical barrier between the serum or plasma and the cells to prevent the cells from metabolizing substances in the serum or plasma.

82. b. Coagulation tests are most affected by tissue thromboplastin contamination because it is a substance found in tissue that is an activator of the coagulation process. Tissue thromboplastin is picked up by the needle as it penetrates the skin during venipuncture and is flushed into the first tube drawn.

83. c. K_2EDTA contains potassium. (K is the chemical symbol for potassium, and K_2EDTA is an abbreviation for dipotassium EDTA.) Carryover of potassium EDTA formulations into tubes for potassium testing have been known to significantly increase potassium levels in the specimen, causing erroneously elevated test results.

84. c. Lavender stoppers contain EDTA and are used to collect hematology specimens. In the NCCLS order of draw for skin puncture, EDTA specimens are collected first because skin puncture blood contains tissue thromboplastin, which activates the coagulation process, causing platelet clumping and microclot formation in the specimen if it is not collected quickly. Platelet clumping and microclots cause erroneous hematology test results.

85. **a.** The intent of the alternate syringe order of draw is to fill tubes for tests that are most affected by microclot formation as soon as possible. In this order of draw the assumption is made that blood that enters the syringe last is the freshest and least affected by microclot formation. Sterile specimens are still filled first, but are immediately followed by anticoagulant tubes because they are most affected by microclot formation. Of the anticoagulant tubes, light blue top coagulation tubes are filled first, followed by lavender tubes for hematology studies, green tops, and gray tops. Red tops, clot activator tubes, and SSTs are filled after all the anticoagulant tubes because blood in these tubes is sup-

posed to clot. To prevent carryover when this method is used, the transfer needle must be kept above the fill level of the tube so that blood mixed with additive does not contaminate it.

86. **a.** A pink top EDTA tube typically has a special label for ID information and is used primarily for blood bank tests.

87. **a.** Prolonged contact with EDTA can change the staining characteristics of white blood cells. This effect is minimized if blood smears are made within 1 hour of specimen collection.

88. **d.** Red top tubes are used to collect serum specimens. Serum is obtained from clotted blood. The insides of plastic tubes are so smooth that platelet aggregation and adhesion are inhibited, resulting in delayed or incomplete clotting of plastic red top tubes. The addition of clot activator to plastic red top tubes solves this problem. This is not a problem for glass tubes because glass has a rougher surface.

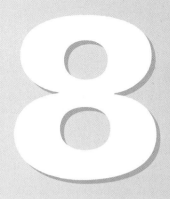

VENIPUNCTURE SPECIMEN COLLECTION PROCEDURES

13. Remove the Cover and Inspect the Needle
14. Anchor the Vein
15. Insert the Needle into the Vein
16. Fill the Tubes
17. Withdraw the Needle
18. Dispose of the Puncturing Unit
19. Label the Tubes
20. Observe Special Handling Instructions
21. Check the Patient's Arm and Apply Bandage
22. Dispose of Contaminated Materials
23. Thank the Patient
24. Remove Gloves and Wash Hands
25. Check Specimen Collection Logs
26. Transport the Specimen to the Lab

H. Procedure for Inability to Obtain a Specimen

I. Butterfly Procedure
  1. Identify Patient and Prepare for Specimen Collection
  2. Select Equipment
  3. Position Patient and Apply Tourniquet
  4. Choose a Vein and Clean the Site
  5. Assemble Equipment
  6. Reapply Tourniquet and Position Equipment
  7. Anchor the Vein
  8. Insert the Needle into the Vein
  9. Fill the Tubes
  10. Withdraw the Needle and Dispose of Collection Equipment
  11. Follow-Up Procedures

J. Syringe Procedure
  1. Identify Patient and Prepare for Specimen Collection
  2. Select Equipment
  3. Position Patient and Apply Tourniquet
  4. Choose a Vein and Clean the Site
  5. Assemble Equipment
  6. Reapply Tourniquet and Position Syringe
  7. Anchor the Vein and Insert the Needle
  8. Fill the Syringe
  9. Withdraw the Needle and Activate Safety Device

10. Transfer Blood to Evacuated Tubes
  a. Syringe Transfer Device
  b. Procedure for Using Syringe Transfer Device
  c. Transferring Blood from a Syringe Without a Transfer Device
11. Follow-Up Procedures

K. Pediatric Venipuncture
  1. Challenges
  2. Dealing with Parents or Guardians
  3. Dealing with the Child
  4. Selecting a Method of Restraint
  5. Equipment Selection
  6. Procedures
    a. Antecubital Vein
    b. Dorsal Hand Vein

L. Geriatric Venipuncture
  1. Challenges
    a. Skin Changes
    b. Hearing Impairment
    c. Visual Impairment
    d. Mental Impairment
    e. Effects of Disease
      1) Arthritis
      2) Coagulation Problems
      3) Diabetes
      4) Parkinson's and Stroke
      5) Pulmonary Function Problems
      6) Other Problems
  2. Safety Issues
  3. Patients in Wheelchairs
  4. Blood Collection Procedures
    a. Patient Identification
    b. Equipment Selection
    c. Tourniquet Application
    d. Select Venipuncture Site
    e. Clean the Site
    f. Perform the Venipuncture
    g. Hold Pressure

M. Dialysis Patients
  1. Hemodialysis
  2. Peritoneal Dialysis

N. Long-Term Care Patients

O. Home Care Patients

P. Hospice Patients

REVIEW QUESTIONS

Match the term with the BEST description.

1. _____ anchor
2. _____ arm/wrist/ID band
3. _____ ASAP
4. _____ barcode
5. _____ bedside manner
6. _____ concentric circles
7. _____ fasting
8. _____ ID card
9. _____ MR number
10. _____ needle sheath
11. _____ NPO
12. _____ palpate
13. _____ patient ID
14. _____ pediatric tube
15. _____ pre-op/post-op
16. _____ requisition
17. _____ STAT

a. special band or bracelet attached to a patient's arm in the area of the wrist that contains identification information

b. before and after an operation, respectively

c. beginning in the center and moving outward in ever-widening circles

d. black and white stripes of varying widths that correspond to letters and numbers

e. cover or cap of a needle

f. clinic- or other healthcare organization-issued identification cards that contain a patient's name and other information identifying them as that organization's patient

g. examine by feel or touch

h. going without food or drink, except water, for 8–12 hours before specimen collection

i. nothing by mouth, or no food or water

j. process by which a patient's identity is verified and matched with the information on a test requisition

k. small-volume evacuated tube designed to be used for small veins or in situations in which only small amounts of blood can be collected

l. term derived from the Latin word *statim*, meaning immediately

m. test collection priority that means results are needed to respond to a serious situation, but the patient is not in critical condition

n. the form on which test orders are entered

o. the way in which an individual conducts himself or herself when interacting with a patient

p. unique number assigned to a patient for identification purposes

q. using the thumb to pull the skin taut below a vein to keep the vein from moving on needle entry

Choose the BEST answer.

18. Which of the following individuals has legal authority to authorize patient testing?
a. laboratory director
b. patient's nurse
c. patient's physician
d. phlebotomist

19. Information on a test requisition *must* include the:
a. ordering physician's name.
b. patient's medical record number.
c. patient's name and date of birth.
d. all of the above

20. Which type of requisition often serves as a test request, report, and billing form?
a. barcode
b. computer
c. manual
d. verbal

21. Using information from the computer requisition (Fig. 8-1), identify the number that points to the type of tube to be drawn.
a. 1
b. 2
c. 3
d. 4

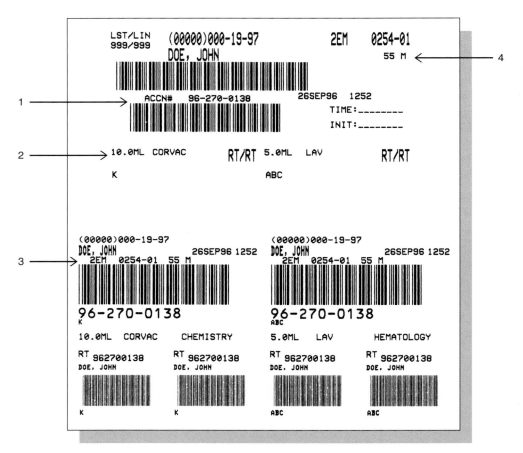

■ FIGURE 8-1 ■
Computer requisition with barcode.

22. Using information from the computer requisition (see Fig. 8-1), identify the number that points to the patient's age,
    a. 1
    b. 2
    c. 3
    d. 4

23. Using information from the computer requisition (see Fig. 8-1), identify the number that points to the accession number.
    a. 1
    b. 2
    c. 3
    d. 4

24. A barcode can represent a(n):
    a. identification number.
    b. laboratory test.
    c. patient's name.
    d. any of the above

25. Outpatient requisitions are typically of this type.
    a. computer
    b. manual
    c. prescription slip
    d. verbal

26. When received by the laboratory, inpatient requisitions are typically sorted according to:
    a. date and time of collection.
    b. location of the patient..
    c. priority of collection.
    d. all of the above

27. Steps taken to unmistakably connect a specimen and the accompanying paperwork to a specific individual are called:
    a. accessioning the specimen.
    b. barcoding.
    c. patient identification.
    d. verification of collection.

28. Which of the following is an example of a common timed test?
    a. blood urea nitrogen (BUN)
    b. complete blood count (CBC)

    c. chemistry profile
    d. cortisol

29. A test that is ordered STAT should be collected:
    a. as soon as possible.
    b. immediately.
    c. on the next scheduled sweep.
    d. within 1 hour.

30. Which of the following tests is commonly ordered STAT?
    a. creatinine clearance
    b. electrolytes
    c. erythrocyte sedimentation rate (ESR)
    d. glucose tolerance test (GTT)

31. If a test is ordered STAT, it means that the patient is in:
    a. critical condition.
    b. serious condition.
    c. surgery.
    d. the emergency room.

32. When a test is ordered ASAP, it means that the:
    a. patient has just returned from surgery.
    b. patient is in critical condition.
    c. results are needed soon to respond to a serious situation.
    d. timing of the test is critical.

33. A pre-op patient:
    a. has just been admitted to the hospital.
    b. has just had an operation.
    c. is an outpatient.
    d. will soon be going to surgery.

34. Tests are classified as routine if they are ordered:
    a. for collection at a specific time.
    b. in the course of establishing a diagnosis.
    c. to assess a patient's condition after surgery.
    d. to specifically eliminate the effects of diet.

35. This term means the same as STAT.
 a. ASAP
 b. med emerg
 c. NPO
 d. pre-op

36. A patient who is NPO:
 a. cannot have food or drink.
 b. cannot have food or drink except water.
 c. is in critical condition.
 d. is recovering from surgery.

37. An example of a test that is commonly ordered fasting is:
 a. blood urea nitrogen (BUN).
 b. electrolytes.
 c. glucose.
 d. hemoglobin and hematocrit (H & H).

38. Which liquid is acceptable to drink when fasting?
 a. black coffee
 b. milk
 c. sugarless tea
 d. water

39. Which is a common post-op test?
 a. creatinine
 b. glucose
 c. hemoglobin and hematocrit (H & H)
 d. partial thromboplastin time (PTT)

40. You arrive to draw a specimen on an inpatient. The patient's door is closed. What do you do?
 a. knock softly and open the door slowly, checking to see if it is all right to enter
 b. knock softly and wait for someone to come to the door
 c. leave to draw another patient and come back later
 d. open the door and proceed into the room

41. There is a sign above the patient's bed that reads, "No blood pressures or venipuncture, right arm" (Fig. 8-2). The patient has an IV in the left forearm.

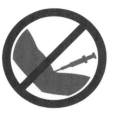

NO BP OR VENIPUNCTURE

RIGHT ARM

■ FIGURE 8-2 ■

Warning sign indicating "No blood pressures or venipuncture in right arm."

You have a request to collect a complete blood count on the patient. How should you proceed?
 a. ask the patient's nurse what to do
 b. ask the patient's nurse to collect the specimen from the IV
 c. collect the specimen from the right arm without using a tourniquet
 d. collect the specimen from the left hand by a fingerstick

42. A code is a way to:
 a. convey important information without alarming the general public.
 b. transmit messages over the public address system.
 c. use numbers or words to represent important information.
 d. all of the above

43. DNR means:
 a. do not call a code if the patient stops breathing.
 b. do not resuscitate.
 c. do not take heroic measures if the patient stops breathing.
 d. all of the above

44. You greet your patient in the following manner: "Hello, my name is John and I am here to collect a blood specimen if that is all right with you." The patient responds by saying, "OK, but I would rather not." Do you have permission to draw the specimen?
    a. yes
    b. no

45. Which of the following is part of informed consent?
    a. explaining why a test was ordered
    b. letting the patient know that you are a student phlebotomist
    c. telling a patient what can happen if you do not clean the site properly
    d. all of the above

46. Your inpatient is asleep when you arrive to draw blood. What do you do?
    a. call out the patient's name softly and shake the bed gently
    b. check the ID and draw the sample quickly before the patient awakens
    c. come back later when the patient is awake
    d. fill out a form that says you were unable to obtain the specimen because the patient was asleep

47. Laboratory results can be negatively affected if the phlebotomist:
    a. collects a specimen in dim lighting conditions.
    b. draws a specimen from an unconscious patient.
    c. startles a sleeping patient when arriving to collect a specimen.
    d. all of the above

48. How would you handle a blood draw on an unconscious patient?
    a. have someone assist you in case the patient moves
    b. identify yourself and inform the patient of your intent

    c. talk to the patient as you would an alert patient
    d. all of the above

49. What do you do if the patient's physician is in the room and the specimen is ordered STAT?
    a. ask the patient's nurse what to do
    b. come back later when the physician has gone
    c. politely introduce yourself, explain why you are there, and ask permission to proceed
    d. say "Excuse me" and proceed to collect the specimen

50. What is the *best* thing to do if family or visitors are with a patient?
    a. ask the patient's nurse to tell the visitors to leave
    b. ask the visitors to step out of the room until you are finished
    c. come back later to collect the specimen
    d. none of the above

51. Your patient is not in the room when you arrive to collect a timed specimen. The patient's nurse states that the patient will be unavailable for several hours. What should you do?
    a. cancel the request
    b. demand to be told where the patient is
    c. fill out a delay slip stating why you were unable to collect the specimen
    d. return to the lab and put the request in the stack for the next sweep

52. Misidentification of a specimen for this test is *most* likely to have fatal consequences.
    a. blood urea nitrogen (BUN)
    b. thyroid-stimulating hormone (TSH)
    c. type and screen
    d. urinalysis (UA)

53. You arrive to collect a specimen on a patient named John Doe in 302B. How do verify that the patient in 302B is indeed John Doe?
    a. ask the patient, "Are you John Doe?" If he says yes, collect the specimen
    b. ask the patient to please state his name and date of birth before proceeding
    c. check the patient's ID band and say, "I see that you are John Doe"
    d. any of the above

54. Which requisition information *must* match information on the patient's ID band?
    a. medical record number
    b. physician's name
    c. room number
    d. test status

55. The medical record number on the ID band matches the number on your requisition, but the patient's name is spelled differently than the one on your requisition. What should you do?
    a. do not collect the specimen until the discrepancy is resolved
    b. collect the specimen since the medical record number is the same
    c. make the correction on your requisition and proceed to collect the specimen
    d. return to the lab and ask your supervisor what to do

56. An unconscious patient does not have an ID band. The name on the door agrees with the requisition. What should you do?
    a. call your supervisor and ask what to do
    b. do not draw the patient until the nurse has applied an ID bracelet
    c. draw the blood and fill out an incident report form
    d. draw the patient and then ask the nurse to verify his identity

57. What would be the system of choice to identify laboratory specimens from an unconscious woman in the emergency room?
    a. assign a name to the patient, such as Jane Doe
    b. assign a number to the patient until admitted
    c. use a three-part identification band with special tube labels
    d. wait to process specimens until the patient can be identified

58. Which type of inpatient is *most* likely to have more than one ID band?
    a. a child
    b. an adult
    c. a newborn
    d. an outpatient

59. What is the most critical error a phlebotomist can make?
    a. collecting a timed specimen late
    b. failing to obtain a specimen from a patient
    c. giving a patient a hematoma
    d. misidentifying a patient specimen

60. Your patient is not wearing an ID band. You see that the ID band is taped to the night stand. The information matches your requisition. What do you do?
    a. ask the patient to state her name; if it matches the requisition, collect the specimen
    b. ask the patient's nurse to attach an ID band before proceeding
    c. go to the nurse's station, make out an ID for the patient, attach it, and proceed to draw the specimen
    d. return to the lab without the drawing the specimen

61. The patient's nurse or a relative may be needed to confirm the identity of this type of patient.
    a. child
    b. mentally incompetent
    c. non–English-speaking
    d. all of the above

62. The laboratory receptionist finishes checking in a patient and hands you the test request. The request is for a patient named Mary Smith. You call the name, and the woman who was just checked in responds. She is also the only patient in the waiting room. How do you verify that she is the correct patient?
    a. ask the woman to state her name and date of birth to confirm her identity
    b. conclude that she must be the right one because she was the only one in the waiting room
    c. conclude that you do not have to verify her identity because the receptionist already did
    d. conclude that she is the right one because she answered when you called the name

63. A cheerful, pleasant bedside manner and exchange of small talk help to:
    a. divert attention from any discomfort associated with the draw.
    b. gain a patient's trust and confidence.
    c. put a patient at ease.
    d. all of the above

64. Your patient is cranky and rude to you. What do you do?
    a. ask the patient's nurse to draw the specimen
    b. be as polite and professional as you can and draw the specimen in your normal way
    c. do not speak to the patient; just get the necessary blood work and leave
    d. refuse to draw the patient and leave

65. All of the following are part of informed consent as related to the phlebotomist EXCEPT:
    a. advising the patient of his or her prognosis
    b. informing the patient that you are a student

    c. telling the patient that you will be drawing a blood specimen
    d. telling the patient the name of the test ordered

66. The patient asks if the test you are about to draw is for diabetes. How do you answer?
    a. explain that it is best to discuss the test with his or her physician
    b. if the test is for glucose say, "Yes it is"
    c. say that you do not know
    d. tell the patient that it is not, even if it is

67. A patient vehemently refuses to allow you to collect a blood specimen. What should you do?
    a. convince the patient to cooperate
    b. have the nurse physically restrain the patient and collect the specimen
    c. notify the patient's nurse
    d. return to the lab and cancel the request

68. You arrive to draw a fasting specimen. The patient is just finishing breakfast. What do you do?
    a. check with the patient's nurse first; if the specimen is collected, write "non-fasting" on the lab slip and the specimen label
    b. collect the specimen anyway since the patient had not quite finished eating
    c. collect the specimen anyway, but write "non-fasting" on the lab slip and the specimen
    d. refuse to collect the specimen, fill out an incident report, and leave a copy at the nurse's station

69. Why is it sometimes best to assemble equipment after selecting and cleaning the blood collection site?
    a. you will be more apt to allow sufficient time for the alcohol to dry
    b. you will have a better idea of what equipment to use

c. you will waste less equipment
d. all of the above

70. When performing venipuncture, hand washing is necessary:
    a. after glove removal only.
    b. after you have drawn your last patient.
    c. before and after each patient.
    d. hand washing is not necessary if you change gloves between patients.

71. Proper hand washing involves:
    a. creating friction to dislodge surface debris and bacteria.
    b. scrubbing downward from wrists to fingertips.
    c. using a clean paper towel to shut off the water faucet.
    d. all of the above

72. You must collect a specimen on a 6 year old. The child is a little fearful. What do you do?
    a. explain what you are going to do in simple terms and ask the child for cooperation
    b. have someone restrain the child and go ahead and draw the specimen without explanation
    c. tell the child not to worry because it won't hurt
    d. tell the child that you will give him a treat if he doesn't cry

73. If the patient asks you if the procedure will hurt, you should say that it:
    a. may hurt a little, but only for a short time.
    b. only hurts if you watch, so look the other way.
    c. won't hurt a bit.
    d. will hurt and the patient had better be prepared for it.

74. What is the proper arm position for routine venipuncture?
    a. in a downward position, but bent at the elbow

b. straight from shoulder to wrist and in a downward position with the palm up
    c. straight from shoulder to wrist with the palm down
    d. the position of the arm does not matter

75. Outpatients who have previously fainted during a blood draw should be:
    a. asked to lie down, or the drawing chair should be reclined if possible.
    b. allowed to sit up, but you should keep ammonia inhaler handy.
    c. allowed to sit up, but watched closely during the draw for signs of fainting.
    d. any of the above

76. Which of the following acts can lead to liability issues?
    a. asking visitors to temporarily leave the room while you collect the specimen
    b. drawing a patient who is talking on the phone
    c. lowering a bed rail to make access to the patient's arm easier
    d. pulling the curtain between the beds while you collect a specimen

77. Never leave a tourniquet on for more than:
    a. 30 seconds.
    b. 1 minute.
    c. 2 minutes.
    d. 3 minutes.

78. Where is the best place to apply the tourniquet?
    a. 3–4 inches above the venipuncture site
    b. directly above the venipuncture site
    c. distal to the venipuncture site
    d. distal to the wrist bone

79. What happens if the tourniquet is too tight?
    a. arterial flow may be stopped
    b. hemoconcentration

c. it hurts the patient
d. all of the above

80. All of the following can be used to enhance the vein selection process EXCEPT:
a. having a patient pump his or her fist
b. lowering the arm
c. palpating the antecubital area
d. using a warm towel to increase blood flow

81. When selecting a venipuncture site, how can you tell a vein from an artery?
a. an artery has a pulse
b. a vein has more resilience
c. a vein looks blue, an artery looks red
d. a vein will feel larger

82. What does a sclerosed vein feel like?
a. bouncy and resilient
b. hard and cord-like
c. pulsating
d. soft and mushy

83. It is acceptable to use an ankle vein if:
a. coagulation tests are ordered.
b. the patient is paralyzed.
c. the patient's physician gives permission.
d. there is no other suitable site.

84. To avoid inadvertently puncturing an artery during venipuncture:
a. do not select a vein that overlies or is close to an artery.
b. do not select a venipuncture site that is near where you feel a pulse.
c. avoid drawing the basilic vein.
d. all of the above

85. You must collect a light blue top for a special coagulation test from a patient who has an IV in the left wrist area and dermatitis all over the right arm and hand. The veins on the right arm and hand are not readily visible. What is the best way to proceed?
a. ask the patient's nurse to collect the specimen from the IV
b. apply a tourniquet on the right arm over a washcloth or towel and proceed as usual
c. collect the specimen by fingerstick on the left hand
d. draw the specimen from the left antecubital area without using a tourniquet

86. What is the *best* thing to do if the vein can be felt but not seen, even with the tourniquet on?
a. insert the needle where you think it is and probe until you find it
b. leave the tourniquet on while cleaning the site
c. look for visual clues on the skin to help you remember where it is
d. mark the spot with a felt tip pen

87. Release the tourniquet after vein selection and before cleaning the site to:
a. allow the vein to return to normal.
b. avoid hemoconcentration of the specimen.
c. help ensure accurate test results.
d. all of the above

88. What is the National Committee for Clinical Laboratory Standards (NCCLS) recommended way to clean a venipuncture site?
a. any way; just scrub as vigorously as you can
b. cleanse with a circular motion from the center to the periphery
c. wipe using concentric circles from the outside to the center
d. any of the above

89. What is the purpose of waiting 30 seconds for the alcohol to dry before needle insertion?
a. to allow the evaporation process to help destroy microbes
b. to avoid a stinging sensation
c. to prevent hemolysis of the specimen
d. all of the above

90. What happens if you advance the tube past the guideline on the holder before needle insertion?
    a. the tube will fail to fill with blood
    b. the vacuum will be lost
    c. you will have to get a new tube
    d. all of the above

91. It is important for the phlebotomist to visually inspect the needle tip before inserting it in a patient's vein to:
    a. check for the presence of bacteria.
    b. check the needle point for imperfections that might damage the patient's vein.
    c. ensure that the bevel is down during insertion.
    d. make certain that the needle is not outdated.

92. Which is the proper way to anchor a vein?
    a. press down on the skin below the site with your thumb
    b. pull the skin taut below the site with your thumb
    c. use your index finger above and thumb below the site
    d. any of the above

93. You are about to draw blood from a patient. You touch the needle to the skin, but change your mind and pull the needle away. What do you do next?
    a. clean the site and try again using the same needle
    b. try again immediately using the same needle
    c. obtain a new needle before trying again
    d. wipe the needle across the alcohol pad and try again

94. What is the best angle to use for needle insertion during routine venipuncture?
    a. less than 15°
    b. 15–30°
    c. 35–45°
    d. angle does not matter

95. When performing venipuncture, the needle is inserted:
    a. bevel up.
    b. bevel down.
    c. bevel sideways.
    d. any of the above

96. How can you tell when the needle is in the vein as you insert it into the patient's arm?
    a. the needle will start to vibrate
    b. you will feel a slight "give"
    c. you will hear a hissing sound
    d. there is no way to tell

97. When is the best time to release the tourniquet during venipuncture?
    a. as soon as blood begins to flow into the tube
    b. as soon as the needle penetrates the skin
    c. after the last tube is collected
    d. after the needle is withdrawn

98. Prolonged tourniquet application or vigorous fist pumping can elevate this analyte.
    a. potassium
    b. protein
    c. red blood cell count
    d. all of the above

99. Proper technique for collecting specimen tubes when using the evacuated tube method includes all of the following EXCEPT:
    a. collect a "clear" tube before special coagulation tests
    b. collect nonadditive tubes before additive tubes
    c. fill each tube until the normal vacuum is exhausted
    d. position the arm to ensure that tubes fill from the stopper end first

100. It is important to fill anticoagulant tubes to the proper level to ensure that:
    a. the specimen clots properly.
    b. there is a proper ratio of blood to anticoagulant.

c. there is adequate volume of blood to perform the test.

d. tissue fluid contamination of the specimen is minimized.

101. It is important to mix anticoagulant tubes immediately after filling them to:
a. avoid microclot formation.
b. encourage coagulation.
c. inhibit hemoconcentration.
d. minimize hemolysis.

102. You are in the middle of drawing a blood specimen using the evacuated tube method when you realize that you just filled an EDTA tube and still have a green top to collect. What do you do?
a. draw the green one next and hope that there is no carryover
b. draw several milliliters into a plain discard tube; then fill the green one
c. remember that it is acceptable to draw the EDTA before the green stopper
d. skip the green tube and come back later to collect it

103. How many times do you mix nonadditive tubes?
a. 0
b. 2 or 3
c. 5–10
d. 8–12

104. What may happen if you mix tubes too vigorously?
a. hemoconcentration
b. hemolysis
c. lipemia
d. no affect

105. Use several layers of gauze during needle removal so that:
a. blood will not contaminate your glove.
b. it will not hurt when you pull out the needle.
c. the patient does not see you pull out the needle.
d. bruising is prevented.

106. It is better to use gauze and not cotton balls for pressure over the site, because cotton balls:
a. are less sterile.
b. may irritate the patient's skin.
c. may pull the platelets away when removed.
d. soak up too little blood.

107. What happens if you put pressure on the gauze while the needle is being removed?
a. it is painful
b. it prolongs needle removal
c. the needle may slit the skin
d. all of the above

108. A needle safety feature, other than a blunting needle, should be activated:
a. after you have asked the patient to hold pressure over the gauze.
b. immediately after needle withdrawal.
c. while the tube is still engaged in the holder.
d. any of the above

109. What may happen if the arm is bent up at the elbow (folded back) to hold pressure on the gauze after venipuncture?
a. bleeding may occur when the arm is lowered
b. bruising may occur
c. the platelets may pull away when the arm is straightened
d. all of the above

110. Proper needle disposal involves:
a. disposing of the needle and tube holder as one unit.
b. ejecting the needle from the tube holder so that the holder can be reused.
c. unscrewing the needle from the holder using a slot in the sharps container.
d. any of the above

111. Labeling of routine inpatient blood specimens should take place:
   a. at the bedside immediately after collection.
   b. before the specimen is collected.
   c. in the laboratory after collection.
   d. outside the patient's room after collection.

112. Mandatory information on a specimen label includes all of the following EXCEPT:
   a. patient's first and last name
   b. phlebotomist's initials
   c. patient's room number and bed
   d. time and date

113. Why is a patient's identification number included on the specimen tube label?
   a. to be used for insurance identification and payment purposes
   b. to be used for an accession number in the laboratory
   c. to avoid confusing multiple specimens from the same patient
   d. to avoid confusing specimens from patients with the same name

114. What precautionary information should an outpatient be given before being allowed to leave after venipuncture?
   a. do not carry a bag or purse on that arm
   b. do not lift heavy objects for at least 1 hour
   c. leave the bandage on for a minimum of 15 minutes
   d. all of the above

115. Which of the following specimens requires special handling?
   a. ammonia
   b. bilirubin
   c. cold agglutinin
   d. all of the above

116. All of the following are valid reasons for failure to obtain a blood specimen EXCEPT:
   a. the patient refused
   b. the patient was not available
   c. you attempted but were unable to obtain the blood
   d. you did not have the right equipment on your tray

117. You have just made two unsuccessful attempts to collect a fasting blood specimen from an outpatient. The patient rotates his arm, and you note a large vein that you had not seen before. How do you proceed?
   a. ask another phlebotomist to attempt to collect the specimen
   b. ask the patient to come back in an hour or two so that you can try again
   c. call the patient's physician and ask what to do
   d. make a third attempt on the newly discovered vein

118. Butterfly is another name for a:
   a. multisample needle.
   b. hypodermic needle.
   c. needle safety feature.
   d. winged infusion set.

119. What is the advantage of using a butterfly?
   a. blood flow is increased
   b. butterflies are less expensive
   c. butterflies make it easier to draw difficult veins
   d. there is a greater choice of needle sizes

120. Where is the tourniquet applied when drawing a hand vein?
   a. distal to the wrist bone
   b. in the antecubital area
   c. proximal to the wrist bone
   d. a tourniquet is not used when drawing a hand vein

121. Although the ETS system is the preferred method of blood collection, it may be necessary to use a syringe when:

a. a large amount of blood is needed for the test.
b. the patient has fragile veins.
c. you are out of butterfly needles.
d. all of the above

122. Hemolysis of the specimen can result from:
a. mixing additive tubes too vigorously.
b. using a large-volume tube with a small-diameter needle.
c. forcing blood from a syringe into a tube by pushing on the syringe plunger.
d. all of the above

123. How can you tell that you are in a vein when using a syringe?
a. a "flash" of blood will appear in the hub of the needle
b. blood will pump into the syringe
c. pull back on the plunger until you see blood in the syringe
d. there is no way to tell

124. When transferring blood from a syringe to evacuated tubes, which is the proper technique?
a. force the blood in the tubes by pushing the syringe plunger
b. hold the tube steady in your hand while the syringe needle penetrates the stopper
c. place the evacuated tube in a rack before penetrating stopper
d. use a syringe transfer device

125. Before obtaining a blood specimen from a child, you must do all of the following EXCEPT:
a. establish rapport with the child and parent.
b. greet parent and child.
c. tell the child it won't hurt.
d. tell the child what to expect.

126. A butterfly and 23g needle is the best choice to use for venipuncture on a young child because:

a. children like the idea of the butterfly.
b. children's veins are often sclerotic.
c. flexibility of tubing allows for the child's movement.
d. it eliminates excessive bleeding tendencies.

127. Success of pediatric blood collection is most dependent on:
a. aseptic technique.
b. order of draw.
c. patient immobilization.
d. tourniquet application.

128. Proper immobilization of the pediatric patient involves all of the following EXCEPT:
a. allowing the child to sit with one arm bracing the other.
b. cradling the child close to the immobilizer.
c. grasping the child's wrist in a palm-up position.
d. using two people—an immobilizer and a blood drawer.

129. When drawing blood from an older child the most important consideration is:
a. assuring the child that it won't hurt.
b. explaining the importance of holding still.
c. explaining the tests that are being collected.
d. offering the child a reward for not crying.

130. Dorsal hand vein procedure on infants involves all of the following EXCEPT:
a. applying a tourniquet.
b. cleansing the area with isopropyl alcohol.
c. identifying the patient.
d. inserting the needle in a superficial vein.

131. The *best* way to collect a phenylke-tonuria (PKU) specimen from a dorsal hand vein is:
  a. allow the blood to drip into an EDTA microcollection tube.
  b. collect the blood with a syringe.
  c. let the blood drip onto the PKU card.
  d. all of the above

132. Tremors associated with this disease can make blood collection difficult.
  a. Alzheimer's
  b. arthritis
  c. diabetes
  d. Parkinson's

133. A diabetic outpatient has had a mastectomy on her right side and cannot straighten her left arm because of arthritis. The best place to collect a blood specimen is:
  a. an ankle or foot vein of either leg.
  b. the lower right arm.
  c. the left arm while a coworker forces it to straighten.
  d. the left arm in a comfortable position for the patient and using a butterfly.

134. Which of the following is proper procedure when dealing with an elderly patient?
  a. apply a pressure bandage in case the patient does not hold adequate pressure
  b. address questions to a relative or attendant in if the patient has a hearing problem
  c. raise the pitch of your voice to make certain you are heard properly
  d. refrain from drawing elderly patients if you have a cold, or wear a mask

135. The most common reason a patient must undergo dialysis treatment is:
  a. arthritis.
  b. coagulation problems.
  c. end-stage renal disease (ESRD).
  d. Parkinson's disease effects.

136. A type of care for patients who are terminally ill is:
  a. elder care.
  b. home care.
  c. hospice.
  d. long-term care.

ANSWERS AND EXPLANATIONS

1. **q.** using the thumb to pull the skin taut below a vein to keep the vein from moving on needle entry

2. **a.** a special band or bracelet attached to a patient's arm in the area of the wrist that contains identification information

3. **m.** as soon as possible; test collection priority that means results are needed to respond to a serious situation, but the patient is not in critical condition

4. **d.** black and white stripes of varying widths that correspond to letters and numbers

5. **o.** the way in which an individual conducts himself or herself when interacting with a patient

6. **c.** beginning in the center and moving outward in ever-widening circles

7. **h.** going without food or drink, except water, for 8–12 hours before specimen collection

8. **f.** clinic- or other healthcare organization-issued identification cards that contain a patient's name and other information identifying them as that organization's patient

9. **p.** medical record number, a unique number assigned to a patient for identification purposes

10. **e.** cover or cap of a needle

11. **i.** from Latin (*nulla per os*) meaning nothing by mouth, or no food or water

12. **g.** examine by feel or touch

13. **j.** process by which a patient's identity is verified and matched with the information on a test requisition

14. **k.** small-volume evacuated tube designed to be used for small veins or in situations in which only small amounts of blood can be collected

15. **b.** before and after an operation, respectively

16. **n.** the form on which test orders are entered

17. **l.** term derived from the Latin word *statim*, meaning immediately

18. **c.** A physician or other legally designated person must authorize all laboratory testing. A laboratory director can request a sample be redrawn if results are in question. The patient's nurse may convey a physician's request for testing but may not, under normal circumstances, initiate the test request. A phlebotomist collects specimens but cannot authorize testing.

19. **d.** Information on the test requisition must include the patient's name and date of birth or age, the patient's medical record number, and the ordering physician's name.

20. **c.** A manual requisition is often a three-part form that serves as a test request, report, and a billing form.

21. **b.** On the sample requisition in Figure 8-1, the type of tube to be collected appears as a mnemonic code with the volume of tube requested preceding the type of tube requested. In the example, the type of tube requested is a 10.0 mL Corvac (type of serum separator tube). A 5.0 mL lavender top is also requested.

22. **d.** On the sample requisition in Figure 8-1, the patient's age and gender are signified by the number "55"

followed by the letter "M," which means that the patient is a 55-year-old male.

23. **a.** A computer requisition has an accession number given to the patient's sample during the data entry phase. On the sample requisition in Figure 8-1, arrow 1 points to the accession number.

24. **d.** A barcode is a series of black and white stripes of varying widths corresponding to letters and numbers. The stripes can be grouped together to represent identification numbers, laboratory tests, or patient names.

25. **b.** Outpatient requisitions are typically manual forms.

26. **d.** After the laboratory receives them, requisitions are sorted according to date and time of collection, location of the patient, and priority of collection.

27. **a.** Steps taken to unmistakably connect a specimen and the accompanying paperwork to a specific individual is called accessioning the specimen.

28. **d.** Cortisol is an example of a timed test. BUN, CBC, and chemistry profiles are not typically timed tests.

29. **b.** STAT comes from the Latin word *statim,* which means immediately. A test that is ordered STAT should be collected immediately.

30. **b.** Abnormal electrolyte levels can lead to death; consequently, electrolyte tests are often ordered STAT.

31. **a.** When a test is ordered STAT, it means that the results are urgently needed on a patient in critical condition. A patient that is critical is in a life or death situation.

32. **c.** ASAP means as soon as possible. If a test is ordered ASAP, it means that test results are needed soon to respond to a serious situation, but the patient is not in critical condition or in danger of dying.

33. **d.** Pre-op means before an operation and indicates that the patient will soon be going to surgery.

34. **b.** Routine tests are those tests that are typically ordered in the course of establishing a diagnosis or monitoring a patient's care.

35. **b.** Medical emergency (med emerg) means the same as STAT. It has replaced STAT in some institutions to identify specimens whose results are needed immediately to respond to critical situations.

36. **a.** NPO comes from Latin (*non per os*) and means nothing by mouth. Patients who are NPO cannot have food or drink, not even water. Patients are typically NPO before surgery, not after.

37. **c.** Glucose levels normally rise with the intake of food and return to normal fasting levels within 2 hours if no more food is eaten. Glucose levels are ordered fasting to see if glucose is being metabolized properly. If glucose is not being metabolized properly, fasting levels will not be normal.

38. **d.** The only liquid that it is acceptable to drink when fasting is water.

39. **c.** Post-op means after an operation. Both hemoglobin and hematocrit are indications of the red blood cell count. H & H levels are a common post-op test to monitor blood levels after surgery.

40. a. If the door to the room is closed, you should knock lightly and proceed with caution. Even if the door is open, it is a good idea to knock lightly to make occupants aware that you are about to enter.

41. d. Because the specimen is a complete blood count (CBC), it can easily be collected by fingerstick from the left hand. The right arm should not be used. Collecting the CBC from the IV is not worth the risk when it can easily be collected from a fingerstick. A competent phlebotomist should be able to decide what to do in this situation without having to ask the nurse.

42. d. Codes are one way healthcare institutions convey important information over a public address system to those who need to know without alarming the general public. Codes use numbers or words to convey information. For example, code "blue" typically means someone has stopped breathing.

43. d. DNR means do not resuscitate. It means no code should be called or heroic measures taken if the patient stops breathing. It is sometimes used when patients are terminally ill.

44. b. If you ask if it is all right to draw a patient's blood and the patient replies, "Yes, but I would rather not," or something similar, they have given permission and taken it back in the same breath. You should not draw the patient until you are certain that you have permission.

45. b. Letting patients know that you are a student before they give permission for blood collection is necessary information for them to have to give informed consent. Letting a patient know why a test is ordered is not a phlebotomist's duty. Telling a patient what can happen if the site is not cleaned properly is unnecessary information that could unduly alarm a patient. The expectation is that the site will be cleaned properly.

46. a. It is acceptable procedure to wake a patient for a blood draw. If an inpatient is asleep, call out his or her name softly and shake the bed gently. Do not shake the patient. You may startle him or her and affect test results. Never attempt to collect a blood specimen from a sleeping patient. Such an attempt can also startle the patient, and you or the patient may be injured. In addition, a startle reflex can affect test results and should be avoided.

47. c. A startle reflex can affect test results and should be avoided. Collecting the specimen in dim lighting or collecting a specimen from an unconscious patient should not affect test results, provided the specimen is collected properly.

48. d. Some patients can hear what is going on around them despite being considered unconscious. Identify yourself and inform the patient of your intent, talking to him or her as you would an alert patient. In addition, an unconscious patient may be able to feel pain and may move during a blood draw, so it is a good idea to have someone assist you by holding the patient's arm still.

49. c. If a physician is with the patient and the test is ordered STAT, it is generally acceptable procedure to politely introduce yourself, explain why you are there, and ask permission to collect the specimen.

50. **b.** It is acceptable and in the best interest of all to ask family or visitors to step out of the room temporarily while you collect a blood specimen. Most will be more than willing to do so.

51. **c.** All specimens and test requests must be accounted for. Generally, if a patient is unavailable for testing, a delay slip is filled out stating why you were unable to collect the specimen. The original is left at the nurse's station, and a copy goes back to the laboratory. It is then up to the patient's nurse to notify the lab when the patient is available for testing.

52. **c.** Misidentification of a type and screen could lead to a patient getting the wrong type of blood and a possible fatal transfusion reaction.

53. **b.** Proper patient identification involves asking the patient to state his or her name and date of birth. This step is followed by checking the ID band and the requisition to see if they match. Verbal statement of identity from the patient is important. An ill or hard of hearing patient may answer, "Yes" to almost anything. It is not unheard of for a patient to be wearing an ID band with incorrect information.

54. **a.** It is important that certain information on the ID band match the information on the requisition exactly. The medical record number is mandatory information and should match exactly. The room number may change during a patient's stay in the hospital and should not be relied on as proper identification. In

addition, the physician may change or the patient may have more than one physician ordering tests. Test status information changes with each order and is not information that is found on the ID band.

55. **a.** Any discrepancy in the patient's name, date of birth, or medical record number between the requisition and the patient's ID band should be addressed and resolved before a specimen is collected.

56. **b.** Identification should never be a based on information on the patient's door. When no ID band can be found, it is necessary to ask the patient's nurse to make positive identification and attach an ID band before the specimen can be drawn.

57. **c.** It is not uncommon for an emergency room to receive an unconscious patient with no identification. Specimens should not be collected without some way to positively connect the specimen with the patient. In many institutions, a phlebotomist will attach a special three-part ID band to the unidentified patient's wrist. The special ID band has a unique number. The same number is on labels that are placed on specimens collected from that patient.

58. **c.** A newborn may have more than one ID band, one with the infant's information and one with the mother's.

59. **d.** The most critical error a phlebotomist can make is misidentifying a patient specimen. A misidentified specimen can have serious or even fatal consequences to the patient, especially if the specimen is for a type and screen for a blood transfu-

sion. Misidentification of a patient's specimen can be grounds for dismissal of the person responsible and could even lead to malpractice lawsuit against that person.

60. b. Identification should never be verified from an ID band that is *not* attached to the patient. An ID band on the night stand could belong to a patient who previously occupied that bed. Even if the ID band and the requisition matches, it is not adequate as proper identification of the patient. If an ID band is not attached to the patient, you must ask the patient's nurse to attach an ID band before you can collect the specimen.

61. d. The patient's nurse or other caregiver, or a relative, may be needed to confirm the identity of a patient who is a child, mentally incompetent, or non–English-speaking.

62. a. Never make assumptions about a person's identity and do not rely on others to identify patients for you. Always verify identification yourself by asking the patient to state his or her name and date of birth.

63. d. A cheerful pleasant bedside manner and exchange of small talk puts both you and the patient at ease, helps you gain the patient's trust and confidence, and helps divert attention from any discomfort associated with the blood draw.

64. b. Most patients understand that blood tests are needed in the course of their treatment. However, illness can be quite stressful and occasionally a patient who is tired of being "poked" will be cranky and rude. It is important to remain polite and professional and draw the specimen in your normal way. You may dis-

cover that the patient will actually apologize to you by the time you have finished.

65. a. Advising a patient of his prognosis is a physician's responsibility. It is not a phlebotomist's duty and is not necessary to informed consent. Informing a patient when you are a student is important to informed consent. A patient has a right to refuse to be drawn by a student. Knowing that you are going to draw a blood specimen is necessary to informed consent. Many patients request to know the name of the test before consenting to a blood draw.

66. a. They are many reasons why a physician will order certain tests. Any attempt at explanation of why a test was ordered may mislead the patient. For example, a glucose test may be ordered because the patient is taking medication that can affect glucose levels, not because diabetes is suspected. Usually such inquiries are handled by explaining that the doctor has ordered the tests as part of the patient's care and that the he or she will be happy to explain the tests if asked.

67. c. When it has been determined that a patient truly refuses to cooperate, you should write on the requisition that the patient has refused to have blood drawn. You should also notify the patient's nurse and the phlebotomy supervisor that the specimen was not obtained because of patient refusal. Some institutions have a special form on which you state that you were unable to collect the specimen and the reason why. The original form is left at the nurse's station and a copy goes to the lab.

68. a. If you determine that the patient has not been fasting, notify the patient's nurse so that a determination can be made regarding whether to proceed with the test. If you are told to proceed with collection, write "non-fasting" on the requisition and specimen label so that testing personnel know the status of the patient.

69. d. If you wait to assemble equipment after selecting the collection site, you will have a better idea of what equipment to use and will ultimately waste less equipment. For example, if you have a multisample needle and holder ready before you select the site, it will have to be thrown away if you later decide to use a butterfly instead. However, if you had waited until after selecting the site to select equipment, you would only be using the butterfly equipment. There is plenty of time to get equipment ready while you are waiting for the alcohol to dry after cleaning the site, and you will be more apt to allow sufficient time for the alcohol to dry.

70. c. When performing a routine blood draw, the hands must be washed before glove application at the beginning of the procedure and at the end after glove removal, before proceeding to the next patient.

71. d. Proper hand washing is an important part of the venipuncture procedure. Hands should be washed in a downward motion, scrubbing from wrists to fingertips to prevent backflow of contaminated soap and water. A circular scrubbing motion that creates plenty of friction is needed to dislodge surface debris and bacteria. If the sink does not have an automatic shut-off, a clean paper towel should be used to turn off the faucet to avoid contaminating clean hands.

72. a. Do everything you can to establish a rapport with the child and his or her parents. Even young children can sense when you are not being honest with them. Tell the child that it may be slightly uncomfortable without being overly blunt. Never tell a child it will not hurt.

73. a. You should never tell a patient that a venipuncture will not hurt, nor should you infer that it will hurt a great deal. Some patients are more sensitive to pain than others. Tell the patient that it may hurt a little, but only for a short time. You should warn the patient just before you slip the needle into the vein to help them prepare for it. You can suggest to a fearful patient that he or she look away as the needle goes in, but do not imply that looking away will keep it from hurting.

74. b. Proper arm position is important for successful venipuncture. An arm in proper position for routine venipuncture is supported firmly and extended downward in a straight line from shoulder to wrist with the palm up. It should not be bent at the elbow. The hand is sometimes turned palm down when accessing the cephalic vein or hand veins.

75. a. An outpatient who has previously fainted during a blood draw should be asked to lie down or the drawing chair should be reclined if possible.

76. c. It is acceptable to lower a bed rail to make blood collection easier; however, you can be held liable if you forget to raise it again after you are finished and the patient falls out of bed and is injured.

77. **b.** Blockage of blood flow (stasis) by the tourniquet causes hemoconcentration, which affects specimen composition and leads to erroneous test results. To minimize these effects, the tourniquet should never be left in place longer than 1 minute.

78. **a.** The best place to apply the tourniquet is 3–4 inches above the intended venipuncture site (Fig. 8-3). If it is too close to the collection site, the vein may collapse as blood is withdrawn; if it is too far away, it may be ineffective. Applying a tourniquet distal or below a venipuncture site would prevent blood flow into the area and result in vein collapse and unsuccessful venipuncture. When drawing a hand vein, the tourniquet is applied proximal to the wrist bone, not distal.

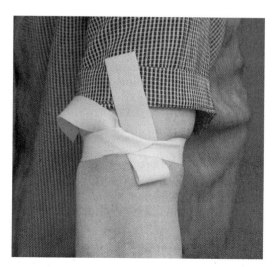

■ FIGURE 8-3 ■
Properly tied tourniquet.

79. **d.** A tourniquet that is too tight may prevent arterial blood flow into the area, resulting in failure to obtain blood. A tourniquet that is too tight increases the effects of hemoconcentration and contributes to erroneous results on the sample. A tourniquet that is too tight will pinch and hurt the patient and cause the arm to turn red or purple.

80. **a.** To enhance vein selection, you are encouraged to palpate the anticubital area, lower the arm, or use a warm towel to increase blood flow. It is not a good idea to have a patient pump (repeatedly open and close) his or her fist because it may cause erroneous results for some tests, most notably potassium levels, as a result of hemoconcentration.

81. **a.** You can easily tell an artery from a vein because an artery has a pulse; a vein does not.

82. **b.** A normal vein feels bouncy and resilient; a sclerosed vein feels hard and cord-like and lacks resiliency. A sclerosed vein is difficult to penetrate, rolls easily, and should not be used for venipuncture.

83. **c.** Ankle veins are sometimes used as a last resort but only after obtaining permission from the patient's physician.

84. **d.** To avoid inadvertently puncturing an artery never select a vein that overlies or is close to an artery or near where you feel a pulse. Avoid drawing from the basilic vein as it is in the area of the brachial artery.

85. **b.** When a person has dermatitis and there is no other site available, it is acceptable to apply the tourniquet over a towel or washcloth placed over the patient's arm. A coagula-

tion test should not be collected from an IV and cannot be collected by fingerstick. The area above an IV must not be used regardless of whether you use a tourniquet.

86. c. If the vein can be felt, but not seen, try to mentally visualize its location. It often helps to note the position of the vein in reference to a mole, hair, or skin crease. Never insert the needle blindly or probe to find a vein as damage to nerves and tissue may result. Never leave the tourniquet on for more than 1 minute as hemoconcentration of the specimen may result. Marking the site with a felt tip pen could contaminate the specimen or transfer disease from patient to patient.

87. d. NCCLS guidelines recommend that if a tourniquet is used for initial vein selection, it should be released and not reapplied for a minimum of 2 minutes to allow the vein to return to normal. This avoids hemoconcentration of the specimen and helps to ensure accurate test results.

88. b. NCCLS venipuncture guidelines recommend cleaning the site with a circular motion from the center to the periphery. In other words, start at the center and wipe outward in ever-increasing circles.

89. d. Alcohol takes around 30 seconds to evaporate completely. The evaporation process helps destroy microbes. Allowing the alcohol to dry before venipuncture also prevents hemolysis of the specimen and a stinging sensation when the needle is inserted.

90. d. When the tube is advanced past the guideline on the holder, the stopper is penetrated causing the tube to

lose its vacuum. A tube that has lost its vacuum will fail to fill with blood, which means you will have to replace it with a new tube.

91. b. Visually inspecting the needle tip before insertion not only ensures that you are entering bevel up, but also prevents damage and unnecessary pain during the procedure should the point or beveled edges have imperfections. Needles are sterile when first opened as long as they are not allowed to touch anything before use. You cannot tell that a needle is outdated by inspecting the tip. The expiration date is typically printed on the label that covers the twist-apart shields or on the packaging as in the case of butterfly needles. Outdated needles must be discarded during regular inventory of the stock.

92. b. The proper and safe way to anchor a vein is to pull the skin taut below the site with your thumb (Fig. 8-4). Simply pressing down on the skin will not anchor the vein. For safety reasons, *do not* use two-finger technique (also called the "C" hold) in which the entry point of the vein is straddled by the index finger above and the thumb below. If the patient pulls the arm back when the needle is inserted, there is a possibility that the needle may recoil as it comes out of the arm and spring back into your index finger.

93. c. If the needle touches the skin and then is withdrawn before piercing the tissue, the needle is considered contaminated and a new needle should be used for the draw to avoid a possible infection.

94. b. For normal venous punctures, the best angle is between 15 and 30°

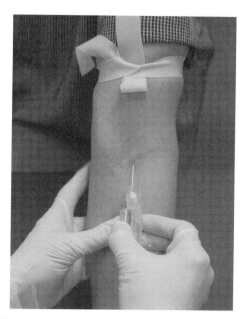

■ FIGURE 8-4 ■

Entering the vein with the needle while the thumb pulls the skin taut.

depending on the depth of the vein. When using a butterfly, the angle will probably be less than 15°.

95. **a.** A venipuncture needle is always inserted bevel up.

96. **b.** When the needle enters the vein, you will feel a slight "give" or decrease in resistance. Some phlebotomists describe this as a "pop." If the needle hisses, the vacuum of the tube is drawing in air, which means that the needle bevel is partially or totally out of the vein and not completely under the skin. If you can feel the needle vibrate, the needle bevel is against the vein wall or a valve causing flapping of tissue against the needle opening.

97. **a.** According to NCCLS guidelines, the best time to release the tourniquet is as soon as blood begins to flow

into the first tube. Releasing the tourniquet as well as having the patient release the fist minimizes the effects of stasis and hemoconcentration on the specimen. A tourniquet should not remain in place longer than 1 minute.

98. **d.** Prolonged tourniquet application or vigorous fist pumping lead to hemoconcentration of the specimen notably affecting potassium, protein levels, and cell counts.

99. **d.** To avoid reflux of tube contents into the patient as well as carryover of additives between tubes, the arm should be in a downward position so that tubes fill from the bottom up and *not* from the stopper end first. Clearing for special coagulation tests, collecting nonadditive tubes before additive tubes, and filling tubes until the normal vacuum is exhausted are all part of proper venipuncture technique.

100. **b.** It is important to fill additive tubes to the proper fill level to ensure a proper ratio of additive to blood. The proper fill level is attained by allowing the tube to fill until the normal vacuum is exhausted and blood ceases to flow into the tube. Tubes will not fill completely as there is always dead space at the top. Blood in an anticoagulant tube does not clot. A partially filled tube would likely have enough specimen to perform the test; however, the results would be inaccurate. Tissue thromboplastin is a problem for some tests, particularly special coagulation tests collected in light blue tops. However, contamination is minimized by first collecting a discard tube to flush the tissue thromboplastin out of the needle.

101. **a.** Lack of or inadequate mixing immediately after filling anticoagulant tubes can lead to microclot formation. Anticoagulant tubes are not supposed to clot, so coagulation would definitely *not* be encouraged. Hemoconcentration is related to dehydration of the patient, fist pumping, and prolonged tourniquet application, not mixing of the tube. Hemolysis can be caused by mixing tubes too vigorously. Nonadditive tubes do not require mixing.

102. **b.** To avoid EDTA contamination of the green top, draw a few milliliters of blood into a plain red top discard tube. Penetrating the stopper of the red top should help clear the outside of the needle of contamination. Drawing a few milliliters of blood into the discard tube should flush any contamination from inside the needle. If the error had been discovered after the green top had started to fill, that green top could be considered the discard tube and another green top collected after it.

103. **a.** Nonadditive tubes should not be mixed. In fact, mixing may cause hemolysis if the sample has already begun to clot.

104. **b.** Vigorous mixing or shaking of the tube can cause hemolysis because red cells are fragile and can rupture easily.

105. **a.** Using several layers of gauze helps create adequate pressure to stop the bleeding and keeps the blood from soaking through and contaminating your glove. The purpose of using gauze as the needle is pulled out has nothing to do with whether the patient sees the needle come out or not. Whether or not it hurts when you pull the needle out depends on

your technique, not the amount of gauze used. You could use several layers of gauze and still have bruising if you did not apply adequate pressure to the site.

106. **c.** Gauze pads are preferred for applying pressure to the puncture site because the loose cotton fibers of cotton balls tend to stick to the site, disrupting the platelet plug when the cotton ball is removed and reinitiating bleeding.

107. **d.** Applying pressure to the gauze while removing the needle causes the needle to slit the skin, slowing down needle removal and causing pain to the patient.

108. **b.** An uncovered used needle is a danger to the phlebotomist. A needle safety feature should be engaged (Fig. 8-5) immediately after needle

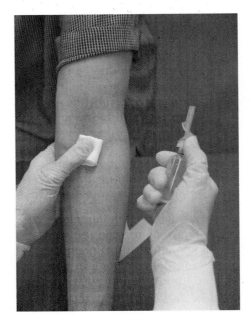

■ Figure 8-5 ■
Needle with safety shield engaged.

removal. Any delay increases the risk of accidental needle injury to the phlebotomist.

109. **d.** Although once standard practice, folding the arm to hold pressure on the site after venipuncture is no longer recommended. When the arm is folded back it sometimes creates a pocket that prevents adequate pressure from being applied to the site. This can lead to continued bleeding and bruising at the site. When the arm is later straightened the platelet plug can be dislodged, causing renewed bleeding and possible bruising.

110. **a.** According to the Occupational Safety and Health Administration (OSHA) regulations, a needle and holder are to be disposed as a single unit. Removing the needle from the holder either by ejection or unscrewing subjects the user to needlestick hazards posed by the exposed rubber sleeve end of the needle.

111. **a.** Inpatient blood specimens should be labeled at the bedside immediately following collection. If tubes are labeled before collection and one of the tubes is not used at that time, another patient's blood could end up in that labeled tube. If tubes are labeled away from the bedside, the specimen can be misidentified.

112. **c.** As a minimum, specimen labels should contain the patient's first and last name, hospital or medical record number, date of birth, date and time of the draw, and phlebotomist's initials. The room number and bed may be found on the label if the label has been generated by a computer, but is not mandatory.

113. **d.** The patient's ID number is included on the specimen label to avoid confusing samples. It is not unusual to have patients with the same or similar names in the hospital at the same time, but two patients will not have the same hospital or medical record number.

114. **d.** Carrying a bag or purse on the venipuncture arm, lifting heavy objects with that arm, or removing the bandage prematurely can all disturb the healing process, reinitiate bleeding, and lead to bruising of the site.

115. **d.** An ammonia specimen is transported on ice, a bilirubin specimen needs to be protected from light, and a cold agglutinin specimen must be transported at body temperature (37 °C).

116. **d.** Patient refusal or unavailability or the fact that you tried but were unsuccessful are all valid reasons for failure to obtain specimen. Not having the right equipment to collect a specimen makes a phlebotomist appear disorganized and unprofessional and is *not* an acceptable reason for failure to collect a specimen. You should check to see that you have the proper equipment for the test before leaving to collect the specimen.

117. **a.** After two unsuccessful attempts at blood collection, *do not* try a third time. Ask another phlebotomist to take over. Unsuccessful venipuncture attempts are frustrating to the patient and the phlebotomist. With the exception of STAT and other priority specimens, if the second phlebotomist is also unsuccessful, it is a good idea to give the patient a rest and come back at a later time.

An outpatient may be given the option of returning another day after consultation with his or her physician.

118. d. A winged infusion set is called a butterfly because it resembles one (see Fig. 7-7).

119. c. The small size of the needle and flexibility afforded by the tubing makes a butterfly a good choice for drawing small, difficult, or hand veins.

120. c. When drawing a hand vein, the tourniquet is applied on the forearm just proximal to the wrist bone.

121. b. A needle and syringe or butterfly and syringe may be used if the patient has small, fragile, or weak veins that collapse easily. The vacuum pressure of the evacuated tube may be too great for such veins. When a syringe is used the pressure can be controlled by pulling slowly on the syringe plunger.

122. d. A number of things can cause hemolysis of a specimen, including mixing tubes too vigorously, using a large-volume tube with a small-diameter needle, and pushing on the plunger to force blood from a syringe into an evacuated tube.

123. a. When a syringe needle is inserted in a vein, a "flash" of blood will usually appear in the hub of the needle.

124. d. The safest and proper way to transfer blood from a syringe into the evacuated tubes is to use a syringe transfer device (Fig. 8-6). If a transfer device is not available, the second best way is to place the tube in a rack before penetrating the tube stopper with the needle. Holding

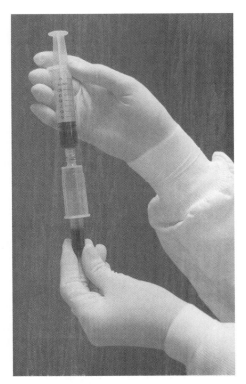

■ FIGURE 8-6 ■

Blood being transferred using a Greiner transfer device attached to a syringe. (Courtesy Greiner Bio-One, Kremsmuenster, Austria.)

the tube with your hand is dangerous because the needle may slip and stick your hand. Never force the blood into the tube by pushing on the syringe plunger. Let the vacuum of the tube draw the blood into it. Pushing on the plunger and forcing blood into the tube can hemolyze the specimen and can also allow blood to spurt out around the needle and contaminate you.

125. c. It is important to greet the parents and the child and try to establish a rapport with each of them. Explain what you are going to do in terms the child can understand so he or

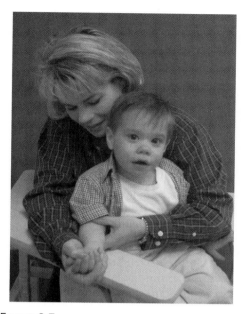

■ FIGURE 8-7 ■
Seated adult restraining a toddler.

she knows what to expect. Answer questions honestly. *Never* tell a child it won't hurt.

126. c. Small children seldom hold still for blood collection. The flexibility of the butterfly tubing enables successful blood collection despite some movement by the child. Children do like the idea of the butterfly, but it is not the reason it is used.

127. c. A big factor in successful blood collection from pediatric patients is proper immobilization. Preventing excessive movement makes the process quicker and safer for the patient and the blood drawer.

128. a. Proper immobilization of a pediatric patient typically involves two people—the phlebotomist and someone to immobilize the child by cradling him or her and grasping the arm at the wrist (Fig. 8-7). Al-lowing a pediatric patient to brace his or her own arm is asking for trouble. Even if it appears that the child understands and will stay still, chances are the he or she will pull away as soon as the needle is seen.

129. b. Older children appreciate honesty and will be more cooperative if you explain what you are going to do and stress the importance of holding still. *Never* tell the child it won't hurt. It is all right to offer the child a reward for being brave, but *do not* put conditions on receiving the reward such as, "You can only have the reward if you don't cry." Some crying is to be anticipated, and it is important to let the child know that it is all right to cry.

130. a. Dorsal hand vein procedure (Fig. 8-8) on infants does not require the use of a tourniquet.

131. c. The *best* way to collect a PKU specimen from a dorsal hand vein is to let the blood drip directly onto the PKU filter paper. Blood collected in an EDTA microcollection tube or in a syringe may have microclots that could cause erroneous results.

132. d. Tremors associated with Parkinson's disease can make blood collection difficult.

133. d. In this scenario it is best to draw the specimen from the left arm in a position that the patient chooses. Using a butterfly will offer the flexibility needed to access veins from an awkward angle. Diabetes can affect circulation and healing in the lower extremities and generally makes venipuncture of leg, ankle, and foot veins off limits. A blood draw should not be performed on the same side as a mastectomy

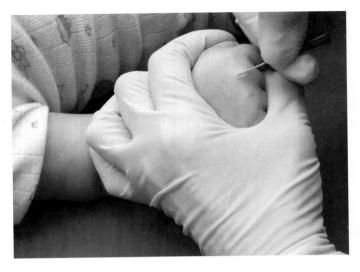

■ FIGURE 8-8 ■
Venipuncture of an infant dorsal hand vein.

without approval of the patient's physician. *Never* use force to extend a patient's arm.

134. d. The effects of colds and influenza are more severe in the elderly. If you have a cold, refrain from drawing elderly patients if possible or wear a mask. *Never* substitute a pressure bandage in lieu of holding pressure. You must hold pressure if the patient is unable to do so. It is discourteous to address questions to a relative or attendant as if a patient were not there. Speak clearly and distinctly but do not raise the pitch of your voice. Raising the pitch of your voice actually makes it harder to understand.

135. c. The most common reason a patient must undergo dialysis is end-stage

renal disease (ESRD), a serious condition in which the kidneys have deteriorated to a point at which they fail (no longer function). The most common cause of ESRD is diabetes and the second most common cause is high blood pressure. Patients with ESRD require ongoing dialysis treatments or a kidney transplant.

136. c. Hospice is a type of care designed for patients who are dying. The majority of hospice patients have incurable forms of cancer. Hospice care allows terminally ill patients to spend their last days in a peaceful, supportive atmosphere that emphasizes pain management to help keep them comfortable.

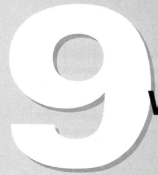

BLOOD COLLECTION VARIABLES, COMPLICATIONS, AND PROCEDURAL ERRORS

A. Introduction

B. Physiologic Variables That Influence Specimen Composition
1. Basal State
2. Factors That Influence Basal State
   a. Age
   b. Altitude
   c. Dehydration
   d. Diet
   e. Diurnal (Daily) Variations
   f. Drug Therapy
   g. Exercise
   h. Fever
   i. Gender
   j. Jaundice
   k. Position
   l. Pregnancy
   m. Smoking
   n. Stress
   o. Temperature and Humidity

C. Site Selection Variables That Influence Specimen Composition
1. Physical Problem Areas to Avoid in Site Selection
   a. Burns, Scars, and Tattoos
   b. Damaged Veins
   c. Edema
   d. Hematomas
   e. Mastectomy

2. Vascular Access Areas and Devices to Avoid in Site Selection
   a. IV Sites
   b. Previously Active IV Sites
   c. Arterial Lines
   d. Arteriovenous Shunts or Fistulas
   e. Heparin or Saline Locks
   f. Vascular Access Devices
      1) Central Venous Catheters
      2) Implanted Ports
      3) Peripherally Inserted Central Catheters

D. Complications and Procedural Errors Associated With Blood Collection
1. Complications Related to Patient Conditions
   a. Allergies to Antiseptics and Adhesives
   b. Allergies to Latex
   c. Excessive Bleeding
   d. Fainting (Syncope)
   e. Nausea/Vomiting
   f. Obesity
   g. Petechiae
   h. Seizures/Convulsions
2. Complications and Procedural Errors That Adversely Affect the Patient
   a. Hematoma Formation
   b. Inadvertent Arterial Puncture
   c. Iatrogenic Anemia
   d. Infection

   e. Nerve Damage
   f. Pain
   g. Reflux of Anticoagulant
   h. Vein Damage
3. Procedural Errors That Affect Specimen
   Quality
   a. Hemoconcentration/Venous Stasis
   b. Hemolysis
   c. Partially Filled Tubes
   d. Specimen Contamination

4. Procedural Errors That Lead to Failure to
   Draw Blood
5. Tube Position and Vacuum
6. Needle Position
   a. Bevel Against the Vein Wall
   b. Too Deep
   c. Not Deep Enough
   d. Beside the Vein
   e. Undetermined
7. Collapsed Vein

REVIEW QUESTIONS

Match the term with the BEST description.

1. ____ basal state	8. ____ hemoconcentration	15. ____ reflux
2. ____ collapsed vein	9. ____ hemolysis	16. ____ sclerosed
3. ____ CVC	10. ____ heparin lock	17. ____ syncope
4. ____ diurnal variations	11. ____ iatrogenic	18. ____ thrombosed
5. ____ edema	12. ____ lipemic	19. ____ VAD
6. ____ fistula	13. ____ patency	20. ____ venous stasis
7. ____ hematoma	14. ____ petechiae	

a. abnormal retraction of blood vessel walls, temporarily shutting off blood blow

b. accumulation of fluid in the tissues

c. backflow of blood from a collection tube into a patient's vein during venipuncture

d. clotted

e. condition in which plasma and filterable components of the blood pass through the walls of the blood vessels into the tissues, concentrating nonfilterable blood components and decreasing blood plasma volume

f. destruction of RBCs and liberation of hemoglobin into the fluid portion of a specimen

g. early in the morning while the body is at rest and approximately 12 hours after last intake of food, exercise, or activity

h. fainting

i. hard, cord-like, and lacking resiliency

j. induced by the effects of treatment

k. internal shunt created by permanent fusion of an artery and a vein

l. normal fluctuations throughout the day

m. small, non-raised red spots that appear on a patient's skin when a tourniquet is applied because of a defect in the capillary walls or platelets

n. special winged needle set or cannula that can be left in a patient's arm for up to 48 hours and used to administer medication and draw blood

o. stagnation or stoppage of normal venous blood flow

p. state of being freely open, as in a patient's veins

q. type of line inserted into a large vein and advanced into the superior vena cava, proximal to the right atrium

r. swelling or mass of blood caused by leakage of blood from a vessel during or after venipuncture or arterial puncture

s. term used to describe cloudy serum or plasma caused by increased fat or lipid content

t. tubing inserted into a main vein or artery and used for administering fluids and medications, monitoring pressures, and drawing blood

Choose the BEST answer.

21. The *best* specimens to use for establishing inpatient reference ranges are:
    a. basal state specimens.
    b. fasting specimens.
    c. steady-state specimens.
    d. 2-hour postprandial specimens.

22. In which instance is the patient closest to basal state? The patient has just:
    a. arrived at the lab after working all night, but was fasting at work.
    b. arrived at the lab for a fasting blood test.
    c. awakened at 0600 hours after fasting since the previous evening meal.
    d. been lying down quietly for 1 hour.

23. Which of the following tests requires the patient's age when calculating results?
    a. calcium
    b. creatine phosphokinase (CPK)
    c. creatinine clearance
    d. glucose

24. Which of the following tests is most affected by altitude?
    a. bilirubin
    b. glucose
    c. pH
    d. red blood count

25. Persistent diarrhea in the absence of fluid replacement may cause:
    a. hemoconcentration of the blood.
    b. hemolysis of red blood cells.
    c. high white blood count.
    d. low iron (Fe) levels.

26. The serum or plasma of a lipemic specimen appears:
    a. cloudy.
    b. dark yellow.
    c. foamy.
    d. pink to red.

27. A lipemic specimen is a clue that the patient was:
    a. dehydrated.
    b. in a basal state.
    c. not fasting.
    d. supine.

28. A 12-hour fast is normally required when testing for this analyte.
    a. bilirubin
    b. calcium
    c. electrolytes
    d. triglycerides

29. This blood component exhibits diurnal variation with peak levels occurring in the morning.
    a. bilirubin
    b. cardiac enzymes
    c. cortisol
    d. iron

30. Tests influenced by diurnal variation are often ordered:
    a. fasting.
    b. postprandial.
    c. STAT.
    d. timed.

31. College of American Pathologists (CAP) guidelines state that drugs known to interfere with blood tests should be discontinued how many hours before the test?
    a. 4–24
    b. 12–24
    c. 24–36
    d. 48–72

32. A falsely decreased test result can be caused by:
    a. a drug that competes with the test reagents for the analyte being tested.
    b. a drug that enhances the color reaction used to detect an analyte.
    c. reflux of anticoagulant during specimen collection.
    d. testing a serum from a partially filled red top tube.

33. Which of the following analytes is *most* affected by muscular activity before specimen collection?
   a. bilirubin
   b. calcium
   c. enzymes
   d. hemoglobin

34. The presence of fever influences the levels of:
   a. insulin.
   b. glucagon.
   c. cortisol.
   d. all of the above

35. Which analyte has higher reference values for males than for females?
   a. cholesterol
   b. glucose
   c. hematocrit
   d. potassium

36. An icteric specimen:
   a. may indicate that the patient has hepatitis.
   b. may yield erroneous test results for some analytes.
   c. will most likely have a high bilirubin level.
   d. all of the above

37. What physical changes occur when a patient goes from supine to standing?
   a. calcium levels decrease
   b. nonfilterable blood elements increase
   c. plasma volume increases
   d. red blood cell counts decrease

38. Why do pregnant patients have lower reference ranges for red blood counts?
   a. body fluid increases in pregnancy have a diluting effect on red blood cells
   b. constant nausea leads to hemoconcentration of red blood cells
   c. poor appetite leads to transient anemia
   d. the growing fetus uses up the mother's iron reserves

39. Which of the following analytes may be increased in smokers?
   a. cortisol
   b. hemoglobin
   c. white blood count
   d. all of the above

40. It is *not* a good idea to collect a complete blood count from a screaming infant because the:
   a. crying can temporarily elevate the white blood count.
   b. platelets are more likely to clump.
   c. specimen may be hemoconcentrated.
   d. specimen may be hemolyzed.

41. Of the following factors known to affect basal state, which would be automatically accounted for when reference ranges are established?
   a. diurnal variation
   b. drug interferences
   c. effects of exercise
   d. geographic environment

42. All of the following are reasons to control temperature and humidity in a laboratory EXCEPT:
   a. to establish reference values under controlled conditions
   b. to ensure proper functioning of equipment
   c. to lessen drug interference
   d. to maintain specimen integrity

43. Why should scarred or burned areas be avoided as blood collection sites?
   a. newly burned sites may be painful and are susceptible to infection
   b. scarred sites may have impaired circulation
   c. veins are difficult to palpate in such areas
   d. all of the above

44. A vein that feels hard and cord-like and lacks resiliency may be:
   a. an artery.
   b. collapsed.

c. superficial.
d. thrombosed.

45. Drawing blood from an edematous extremity may cause:
a. erroneous results.
b. hemolysis of the specimen.
c. premature clotting of the specimen.
d. none of the above

46. If you have no choice but to collect a specimen from an arm with a hematoma, collect the specimen:
a. above the hematoma.
b. distal to the hematoma.
c. in the area of the hematoma.
d. any of the above

47. A venipuncture made through a hematoma:
a. can result in the collection of hemolyzed blood.
b. is painful to the patient.
c. may result in inaccurate test results on the specimen.
d. all of the above

48. Avoid collecting a specimen from an arm on the same side as a mastectomy because the:
a. arm is usually edematous.
b. effects of lymphostasis may cause erroneous results.
c. veins in that arm may collapse more easily.
d. all of the above

49. You must collect a protime specimen from a patient with IVs in both arms. The *best* place to collect the specimen is:
a. above one of the IVs.
b. below one of the IVs.
c. from an ankle vein.
d. from one of the IVs.

50. A phlebotomist must collect a hemoglobin on a patient in the intensive care unit. There is an IV in the patient's left arm. There is no suitable antecubital vein or hand vein in the right arm. What should the phlebotomist do?
a. ask another phlebotomist to collect the specimen
b. attempt to draw a hand vein below the IV
c. collect the specimen by skin puncture of a finger of the right hand
d. draw the specimen from an ankle vein

51. Which of the following should be avoided when selecting a venipuncture site?
a. a previous IV site within 24 hours of IV removal
b. an arm that has a heparin lock in the wrist area
c. an arm with an arteriovenous (AV) shunt in the forearm
d. all of the above

52. A type of line that is commonly used to collect blood gas specimens.
a. arterial line
b. central venous catheter (CVC)
c. intravenous (IV)
d. peripherally inserted central catheter (PICC)

53. A vascular access pathway that is surgically created to provide access for dialysis is called a(n):
a. arteriovenous (AV) shunt.
b. central venous catheter (CVC).
c. heparin lock.
d. implanted port.

54. When a blood specimen is collected from a heparin lock, it is important to draw:
a. a 5 mL discard tube before collecting the specimen.
b. an extra tube for each test requested.
c. coagulation specimens first.
d. all of the above

55. Central venous catheters include all the following EXCEPT:
   a. Broviac.
   b. Groshong.
   c. Hep-lok.
   d. Hickman.

56. A subcutaneous vascular access device consisting of a small chamber attached to an indwelling line that is implanted under the skin and located by palpating the skin.
   a. central venous catheter
   b. implanted port
   c. peripherally inserted central catheter
   d. saline lock

57. How do you bandage a venipuncture site if the patient is allergic to the glue in adhesive bandages?
   a. use paper tape over a folded gauge square placed over the site
   b. wrap self-adhering bandage over a folded gauze square
   c. have the patient hold pressure longer in lieu of a bandage
   d. any of the above

58. You may have to be careful about what type of equipment is brought into the room if a patient is severely allergic to:
   a. adhesive bandages.
   b. latex.
   c. perfume.
   d. any of the above

59. If a blood collection site continues to bleed after 5 minutes:
   a. bandage the site and tell the patient to hold pressure over the bandage.
   b. notify the patient's physician or nurse.
   c. wrap a pressure bandage around the site.
   d. none of the above

60. Which patient should be asked to lie down during a blood draw? A patient with a:

a. coagulation disorder.
b. history of syncope during blood draws.
c. central venous catheter.
d. latex allergy.

61. What should a phlebotomist do if a patient feels faint during a blood draw?
   a. lower the patient's head and continue the draw
   b. immediately discontinue the draw and lower the patient's head
   c. remove the needle and shake the patient to revive him or her
   d. use one hand to hold the patient upright and continue the draw

62. An outpatient becomes weak and pale following blood collection. What should the phlebotomist do?
   a. have someone accompany the patient to his or her car
   b. have the patient lie down
   c. offer the patient a drink of water
   d. tell the patient to go and get something to eat right away

63. If an outpatient tells you that she is feeling nauseous, you should:
   a. give her an emesis basin in case she vomits.
   b. hold a cold, damp washcloth to her forehead.
   c. tell her to breathe slowly and deeply.
   d. all of the above

64. Of the following veins, which is often the one that is easiest to feel on obese patients?
   a. basilic
   b. brachial
   c. cephalic
   d. ulnar

65. All of the following would be reasons to eliminate a potential venipuncture site EXCEPT:

a. petechiae appear when the tourniquet is applied
b. massive scarring is present
c. the arm is edematous
d. the only vein feels hard and cord-like

66. A patient goes into convulsions while you are in the middle of a venipuncture. All of the following would be appropriate actions to take EXCEPT:
a. complete the draw as quickly as you can
b. remove the needle as soon as possible
c. prevent the patient from injuring himself or herself
d. notify appropriate first aid personnel

67. You are in the process of collecting a blood specimen on a patient with difficult veins. You had to redirect the needle but it is now in the vein, and you have just started to fill the first tube. The blood is filling the tube slowly. The skin around the venipuncture site starts to swell. What should you do? You have several tubes to fill.
a. ask the patient if it is hurts; if not, continue the draw
b. push the needle deeper and continue the draw
c. pull back the needle slightly and continue the draw
d. remove the tourniquet and discontinue the draw immediately

68. All of the following can cause hematoma formation during venipuncture EXCEPT:
a. inadequate pressure is applied to site after needle removal
b. the needle has penetrated through the back of the vein
c. the needle bevel is centered in the lumen of the vein
d. the needle bevel is only partially inserted in the vein

69. Which of the following is the *best* indication that you have accidentally punctured an artery?
a. a hematoma starts to form instantly
b. the blood obtained is dark red
c. the blood pulses into the tube
d. there is no way to tell

70. Term used to describe anemia brought on by withdrawal of blood for testing purposes.
a. hemolytic
b. iatrogenic
c. icteric
d. neutropenic

71. If you suspect that you have accidentally collected an arterial specimen instead of a venous specimen:
a. apply a pressure bandage to the site.
b. ask another phlebotomist to recollect the specimen.
c. discard the specimen and collect a new one at another site.
d. keep the specimen and label it as a possible arterial specimen.

72. Infection at the site following venipuncture can result from:
a. following the wrong order of draw.
b. leaving the tourniquet on throughout the draw.
c. touching the site after it has been cleaned.
d. all of the above

73. Excessive or blind probing for a vein can cause:
a. diurnal variation.
b. lipemia.
c. nerve damage.
d. petechiae.

74. A patient complains of significant pain when you insert the needle. The pain does not subside and radiates down his arm. What should you do?
a. ask the patient if it is alright to continue the draw

b. discontinue the draw immediately
c. collect the specimen as quickly as you can
d. tell the patient to hang in there so that you do not have to stick him again

75. A stinging sensation when the needle is first inserted is *most* likely the result of:
a. a dull needle.
b. not allowing the alcohol to dry properly.
c. pushing down on the needle as it is inserted.
d. tying the tourniquet too tightly.

76. Which is the *best* way to avoid reflux?
a. do not release the tourniquet until the last tube is filled
b. draw the specimen while the patient is supine
c. keep the patient's arm straight
d. make certain that tubes fill from the bottom up

77. Which of the following is *least* likely to impair vein patency?
a. improperly redirecting the needle
b. leaving the tourniquet on for 2 minutes
c. performing numerous venipunctures in the same area
d. probing for a deep vein

78. Prolonged tourniquet application may cause a change in blood composition primarily because of:
a. hemoconcentration.
b. hemoglobin.
c. hemolysis.
d. homeostasis.

79. The serum or plasma of a hemolyzed specimen appears:
a. clear light yellow.
b. cloudy white.
c. dark greenish yellow.
d. pink or reddish.

80. Which action is *least* likely to cause hemolysis of a specimen?
a. collecting more than one tube of blood
b. mixing tubes vigorously
c. pulling blood into a syringe too quickly
d. using a small-bore needle and a large-volume tube

81. The ratio of blood to anticoagulant is *most* critical for which of the following tests?
a. bilirubin
b. complete blood count
c. prothrombin time
d. sodium

82. A phlebotomist has tried twice to collect a light blue top on a patient with difficult veins. Both times the phlebotomist has been able to collect only a partial tube. What should the phlebotomist do?
a. collect the specimen by skin puncture
b. have another phlebotomist collect the specimen
c. pour the two tubes together and mix well
d. send the tube with the most blood to the lab with a note that it was a difficult draw

83. Which of the following situations is *least* likely to cause contamination of the specimen?
a. cleaning with isopropyl alcohol before performing a fingerstick
b. drawing a blood culture specimen while the povidone-iodine is still damp
c. touching the filter paper with your gloves when collecting a phenylketonuria (PKU) specimen
d. using povidone-iodine to clean a heel puncture site

84. You are in the process of collecting a blood specimen. Blood flow has been established. As the tube is filling, you hear a hissing sound and there is a spurt of blood into the tube and the flow then stops. What has *most* likely happened is the:
   a. needle bevel came partly out of the skin and the vacuum escaped from the tube
   b. needle penetrated all the way through the vein and out the other side
   c. patient's blood pressure dropped
   d. tube had a crack in it and there was no more vacuum

85. Which of the following situations could indicate that the needle has gone through the back of the vein? You
   a. fail to get blood flow until you pull back on the needle
   b. felt the needle go into the vein but you fail to get blood flow
   c. filled one tube but the second one failed to fill with blood
   d. all of the above

86. When a vein rolls, the needle typically:
   a. ends up in the lumen of the vein.
   b. lands up against an inside wall of the vein.
   c. penetrates all the way through the vein.
   d. slips beside the vein.

87. You are in the process of collecting a specimen. The needle is inserted but the blood is filling the tube very slowly. You see a hematoma forming very rapidly. What has *most* likely happened is the:
   a. needle is only partly inserted in the vein.
   b. needle is up against the vein wall.

   c. patient has a coagulation problem.
   d. tube is loosing vacuum.

88. You are performing a multi-tube blood draw. You collect the first tube without a problem. The second tube fails to fill with blood. You pull the needle back and nothing happens. You push the needle deeper and nothing happens. You remove the tube, pull back the needle a little, rotate the bevel, and reset the tube. Still nothing happens. Which of the following actions should you take?
   a. discontinue the draw and try at another site
   b. redirect the needle until you get blood flow
   c. try a new tube
   d. none of the above

89. You insert the needle into the vein during blood collection. When you advance the tube onto the needle in the holder you do not get blood flow. You can see that the needle is beside the vein. You redirect the needle two times and still do not get blood flow. What should you do next?
   a. anchor the vein and try again
   b. ask a co-worker to redirect the needle for you
   c. discontinue the draw and try again at a new site
   d. push the needle deeper

90. A vein may collapse because the:
   a. tourniquet is applied too tightly.
   b. tourniquet is too close to the venipuncture site.
   c. tube vacuum is too much for the size of the vein.
   d. any of the above

ANSWERS AND EXPLANATIONS

1. **g.** early in the morning while the body is at rest and approximately 12 hours after the last intake of food, exercise, or activity

2. **a.** abnormal retraction of blood vessel walls, temporarily shutting off blood flow

3. **q.** central venous catheter, a type of line inserted into a large vein and advanced into the superior vena cava, proximal to the right atrium

4. **l.** normal fluctuations throughout the day

5. **b.** accumulation of fluid in the tissues

6. **k.** internal shunt created by permanent fusion of an artery and a vein

7. **r.** swelling or mass of blood caused by leakage of blood from a blood vessel during or after venipuncture or arterial puncture

8. **e.** condition in which plasma and filterable components of the blood pass through the walls of the blood vessels into the tissues, concentrating nonfilterable blood components and decreasing blood plasma volume

9. **f.** destruction of RBCs and liberation of hemoglobin into the fluid portion of a specimen

10. **n.** special winged needle set or cannula that can be left in a patient's arm for up to 48 hours and used to administer medication and draw blood

11. **j.** induced by the effects of treatment

12. **s.** term used to describe cloudy serum or plasma caused by fat or lipid content

13. **p.** state of being freely open, as in a patient's vein

14. **m.** small, non-raised red spots that appear on a patient's skin when a tourniquet is applied because of a defect in the capillary walls or platelets

15. **c.** backflow of blood from a collection tube into a patient's vein during venipuncture

16. **i.** hard, cord-like, and lacking resiliency

17. **h.** fainting

18. **d.** clotted

19. **t.** vascular access device, tubing inserted into a main vein or artery and used for administering fluids and medications, monitoring pressures, and drawing blood

20. **o.** stagnation or stoppage of normal venous blood flow

21. **a.** Inpatient reference ranges for laboratory tests are typically established using basal state specimens to eliminate the effects of diet, exercise, and other factors on results.

22. **c.** Basal state refers to the condition of the body early in the morning when a patient is still at rest and fasting (approximately 12 hours after the last intake of food). The patient who has just awakened at 0600 hours (6 AM) and has not eaten since the previous evening meal is closest to basal state.

23. **c.** Some physiologic functions, such as the amount of creatinine cleared by the kidneys, decrease with age, and the patient's age is required when calculating the results.

24. **d.** The red blood cell count is most affected by altitude because the decrease in oxygen content at higher altitudes causes the body to produce more red blood cells to fulfill the body's oxygen requirements. Aspirin can cause decreased bilirubin levels. Glucose levels are affected by diet. Hyperventilation affects pH levels.

25. **a.** Persistent diarrhea without fluid replacement causes dehydration or a decrease in total body fluid leading to hemoconcentration, a condition in which blood components that cannot easily leave the blood stream become concentrated in the smaller plasma volume.

26. **a.** Serum or plasma that has fatty substances (lipids) dissolved in it appears cloudy or turbid. The term used to describe the condition is *lipemia,* and the term used to describe how the specimen looks is *lipemic.*

27. **c.** A cloudy or lipemic specimen indicates that the patient was probably not fasting before specimen collection. Lipemia results from ingestion of fatty substances (lipids). Lipids are insoluble in water, causing the liquid portion (serum or plasma) of a blood specimen to appear cloudy or turbid for up to 10 hours. A 12-hour fast is generally required to remove the effects of lipids from the blood.

28. **d.** Triglycerides are a type of lipid. A 12-hour fast is required to remove the effects of food ingestion on the triglyceride content of the blood (see answer to question 27).

29. **c.** Diurnal variations are normal fluctuations throughout the day. Cortisol levels exhibit diurnal variation

with highest levels occurring in the morning.

30. **d.** For consistency in evaluating or comparing results, tests that exhibit diurnal variation or fluctuations throughout the day are often ordered for a specific time of day.

31. **a.** According to the CAP, a drug known to interfere with a particular blood test should be stopped or avoided for 4–24 hours before obtaining a blood specimen for that test.

32. **a.** A drug that competes with a test reagent for an analyte being tested will result in false low values for the analyte being tested. A drug that enhances a color reaction during testing will falsely elevate test results. Reflux of anticoagulant during specimen collection may cause an adverse patient reaction. Testing serum from a partially filled red top should have no effect on test results provided there is adequate specimen to perform the test.

33. **c.** Muscular activity elevates blood levels of a number of components, including enzymes. Some enzymes, such as creatine kinase and lactate dehydrogenase, may stay elevated for 24 hours or more.

34. **d.** Hypoglycemia caused by fever increases insulin levels followed by a rise in glucagon levels. Fever also increases cortisol levels and may disrupt its normal diurnal variation.

35. **c.** A patient's gender has a determining effect on the concentration of a number of blood components. These differences are reflected in separate normal ranges for males and females for certain analytes. Males tend to have greater muscle

mass and need more red blood cells to supply oxygen to the muscle. They consequently have higher red blood cell counts and higher reference ranges for red blood counts as well as tests related to red blood counts such as hemoglobin and hematocrit. The hematocrit is a measure of the percentage of a specimen that is red blood cells.

36. **d.** Jaundice, also called icterus, is a condition characterized by increased bilirubin in the blood and deposits of yellow pigment in the skin, mucous membranes, and sclera or whites of the eyes, giving the patient a yellow appearance. Serum, plasma, or urine specimens that have high bilirubin levels have an abnormal deep yellow to yellow-brown color, and the specimen is referred to as icteric. One cause of increased bilirubin levels is hepatitis or liver inflammation. The abnormal color may interfere in the color reactions of a number of chemistry tests including chemical reagent strip analyses on urine.

37. **b.** When a patient stands up after being supine (lying down), blood plasma filters into the tissues, *decreasing* plasma volume and *increasing* nonfilterable elements such as calcium, iron, proteins, and red blood cells.

38. **a.** Normal body fluid increases in pregnancy have a diluting effect on red blood cells. Therefore, red blood count reference ranges for pregnant women are lower. Reference ranges for pregnant women are established using specimens from normal pregnant women. Anemia from poor appetite or inadequate iron reserves represent situations that may result

in patient values that are lower than normal reference ranges. Hemoconcentration would most likely elevate red blood counts.

39. **d.** Nicotine affects a number of blood components. The extent of the effect depends on the number of cigarettes smoked. Patients who smoke before specimen collection may have increased cortisol levels and white blood counts. Chronic smoking often leads to decreased pulmonary function and increased hemoglobin levels.

40. **a.** Emotional stress has been shown to cause short-lived elevations in white blood counts. A white blood count is a part of a complete blood count. Studies performed on crying infants demonstrated significant increases in white blood counts. Counts returned to normal within 1 hour after crying stopped. For this reason, it is best if complete blood count or white blood count specimens are obtained after the infant has been sleeping or resting quietly for at least 30 minutes. If a specimen is collected while an infant is crying, it should be noted on the report.

41. **d.** Reference ranges for specimens are established using basal state specimens. Environmental factors associated with geographic location will affect basal state. However, because all the specimens used to calculate reference range values come from patients in a particular location, the geographical factors will be the same for all specimens and will automatically be reflected in the results.

42. **c.** Temperature and humidity are known to affect test values. There-

fore, these environmental factors are closely controlled in a clinical laboratory to ensure specimen integrity and proper functioning of equipment. Environmental factors have no effect on drug interference.

43. **d.** Scarred and burned areas should be avoided as blood collection sites because they are painful and susceptible to infection, can yield erroneous results because of impaired circulation, and can be difficult to palpate.

44. **c.** A vein will feel hard and cord-like if it is thrombosed (clotted) or sclerosed (hardened).

45. **a.** Edema impairs circulation and may disrupt exchange of oxygen and nutrients between the blood and tissues. In addition, specimens may be contaminated with tissue fluids and yield inaccurate test results. Test results of specimens collected from edematous areas should therefore be considered erroneous. In addition, edematous tissue is often fragile and easily injured.

46. **b.** If you have no other choice of collection site, it is acceptable to collect a blood specimen distal or below the hematoma where blood flow is least affected by the presence of the hematoma. A venipuncture above the hematoma would yield erroneous results from the effects of venous stasis caused by obstruction of blood flow by the hematoma. A venipuncture through or in the area of a hematoma is painful to the patient and can result in collection of a specimen from outside the vein that is contaminated and possibly hemolyzed.

47. **d.** A venipuncture made through a hematoma is painful to the patient and can result in collection of a specimen from outside the vein that is contaminated and possibly hemolyzed. Test results on such a specimen would be inaccurate.

48. **b.** Blood should never be collected from an arm on the same side as a mastectomy (breast removal) without first consulting the patient's physician. Lymphostasis (stoppage of lymph flow) that occurs if lymph nodes have been removed as part of the procedure leaves the area susceptible to infection and can also change the composition of blood in the area, leading to erroneous test results. Tourniquet application can also injure the arm.

49. **b.** It is preferred that blood specimens not be drawn from an arm with an intravenous (IV) line. However, according to the National Committee for Clinical Laboratory Standards (NCCLS), a specimen can be drawn below an IV (Fig. 9-1) after the IV off has been shut off for a minimum of 2 minutes. The patient's nurse must shut off the IV; a phlebotomist should *never* shut off an IV. It should be noted on the requisition that the specimen was drawn below the IV after it was shut off. Never draw above an IV as the specimen may be contaminated with fluid from the IV. Drawing blood specimens from ankle veins requires permission from the patient's physician and is not recommended for coagulation specimens or on patients who have coagulation problems. Only nurses and other specially trained personnel

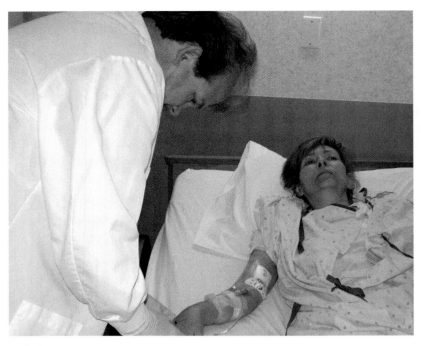

■ FIGURE 9-1 ■

A phlebotomist correctly collects a coagulation specimen from a hand vein below the site of an intravenous (IV) line.

are allowed to collect specimens from an IV.

50. c. The most expedient thing to do in this situation is to collect the specimen by skin puncture. A skin puncture can be collected and on its way to the lab in the time it would take to call another phlebotomist to come and collect the specimen, the IV to be shut off for 2 minutes to collect the specimen below it, or permission obtained to collect the specimen from an ankle vein.

51. d. A previously active IV site within 24 hours of IV removal, an arm with an AV shunt (Fig. 9-2), or a wrist with a heparin lock (Fig. 9-3) should all be avoided as collection sites.

52. a. An arterial line or catheter is most commonly located in the radial artery and is used to provide continuous measurement of a patient's blood pressure. It is also commonly used for collection of blood gas specimens.

53. a. A surgically created graft or connection of an artery and a vein in the forearm is called an AV shunt or fistula (see Fig. 9-2) and is most commonly created to provide access for dialysis. A CVC is a line inserted into a large vein and used to administer medications and sometimes draw blood specimens. A heparin lock is a special winged needle set or cannula that can be left in a patient's arm for up to 48 hours and used to administer med-

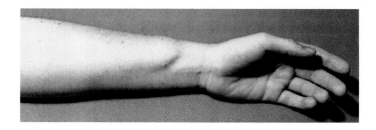

■ FIGURE 9-2 ■
Internal arteriovenous (AV) shunt (fistula).

ications and draw blood. An implanted port is a special device attached to an indwelling line that is surgically implanted under the skin.

54. a. When a blood specimen is collected from a heparin lock (see Fig. 9-3), a 5-mL discard tube must be drawn first to eliminate residual heparin used to flush the lock and keep it from clotting. The only extra tube collected is the clear tube. Drawing coagulation specimens from a heparin lock is not recommended.

55. c. A CVC (Fig. 9-4) is an indwelling line inserted into a main vein, such as the subclavian, and advanced into the vena cava. Broviac, Groshong, and Hickman are all types of CVCs. A heparin lock (Hep-lok) is a special winged needle set or cannula that is typically inserted

into a vein in the lower arm above the wrist area.

56. b. A subcutaneous vascular access device (SVAD), also called an implanted port (Fig. 9-5), is a small chamber that is attached to an indwelling line. The chamber is surgically implanted under the skin in the upper chest or arm. It is located by palpating the skin, and access is gained by inserting a special noncoring needle through the skin into the self-sealing septum (wall) of the chamber. (See explanation of question 55 for a description of a CVC.) A peripherally inserted central catheter (PICC) (Fig. 9-6) is inserted into the peripheral venous system (veins of the extremities) and threaded into the central venous system (main veins leading to the

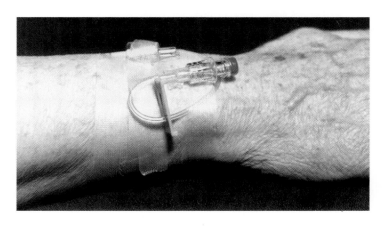

■ FIGURE 9-3 ■
Peripheral heparin lock with extension tubing added for accessibility.

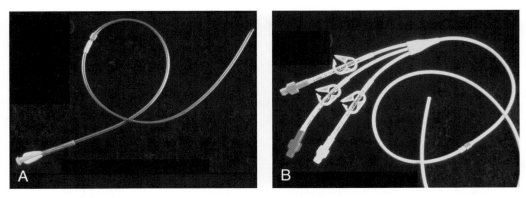

■ FIGURE 9-4 ■

Central venous catheters. **A.** Groshong. **B.** Hickman. (Courtesy Bard Access Systems, Inc., Salt Lake City, UT.)

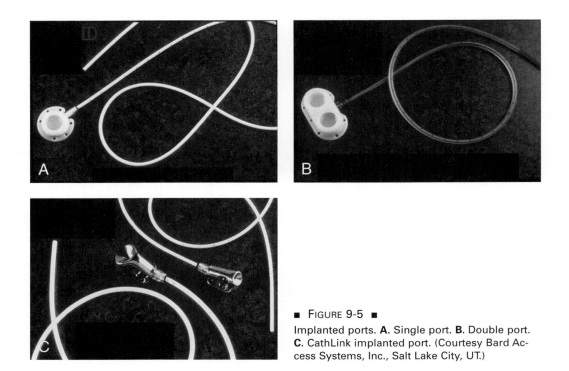

■ FIGURE 9-5 ■

Implanted ports. **A.** Single port. **B.** Double port. **C.** CathLink implanted port. (Courtesy Bard Access Systems, Inc., Salt Lake City, UT.)

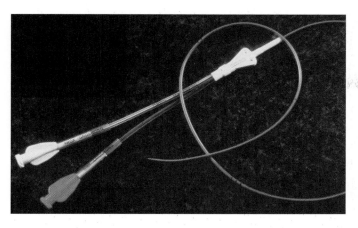

■ FIGURE 9-6 ■

Groshong peripherally inserted central catheter. (Courtesy Bard Access System, Inc., Salt Lake City, UT.)

heart). A saline lock is similar to a heparin lock, which is explained in the explanation of question 53.

57. d. Some patients are allergic to the glue used in adhesive bandages. Paper tape placed over a folded gauze square can usually be used instead. If the patient is also allergic to paper tape, the area can be wrapped with bandaging material such as Coban that sticks to itself, eliminating the need for tape. The patient may also be asked to hold pressure until bleeding stops in lieu of bandaging the site.

58. b. Increasing numbers of individuals are developing allergies to latex. Some allergies are so severe that being in the same room where latex materials are used can set off a life-threatening reaction. If a patient is known to have a severe allergy to latex, there may be a warning sign on the patient's door. It is important that no items made of latex be brought into the room. This means the phlebotomist must wear non-latex gloves, use a non-latex tourniquet, and use non-latex bandages when in the room, whether collect-

ing blood from the patient or the patient's roommate.

59. b. Notify the patient's nurse or physician if a patient continues to bleed after 5 minutes. Do not bandage a site until you are certain that bleeding has stopped. Never wrap a pressure bandage around a site in lieu of holding pressure.

60. b. A patient with a history of syncope (fainting) during blood collection should be asked to lie down during a blood draw.

61. b. If an outpatient feels faint during blood collection, discontinue the draw immediately and lower his or her head. Do not continue the draw or slap or shake the patient to revive him or her.

62. b. An outpatient who becomes weak and pale following a draw may faint and should be encouraged to lie down until he or she recovers. Offer the patient juice or crackers once he or she has recovered. The patient should not drive for at least 30 minutes.

63. d. A feeling of nausea often precedes vomiting, so it is a good idea to give the patient an emesis basin to hold as a precaution. Apply a cold, damp washcloth or other cold compress to the patient's forehead and ask him or her to breathe slowly and deeply.

64. c. Veins on obese patients may be deep and difficult to find. The cephalic vein is sometimes the easiest vein to palpate. To locate it, rotate the patient's arm so that the hand is prone. In this position, the weight of excess tissue often pulls downward, making the cephalic vein easy to feel and penetrate with a needle.

65. a. Petechiae (small, red, non-raised spots) appear with tourniquet application on some patients with platelet or capillary wall defects. They do not compromise test results and may not be avoidable because they will probably occur at any site that is chosen. Sites with massive scarring, edema, or veins that feel har and cord-like should be avoided.

66. a. Do not attempt to complete the draw on a patient who goes into convulsions during venipuncture. Discontinue the draw immediately and remove the needle as soon as possible. Try to prevent the patient from injuring himself or herself and notify the appropriate first aid personnel as soon as possible.

67. d. A hematoma caused by blood leaking into the tissues and identified by swelling at or near the venipuncture site is the most common complication of venipuncture. It is painful to the patient, results in unsightly bruising, and can cause compression injuries to nerves which lead to lawsuits. If a

hematoma starts to form during blood collection, immediately release the tourniquet, withdraw the needle, and hold pressure over the site for a minimum of 2 minutes.

68. c. Hematoma formation can be caused by a number of different errors in phlebotomy technique including failure to apply adequate pressure to the site after a blood draw, leakage of blood from a hole made by a needle that penetrated out the back of the vein during needle entry or the collection process, or leakage of blood from a vein because the needle is only partly inserted in the vein. A needle bevel that is centered in the lumen is right where it should be and would not be the cause of hematoma formation.

69. c. Blood pulsing or spurting into the tube is an indication that you may have accidentally hit an artery. A hematoma *may* start to form if you hit an artery, but there are a number of other reasons that hematomas form. Color is not a good way to identify arterial blood. Normal venous blood is typically dark red. Arterial blood in normal individuals is bright red, but it may look as dark as venous blood if the patient has a pulmonary problem.

70. b. Iatrogenic is an adjective used to describe an adverse condition brought on by the effects of treatment. Blood loss as a result of removal for testing purposes is called iatrogenic blood loss. Removal of blood on a regular basis or in large quantities can lead to anemia in some patients, especially infants.

71. d. An inadvertently collected arterial specimen can usually be submitted for testing, rather than redrawing the patient. However, the specimen should be labeled as arterial since some test values are different for arterial specimens. If you suspect that you have accidentally punctured an artery, you must hold pressure over the site for 3 to 5 minutes. Do not have the patient hold pressure or apply a pressure bandage in lieu of holding pressure.

72. c. Infection at the site following venipuncture is rare but not unheard of. Using proper aseptic technique including not touching the site after it has been cleaned, minimizing the time between removing the needle cap and venipuncture, not opening adhesive bandages ahead of time, and reminding the patient to keep the bandage on for at least 15 minutes after specimen collection should minimize the risk of infection.

73. c. Excessive or blind probing during venipuncture can injure nerves and may cause permanent damage. If initial needle insertion does not result in successful vein entry and proper redirection of the needle does not result in blood flow, the needle should be removed and venipuncture attempted at an alternate site, preferably the opposite arm.

74. b. Extreme or significant pain, numbness of the arm, and pain that radiates down the arm are signs of nerve involvement and all require immediate removal of the needle.

75. b. Performing venipuncture before the alcohol has dried completely is the most common cause of a stinging sensation to the patient and can also cause slight hemolysis of the specimen. Blood collection needles

are used only once and are not likely to be dull, but should be examined when first opened to detect defects that could cause pain or even injure the patient. Pushing down on the needle as it is inserted can be painful but does not normally produce a stinging sensation. A tourniquet that is tied too tightly is typically described as a pinching sensation.

76. d. Reflux is a term used to describe the backflow of blood from a collection tube into a patient's vein during venipuncture. It can occur if blood in the tube is in contact with the needle during venipuncture. Reflux of blood mixed with an additive such as EDTA can cause an adverse patient reaction. Keeping the arm in a downward position so that tubes fill from the bottom up and avoiding back and forth movement of contents of the tube during blood collection prevent blood from being in contact with the needle and therefore prevent reflux.

77. b. Leaving the tourniquet on for 2 minutes is not likely to impair vein patency or the state of being freely open. It may, however, lead to erroneous test results caused by hemoconcentration brought on by prolonged blockage of blood flow. Improperly redirecting the needle, probing for deep veins, and performing numerous venipunctures in the same area are all actions that can impair vein patency.

78. a. Prolonged tourniquet application causes stagnation of blood flow (venous stasis), which causes the plasma portion of the blood to filter into the tissues resulting in an increase in non-filterable blood com-

ponents or hemoconcentration. To minimize the effects of hemoconcentration, release the tourniquet within 1 minute of applying it and do not allow the patient to continuously make and release a fist.

79. **d.** Hemolysis is the destruction of red blood cells and the liberation of hemoglobin into the serum or plasma portion of the specimen, causing it to appear pink to reddish depending on the degree of hemolysis. The specimen is described as being hemolyzed.

80. **a.** Mixing tubes vigorously instead of gently inverting them, pulling blood into a syringe too quickly, and using a small-bore needle to collect blood into a large-volume tube can all result in hemolysis of the specimen. Blood collection systems are designed to collect multiple tubes of blood.

81. **c.** A prothrombin time is a coagulation test. The ratio of blood to anticoagulant is *most* critical for coagulation tests because a ratio of nine parts blood to one part anticoagulant must be maintained for accurate test results. The excess anticoagulant in a short draw dilutes the plasma portion of the specimen used for testing, causing erroneously prolonged test results.

82. **b.** There is no skin puncture container for collecting plasma specimens for coagulation tests because, except for those that can be performed with special point of care instruments, coagulation tests cannot be performed by skin puncture. Partially filled coagulation tubes are unacceptable for testing. Pouring two partially filled tubes together would still cause an improper ratio of blood to anticoag-

ulant and is also unacceptable. A phlebotomist should never make more than two attempts at venipuncture on a patient at one time. After the second attempt another phlebotomist should be asked to collect the specimen.

83. **a.** Cleaning a skin puncture site with isopropyl alcohol is accepted technique. Drawing a blood culture while the povidone-iodine is still damp can contaminate the specimen with povidone-iodine residue, which can inhibit growth of microorganisms and lead to false-negative results. Touching the filter paper while collecting a phenylketonuria (PKU) specimen can be a source of contamination that leads to erroneous results. Povidone-iodine should not be used to clean skin puncture sites because it interferes with "BURP" tests: bilirubin, uric acid, phosphorous, and potassium.

84. **a.** When the vacuum escapes from an evacuated tube during blood collection it sometimes makes a hissing sound. This can happen if the needle backs out of the skin slightly, allowing the tube to draw air instead of blood. If the needle penetrates all the way through a vein, the tube will not draw blood but the vacuum will be still intact because the bevel is under the skin. A drop in a patient's blood pressure would not cause a hissing sound. A tube with a crack in it would not draw blood or make a hissing sound because the vacuum would already be gone.

85. **d.** If you fail to get blood flow until you pull back on the needle, the needle most likely went too deep and through the back of the vein.

Being certain that the needle entered the vein but failing to get blood flow could also indicate that the needle has gone through the vein, and you will need to pull back on the needle. In addition, if you fill one tube but the second does not fill, it is possible that the needle pushed through the vein as you pushed the second tube onto the needle, and you will have to pull the needle back to get blood flow.

86. **d.** Veins are fairly tough. If a vein is not anchored well, it may roll (move away) slightly and the needle may slip beside the vein (Fig. 9-7) instead of penetrating it. A needle is supposed to end up in the lumen of the vein during venipuncture. The needle can end up against an inside wall of the vein if it enters it at an angle that is too shallow, if there is a bend in the vein, or if the bevel is down on entry.

87. **a.** If the needle is only partially inserted in the vein during blood collection (Fig. 9-8), the tube will fill very slowly and blood will leak into the tissue around the vein, causing a hematoma.

88. **c.** Although the first tube filled without a problem, the needle position could have changed slightly when

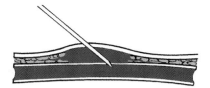

Needle partially inserted and causes blood leakage into tissue

■ FIGURE 9-8 ■

Partially inserted needle causes blood to leak into tissue.

the tube was removed and replaced. However, if this had been the case, blood flow would have been reestablished with slight manipulation of the needle. This suggests there could be a problem with the tube. Always try using a new tube before giving up on a blood draw. Further redirections of the needle would amount to probing and should not be done.

89. **c.** Multiple redirections of the needle while attempting venipuncture amount to probing, which is dangerous and should not be done, even if a second phlebotomist takes over for you. If you cannot obtain blood flow with one or two redirections of the needle, discontinue the draw and try again at a new site.

90. **d.** A vein may collapse (Fig. 9-9) if the tourniquet is applied too tightly or too close to the venipuncture site, or if the tube has too much vacuum for the size of the vein.

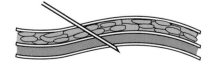

When a vein rolls, the needle may slip to the side of the vein without penetrating it

■ FIGURE 9-7 ■

Needle slipped beside the vein, not into it; caused when a vein rolls to the side.

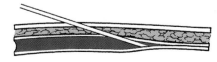

Collapsed

■ FIGURE 9-9 ■

Collapsed vein prevents blood flow.

10

SKIN PUNCTURE EQUIPMENT AND PROCEDURES

REVIEW QUESTIONS

Match the term with the BEST description.

1. _____ arterialized
2. _____ blood smear
3. _____ calcaneus
4. _____ capillary blood gases
5. _____ clay sealant
6. _____ cyanotic
7. _____ differential
8. _____ feather
9. _____ interstitial fluid
10. _____ intracellular fluid
11. _____ lancet
12. _____ microcollection containers
13. _____ microhematocrit tubes
14. _____ newborn screening
15. _____ osteochondritis
16. _____ osteomyelitis
17. _____ PKU
18. _____ plantar surface
19. _____ reference values
20. _____ whorls

a. heredity disease caused by inability to metabolize phenylalanine because of a defective enzyme
b. arterialized skin puncture blood gases
c. blood film made from a drop of blood on a glass slide
d. bottom or sole of the foot
e. determination of the number and characteristics of cells on a blood smear by staining and examining it under a microscope
f. disposable, narrow-bore, plastic-clad glass or plastic tubes used for manual packed cell volume determination
g. fluid found between cells or in spaces within an organ or tissue
h. fluid found within cell membranes
i. grooves of the fingerprint
j. heel bone
k. increased arterial composition due to warming the collection site
l. inflammation of bone and cartilage
m. inflammation of bone, especially the marrow, caused by bacterial infection
n. normal values for lab tests, usually established using basal state specimens
o. performing tests on neonates to check for genetic or inherited diseases
p. small plastic tubes with color-coded bodies or stoppers corresponding to evacuated tubes that are used to collect drops of skin puncture blood
q. sterile, disposable, sharp-pointed instrument used to pierce the skin to obtain droplets of blood for testing
r. substance used to plug one end of a microhematocrit tube
s. pertaining to blue-gray discoloration of skin due to lack of oxygen
t. thinnest area of a blood smear where a differential is performed

Choose the BEST answer.

21. All of the following are desirable charac-
    teristics of skin puncture lancets
    EXCEPT:
    a. controlled puncture depth
    b. permanently retractable blade
    c. reusable
    d. sterile

22. Which of the following equipment is
    used to perform a manual packed cell
    volume test?
    a. magnet
    b. microhematocrit tube
    c. micropipette dilution device
    d. stirring device

23. Which of the following equipment may
    be required to collect capillary blood
    gases?
    a. magnet
    b. metal "fleas"
    c. special capillary tube
    d. all of the above

24. An example of a microcollection con-
    tainer that contains a fluid for direct di-
    lution of the specimen is a:
    a. capillary tube.
    b. microhematocrit tube.
    c. Microtainer.
    d. Unopette.

25. Which of the following statements most
    accurately describes skin puncture
    blood?
    a. a mixture of venous, arterial, and
       capillary blood
    b. mostly tissue fluid mixed with arter-
       ial blood
    c. mostly venous blood and tissue fluid
    d. nearly identical to venous blood

26. The composition of skin puncture blood
    more closely resembles:
    a. arterial blood.
    b. lymph fluid.
    c. tissue fluid.
    d. venous blood.

27. If venous blood is placed in skin punc-
    ture collection devices, it is important to:
    a. label it as venous blood.
    b. mix the specimen vigorously.
    c. transport it to the laboratory ASAP.
    d. all of the above

28. Why should a laboratory report form in-
    dicate the fact that a specimen has been
    collected by skin puncture?
    a. for liability and insurance purposes
    b. some test results may vary depending
       on the source of the specimen
    c. so that subsequent specimens will be
       collected by skin puncture also
    d. so that the patient's nurse can check
       the site for signs of infection

29. Skin puncture blood is sometimes called
    capillary blood because:
    a. collection containers fill by capillary
       action
    b. it is collected in capillary tubes
    c. it is obtained from the capillary bed
    d. tiny amounts of blood are collected

30. Skin puncture blood is the preferred
    specimen for this test.
    a. bilirubin
    b. glucose
    c. phenylketonuria
    d. all of the above

31. Reference values for skin puncture
    blood are higher for:
    a. calcium.
    b. glucose.
    c. phosphorous.
    d. total protein.

32. You need to collect blood cultures, a
    gray top, and a lavender top on an adult
    with difficult veins. Which specimens
    can be collected by skin puncture?
    a. all of them
    b. blood cultures and gray top only
    c. gray top and lavender top only
    d. none of them

33. Which skin puncture specimen is typically collected in an amber microcollection container (Fig. 10-1)?
   a. bilirubin
   b. glucose
   c. phenylketonuria (PKU)
   d. thyroxine (T_4)

34. A skin puncture can be done rather
than a venipuncture in all of the following situations EXCEPT when:
   a. a child is younger than 2 years old.
   b. a light blue top is ordered.
   c. an adult has difficult veins.
   d. veins need to be saved for
      chemotherapy.

35. It is not a good idea to perform skin
puncture if the patient is/has:
   a. dehydrated.
   b. in shock.
   c. poor circulation.
   d. all of the above

36. Which of the following is a proper site
for finger puncture on an adult?
   a. distal segment of the middle or ring
      finger
   b. end segment of the thumb

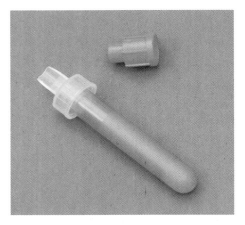

■ FIGURE 10-1 ■

Amber-colored microcollection container used to protect a bilirubin specimen from effects of ultraviolet
light.

   c. medial segment of the right index
      finger
   d. proximal phalanx of the middle or
      ring finger

37. Skin puncture is the preferred method
to obtain blood from infants and children because:
   a. they can be injured by restraining
      methods used during venipuncture.
   b. they have small blood volumes.
   c. venipuncture may damage veins and
      surrounding tissue.
   d. all of the above

38. Which of the following sites would normally be eliminated as a skin puncture
site?
   a. an edematous extremity
   b. a site below an IV
   c. the lateral plantar surface of a baby's
      heel
   d. the middle or ring finger of a warm,
      adult hand

39. It is necessary to control the depth of
lancet insertion during skin puncture to
avoid:
   a. bacterial contamination.
   b. bone injury.
   c. excessive bleeding.
   d. puncturing an artery.

40. The maximum depth of heel puncture
recommended by the (National Committee for Clinical Laboratory Standards)
NCCLS is:
   a. 1.5 mm.
   b. 2.0 mm.
   c. 2.4 mm.
   d. 4.9 mm.

41. Which of the following can be a complication resulting from deep skin punctures of an infant's heel?
   a. anemia
   b. hepatitis
   c. osteochondritis
   d. phenylketonuria

42. Which of the following is a safe area for infant heel puncture?
 a. area of the arch
 b. central area
 c. lateral plantar surface
 d. posterior curvature

43. A recommended site for skin puncture on children 2 years of age or older is the:
 a. bottom of the ear lobe.
 b. fleshy side of the thumb.
 c. palmar fleshy portion of the middle finger.
 d. plantar medial or lateral surface of the heel.

44. In which of the following areas does skin puncture differ from routine venipuncture?
 a. antiseptic used
 b. patient identification
 c. stopper color of collection tubes
 d. none of the above

45. The distance between the skin surface and the bone in the end segment of a finger is:
 a. less at the side and tip than the center.
 b. the same throughout the fingertip.
 c. thickest in the fifth finger.
 d. thinnest in the middle finger.

46. The major blood vessels of the skin are located in/at the:
 a. dermal-subcutaneous junction.
 b. epidermis and dermis.
 c. lower epidermis.
 d. subcutaneous only.

47. A skin puncture that parallels the whorls of the fingerprint will:
 a. allow the blood to run down the finger.
 b. cause the blood to form a round drop.
 c. clot faster.
 d. continue to bleed longer.

48. Skin puncture equipment includes all of the following EXCEPT:
 a. evacuated tube
 b. lancet
 c. microcollection tube
 d. microhematocrit tube

49. Which color-coded microcollection container would be used to collect a complete blood count?
 a. gray
 b. green
 c. lavender
 d. red

50. If the following tests are to be collected during a multisample skin puncture, which test specimen is collected first?
 a. bilirubin
 b. complete blood count
 c. electrolytes
 d. glucose

51. What is the purpose of warming the site before skin puncture?
 a. increasing blood flow up to 7 times
 b. making the veins more visible
 c. preventing hemolysis of the sample
 d. comforting the patient

52. This test requires warming of the heel before specimen collection for accurate test results.
 a. bilirubin
 b. blood gases
 c. electrolytes
 d. phenylketonuria (PKU)

53. The typical antiseptic used to clean a skin puncture site is:
 a. 70% isopropanol.
 b. povidone-iodine.
 c. soap and water.
 d. any of the above

54. The antiseptic must be completely dried before performing skin puncture to avoid:
 a. hematoma formation.
 b. hemoconcentration.

c. hemolysis.

d. hemostasis.

55. Povidone-iodine contamination of a skin puncture specimen affects:

a. bilirubin.

b. potassium.

c. uric acid.

d. all of the above

56. Errors in glucose results have been attributed to:

a. blood collected from punctures that are too deep.

b. failure to collect the first drop of blood.

c. isopropyl alcohol contamination of the specimen.

d. warming the site before skin puncture.

57. The purpose of wiping away the first drop of blood during skin puncture (Fig. 10-2) is to:

a. avoid bacterial contamination.

b. eliminate tissue fluid contamination.

c. improve blood flow

d. minimize effects of platelet aggregation.

58. Contamination of a skin puncture specimen with residual alcohol can erroneously elevate results for this test.

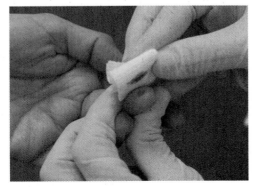

■ FIGURE 10-2 ■

Wiping the first drop with gauze.

a. blood urea nitrogen (BUN)

b. capillary blood gases (CBGs)

c. hemoglobin

d. potassium

59. Proper finger puncture technique includes all of the following EXCEPT:

a. avoid squeezing or vigorous massaging of the finger.

b. puncture parallel to the whorls of the fingerprint.

c. puncture the middle or ring finger.

d. wipe away the first drop of blood.

60. It is inappropriate to apply a bandage to a skin puncture site on an infant younger than 2 years of age because:

a. an adhesive bandage can irritate an infant's tender skin.

b. the bandage can come off and present a chocking hazard.

c. the bandage can tear the skin when removed.

d. all of the above

61. Proper technique for filling microcollection tubes includes all of the following EXCEPT:

a. touching the scoop of the collection tube to the blood drop

b. tapping the tube gently to encourage blood to settle to the bottom

c. scooping up blood that runs down the finger

d. none of the above

62. Which of the following activities can introduce tissue fluid into a skin puncture specimen?

a. milking and massaging

b. squeezing

c. applying strong repetitive pressure

d. all the above

63. During multisample skin puncture collections, blood smears and EDTA specimens are obtained before other specimens to:

a. avoid hemoconcentration.

b. minimize the effects of platelet clumping.

c. minimize tissue fluid contamination.
d. reduce effects of hemolysis.

64. A blood smear is required for this test.
 a. glucose
 b. hemoglobin
 c. manual differential
 d. neonatal bilirubin

65. An acceptable blood smear:
 a. covers the entire surface of the slide.
 b. forms a bullet shape.
 c. has a feathered uniform edge.
 d. is short and thick.

66. A blood smear prepared from an EDTA specimen should be made:
 a. after the blood has settled in the tube.
 b. anytime after specimen collection.
 c. before the specimen is thoroughly mixed.
 d. within 1 hour of collection.

67. When making a blood smear by hand using two glass slides, the typical angle required of the spreader slide is:
 a. 15°.
 b. 20°.
 c. 30°.
 d. 45°.

68. If the phlebotomist makes a blood smear that is too short, he or she should try again and:
 a. exert more pressure with the spreader slide.
 b. decrease the angle of the spreader slide.
 c. increase the angle of the spreader slide.
 d. use a smaller drop of blood.

69. Holes in a blood smear can be caused by:
 a. dirt on the slide.
 b. fingerprints on the slide.
 c. lipids in the blood.
 d. all of the above

70. Collection of a thick blood smear may be requested to detect:
 a. hypothyroidism.
 b. malaria.
 c. phenylketonuria.
 d. all of the above

71. Iron fillings used in capillary blood gas collection:
 a. aid in mixing the anticoagulant.
 b. keep the blood from sticking to the sides of the tube.
 c. prevent air bubble formation.
 d. react with oxygen to stabilize the specimen.

72. All of the following statements are true of capillary blood gases EXCEPT that they:
 a. are less dangerous to perform on infants than arterial blood gases (ABGs).
 b. are more desirable than ABGs.
 c. contain both venous and arterial blood.
 d. employ an open collection system.

73. An infant may require a blood transfusion if blood levels of this substance exceed 18 mg/dL.
 a. bilirubin
 b. glucose
 c. phenylalanine
 d. all of the above

74. Phenylketonuria (PKU) is a(n):
 a. acquired condition caused by too much phenylalanine.
 b. contagious condition caused by lack of phenylalanine.
 c. hereditary inability to metabolize phenylalanine.
 d. temporary condition caused by lack of thyroid hormone.

75. Which of the following is a newborn screening test?
 a. bilirubin
 b. hemoglobin

c. phenylketonuria (PKU)
d. white blood count (WBC)

76. Falsely decreased bilirubin results can be caused by:
   a. specimen collection that was too slow.
   b. hemolysis of the specimen.
   c. failure to protect the specimen from light.
   d. all of the above

77. Contamination of a phenylketonuria (PKU) test can result from:
   a. failure to discard the first drop of blood.
   b. gloves or hands touching the blood spot circles.
   c. stacking specimen slips together after collection.
   d. all of the above

78. Erroneous newborn screening results can be caused by:
   a. applying blood drops to both sides of the filter paper.
   b. hanging specimen slips to dry.
   c. layering successive drops in the same collection circle.
   d. all of the above

79. Neonatal blood screening for this disorder is required by law in the United States.
   a. diabetes
   b. hemolytic disease of the newborn (HDN)
   c. hepatitis B
   d. phenylketonuria (PKU)

80. Jaundice in a newborn is associated with high levels of:
   a. bilirubin.
   b. glucose.
   c. phenylketonuria (PKU).
   d. thyroid hormone.

Chapter 10 / Skin Puncture Equipment and Procedures

ANSWERS AND EXPLANATIONS

1. **k.** increased arterial composition due to warming the site

2. **c.** blood film made from a drop of blood on a glass slide

3. **j.** heel bone

4. **b.** arterialized skin puncture blood gases

5. **r.** substance used to plug one end of a microhematocrit tube

6. **s.** pertaining to blue-gray discoloration of the skin due to lack of oxygen

7. **e.** determination of the number and characteristics of cells on a blood smear by staining and examining it under a microscope

8. **t.** thinnest area of a blood smear where a differential is performed

9. **g.** fluid found between cells or in spaces within an organ or tissue

10. **h.** fluid found within cell membranes

11. **q.** sterile, disposable, sharp-pointed instrument used to pierce the skin to obtain droplets of blood for testing

12. **p.** small plastic tubes with color-coded bodies or stoppers corresponding to evacuated tubes, which are used to collect drops of skin puncture blood

13. **f.** disposable, narrow-bore, plastic-clad glass or plastic tubes used for manual packed cell volume determinations

14. **o.** performing tests on neonates to check for genetic or inherited diseases

15. **l.** inflammation of bone and cartilage

16. **m.** inflammation of bone, especially the marrow, caused by bacterial infection

17. **a.** phenylketonuria, heredity disease caused by inability to metabolize phenylalanine because of a defective enzyme

18. **d.** bottom or sole of the foot

19. **n.** normal values for lab tests, usually established using basal state specimens

20. **i.** grooves of the fingerprint

21. **c.** Skin puncture lancets should be sterile, disposable, and have a controlled puncture depth and a retractable blade for safety. They should not be reusable.

22. **b.** A plastic or plastic-clad glass microhematocrit tube is used to collect and perform a manual hematocrit (packed cell volume) test (Fig. 10-3).

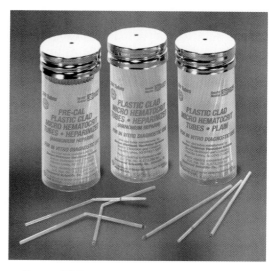

■ FIGURE 10-3 ■

Microhematocrit tubes. (Courtesy Becton Dickinson, Franklin Lakes, NJ.)

23. **d.** Capillary blood gas equipment (Fig. 10-4) typically includes a special capillary tube, magnet, and iron fillings (referred to as fleas) or metal bar to aid in mixing the specimen. In addition, a warming device is needed to warm the site and arterialize the specimen.

24. **d.** The Becton Dickinson Unopette is an example of a micropipet dilution system. The system consists of a sealed plastic reservoir that contains a premeasured amount of diluting fluid; a detachable glass, self-filling capillary pipet; and a pipet shield, which also serves as a device to puncture the reservoir covering or diaphragm before adding the sample.

25. **a.** Skin puncture blood is a mixture of arterial blood (from arterioles), venous blood (from venules), and capillary blood, along with interstitial and intracellular fluids from the surrounding tissues.

26. **a.** Skin puncture blood contains a higher proportion of arterial blood than venous blood because arterial blood enters the capillaries under pressure. The composition of skin puncture blood, therefore, more closely resembles arterial blood than venous blood. This is especially true if the area has been warmed, because warming increases arterial flow into the area.

27. **a.** Sometimes venous blood obtained by syringe during difficult draw situations is put into microcollection containers. When this is done it is important to label the specimen as venous. Otherwise, it will be assumed to be a skin puncture specimen, which may have different normal values.

28. **b.** Test results vary depending on the source of the specimen. A laboratory report form should indicate the fact that a specimen was collected by skin puncture, because skin puncture blood differs in composition from venous blood and may have different reference ranges for some tests.

29. **a.** Skin puncture blood contains a mixture of arterial blood and venous blood with small amounts of tissue fluids. It contains a higher proportion of arterial blood than venous blood, because arterial blood enters the capillaries under pressure.

30. **c.** Skin puncture blood is the preferred specimen for newborn screening tests for phenylketonuria (PKU) and several other inherited diseases. These tests were designed to be performed on skin puncture specimens.

31. **b.** Reference values for glucose are higher in skin puncture specimens.

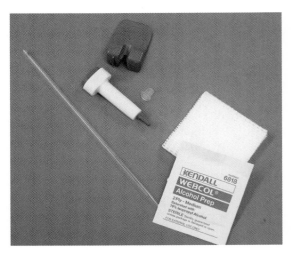

■ FIGURE 10-4 ■

Capillary blood gas collection equipment.

They are lower for calcium, phosphorous, and total protein.

32. c. Blood cultures cannot be collected by skin puncture because of the volume of blood required for testing and skin contamination issues. There are gray top and lavender top microcollection containers available.

33. a. Infant bilirubin specimens are collected in amber microcollection containers (see Fig. 10-1) to help protect them from light. Light breaks down bilirubin and leads to false low values.

34. b. Specimens cannot be collected by skin puncture for coagulation testing later in the laboratory; consequently, there is no microcollection container that corresponds to a light blue top tube. There are, however, some point-of-care testing instruments that directly perform coagulation tests from a drop of blood obtained by skin puncture that is immediately placed in the instrument and tested.

35. d. Skin puncture is generally *not* appropriate for patients who are dehydrated or have poor circulation to the extremities from other causes, such as shock, as specimens may be hard to obtain and may not be representative of blood elsewhere in the body.

36. a. The palmar surface of the distal or end segment of the middle or ring finger (Fig. 10-5) is the recommended site for routine skin puncture on an adult.

37. d. Skin puncture is the preferred method to obtain blood from infants and children for a number of reasons. Restraining methods used during venipuncture can injure them. They have such small blood volumes that removing larger quantities of blood typical of venipuncture can lead to anemia. Removal

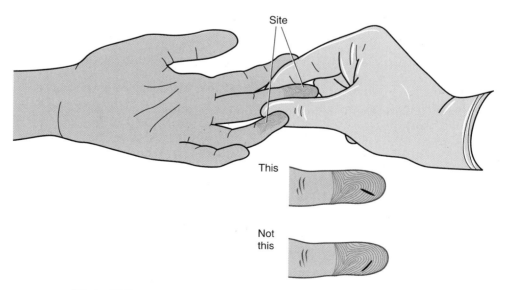

■ FIGURE 10-5 ■

Recommended site and direction of finger puncture.

of more than 10% of an infant's blood volume at one time can lead to cardiac arrest. In addition, venipuncture in infants and children is difficult and may damage veins and surrounding tissues.

38. a. Skin puncture should not be performed on an edematous extremity. Like venipuncture, a skin puncture can be performed below an IV. The lateral plantar surface of a baby's heel and the middle or ring finger of a warm, adult hand are recommended skin puncture sites.

39. b. The depth of lancet insertion must be controlled to avoid injuring the bone.

40. b. Studies have shown that heel punctures deeper than 2.0 mm risk injuring the calcaneus or heel bone. For this reason, the latest NCCLS skin puncture standards document (H4-A4) states that heel puncture depth should not exceed 2.0 mm. In the previous document the maximum depth of puncture was 2.4 mm.

41. c. Deep skin punctures of an infant's heel can penetrate the calcaneus (heel bone) leading to painful osteochondritis (inflammation of the bone and cartilage) or osteomyelitis (inflammation of the bone including the marrow) caused by bacterial infection.

42. c. According to the National Committee for Clinical Laboratory Standards (NCCLS) skin puncture standard H4-A4, the safest areas for performing heel puncture are on the plantar surface of the heel, medial to an imaginary line extending from the middle of the great (big) toe to the heel or lateral to an imaginary line extending from between the fourth and fifth toes to the heel (Fig. 10-6).

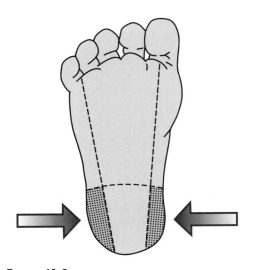

■ FIGURE 10-6 ■

Infant heel. Shaded areas indicated by arrows represent recommended safe areas for heel puncture.

In other words, safe areas are on the medial or lateral plantar surface of the heel. Punctures should not be performed in the area of the arch, the central portion of the heel, or the posterior curvature of the heel as bone, nerves, tendons, and cartilage could be injured.

43. c. The recommended site for skin puncture on older children and adults (see Fig. 10-6) is the fleshy portion of the palmar surface of the distal or end segment of the middle or ring finger.

44. d. The same antiseptic, isopropyl alcohol (isopropanol or ETOH), is used for routine skin puncture and venipuncture. Patient identification is the same regardless of the method of specimen collection. Stopper color of microcollection tubes corresponds to that of evacuated tubes.

45. a. The distance between the skin surface and the bone in the end segment of the finger varies. It is less

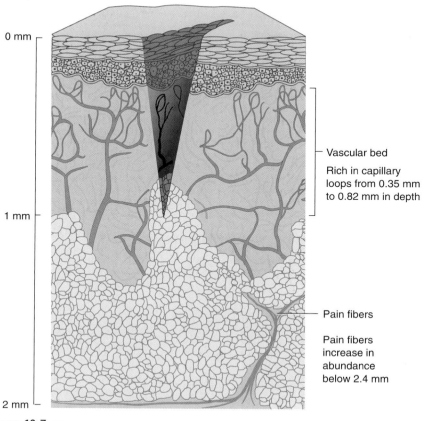

0 mm

1 mm

2 mm

Vascular bed

Rich in capillary
loops from 0.35 mm
to 0.82 mm in depth

Pain fibers

Pain fibers
increase in
abundance
below 2.4 mm

■ FIGURE 10-7 ■
Cross-section of full-term infant's heel showing lancet penetration depth needed to access the
capillary bed.

at the side and tip of the finger than
at the center. It is thinnest in the
fifth or little finger.

46. **a.** The major blood vessels of the skin
are located at the dermal-subcutaneous junction, which in a newborn's heel is located between 0.35
and 1.6 mm below the surface of
the skin (Fig. 10-7).

47. **a.** If a skin puncture is made parallel
to the whorls of the fingerprint (see
Fig. 10-6), blood will run down the
grooves of the fingerprint rather
than form round drops that are
easy to collect.

48. **a.** Evacuated tubes are used for
venipuncture and syringe collections, not skin puncture.

49. **c.** A lavender color-coded microcollection container is used to collect a
complete blood count.

50. **b.** A complete blood count is a hematology specimen. When collected by
skin puncture, slides, platelet
counts, and other hematology specimens are collected first to avoid the
effects of platelet aggregation
(clumping). Other anticoagulant
containers are collected next, and
serum specimens are collected last.

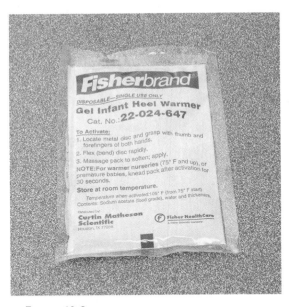

■ FIGURE 10-8 ■
Infant heel warmer.

51. **a.** Warming the site before skin puncture increases blood flow up to 7 times. Because warming increases arterial blood flow, it is said to *arterialize* the specimen. Making the veins more visible is not necessary for skin puncture. Hemolysis occurs primarily from squeezing the site, puncturing before the alcohol is dry, or using the first drop of blood rather than wiping it away and can still occur under these circumstances regardless of whether the site was warmed.

52. **b.** One of the steps in collection of capillary blood gases is to *arterialize* the specimen by warming the site for 5 to 10 minutes to increase arterial blood flow. This increases arterial content of the specimen and makes it more similar to arterial blood. Special warming devices are available (Fig. 10-8).

53. **a.** A skin puncture site is typically cleaned using 70% isopropyl alcohol (isopropanol or ETOH).

54. **c.** The typical antiseptic used to clean a skin puncture site is isopropyl alcohol. If not completely dried before skin puncture, the alcohol can cause hemolysis of the specimen and lead to erroneous test results.

55. **d.** Povidone-iodine contamination of skin puncture blood affects the results of "BURP" tests: bilirubin, uric acid, phosphorous, and potassium.

56. **c.** Errors in glucose results have been attributed to isopropyl alcohol contamination of the specimen. Deep punctures can injure bone but do not affect test results. The first drop of blood should be wiped away to eliminate alcohol residue and tissue fluid contamination. Errors in glucose results have not been attributed to warming the site.

57. **b.** Always wipe away the first drop of skin puncture (see Fig. 10-2) because excess tissue fluid usually contained in the first drop can affect test results. Omitting the first drop from the sample also eliminates alcohol residue that could hemolyze the specimen and also keep the blood from forming a well-rounded drop.

58. **d.** Blood cells contain potassium. Residual alcohol can hemolyze blood cells, releasing potassium and erroneously elevating potassium results.

59. **b.** Skin puncture should be made perpendicular to the whorls or grooves of the fingerprint (see Fig. 10-6) so

that the blood forms round drops (Fig. 10-9) that can be easily collected. A puncture parallel to the whorls will allow the blood to run down the finger and make collection difficult.

60. **d.** Adhesive bandage should not be used on infants younger than 2 years of age. Adhesive bandages can irritate the tender skin of infants, come off and become a chocking hazard, or tear the skin when removed.

61. **c.** Scooping up blood as it runs down the finger should be avoided because it introduces contaminates, activates platelets, and may cause hemolysis.

62. **d.** Milking and massaging, squeezing, and applying strong repetitive pressure can all introduce excess tissue fluid into the specimen and affect test results. They can also cause hemolysis.

63. **b.** Blood smears and EDTA specimens are obtained before other specimens to minimize the effects of platelet aggregation (clumping). When tissue is disrupted by skin puncture,

the coagulation process is set in motion and platelets start to aggregate (stick or clump together) and adhere to the site to seal off the injury. This can lead to erroneously low platelet counts. Platelets are evaluated and their numbers estimated as part of a differential performed on a blood smear. A platelet count is part of a complete blood count performed on an EDTA specimen.

64. **c.** A manual differential is performed on a stained blood smear. Glucose testing is performed on serum, plasma, or whole blood. Hemoglobin requires a whole blood specimen. Neonatal bilirubin is typically performed on serum.

65. **c.** An acceptable smear (Fig. 10-10) will cover about one half to three fourths of the surface of the slide and have the appearance of a feather, in that there will be a smooth gradient from thick to thin when held up to the light. The thinnest area of a properly made smear, often referred to as the "feather," is one cell thick and is the

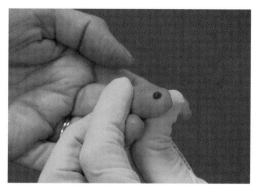

■ FIGURE 10-9 ■
Round blood drop forming at the puncture site.

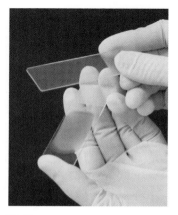

■ FIGURE 10-10 ■
Completed blood smear.

most important area because that is where a differential is performed.

66. d. A blood smear prepared from an EDTA specimen should be made within 1 hour of collection to prevent cell distortion caused by prolonged contact with the anticoagulant.

67. c. When a blood smear is prepared using the two-slide method, one slide holds the drop used to make the smear and a second slide, placed on the first slide at an angle of approximately 30° (Fig. 10-11), spreads the drop of blood across the slide to create the blood film.

68. b. Blood smears that are too long or too short are not acceptable. The length of a blood smear can be controlled by adjusting the angle of the spreader slide or the size of the drop of blood. If a smear is too short, decreasing the angle of the spreader slide or using a larger drop of blood on the next attempt should result in a longer smear. Exerting more pressure will only distort the smear. Increasing the angle of the spreader

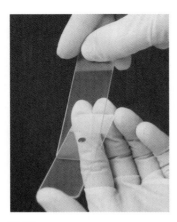

■ FIGURE 10-11 ■
Drop of blood on slide with pusher slide placed in front.

slide or using a smaller drop will make an even shorter slide.

69. d. Dirt or fingerprints on the slide and fat globules or lipids in the specimen can result in holes in a blood smear.

70. b. Malaria is diagnosed by detecting the presence of the organism that causes it in a peripheral blood smear. Diagnosis often requires the evaluation of both regular and thick blood smears. Presence of the organism is observed most frequently in a thick smear; however, identification of the species requires evaluation of a regular blood smear.

71. a. Capillary blood gases are commonly collected in a heparinized capillary tube. After the specimen is collected, one end of the tube is quickly sealed and iron filings, often called "fleas," or a metal bar are inserted into the specimen. The other end of the tube is quickly sealed to prevent exposure to air, and the specimen is mixed by running a magnet along the outside of the tube. The magnet drags the fleas or metal bar back and forth, mixing the specimen with the heparin to prevent clotting.

72. b. Skin puncture blood is less desirable for blood gas analysis because of its partial arterial composition and because the open system of collection temporarily exposes it to air, which can alter test results.

73. a. Bilirubin can cross the blood–brain barrier in infants, accumulating to toxic levels that can cause permanent brain damage or even death. A transfusion may be needed if levels increase at a rate equal to or greater than 5 mg/dL per hour or when levels exceed 18 mg/dL.

74. **c.** Phenylketonuria (PKU) is a hereditary disorder caused by an inability to metabolize the amino acid phenylalanine. Patient's with PKU lack the enzyme necessary to convert phenylalanine to tyrosine. Phenylalanine accumulates in the blood and can rise to toxic levels. PKU cannot be cured but it can normally be treated with a diet low in phenylalanine. If left untreated or not treated early, PKU can lead to brain damage and mental retardation.

75. **c.** Newborn screening is the term used to describe testing of newborns for the presence of genetic, or inherited, diseases such as phenylketonuria (PKU), hypothyroidism, galactosemia, homocystinuria, maple syrup urine disease, and sickle cell disease.

76. **d.** Bilirubin is broken down in the presence of light. Collecting the specimen too slowly or failing to protect the specimen from light after collection allows the specimen to be exposed to light for longer than necessary and leads to falsely decreased results. Hemolysis also falsely decreases bilirubin results.

77. **d.** PKU specimens are collected by placing large drops of blood within circles on special filter paper that is part of the test requisition (Fig. 10-12). Using the first drop of blood can contaminate an entire blood spot with tissue fluid and lead to erroneous results. The blood spots can also be contaminated by hands or gloves that touch the spots before or after specimen collection. Stacking specimen slips together after collection can lead to cross-contamination between several different patient specimens.

78. **d.** Newborn screening blood spots must be collected properly to prevent erroneous results. Applying blood to both sides of the filter paper or layering successive drops in the same circle increase the amount of blood in the test area and can lead to erroneously increased results. Hanging specimens to dry can cause the blood to migrate and concentrate toward the lower end of the filter paper. This leaves the upper areas of the circle with less blood and the lower areas with more blood than required for testing. In this case, the results will be erroneous on any area that is used for testing.

79. **d.** Newborn screening to detect PKU and hypothyroidism are required by law in the United States.

80. **a.** High levels of bilirubin in the blood result in jaundice, a condition characterized by yellow color of the skin, whites of the eyes, mucous membranes, and body fluids.

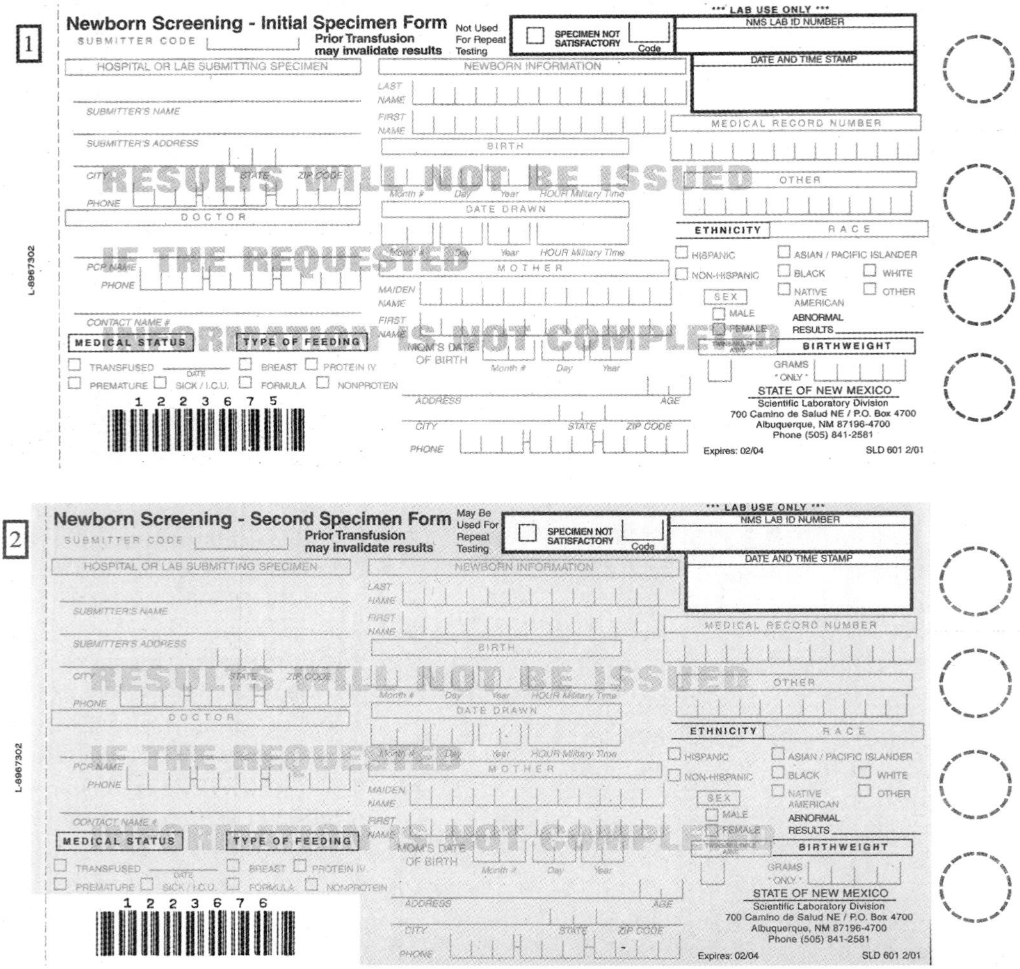
1

L-6967302

Newborn Screening - Initial Specimen Form

SUBMITTER CODE

Prior Transfusion may invalidate results

Not Used For Repeat Testing

*** LAB USE ONLY ***

SPECIMEN NOT SATISFACTORY Code

NMS LAB ID NUMBER

DATE AND TIME STAMP

HOSPITAL OR LAB SUBMITTING SPECIMEN

SUBMITTER'S NAME

SUBMITTER'S ADDRESS

CITY STATE ZIP CODE

PHONE

DOCTOR

PCP NAME

PHONE

CONTACT NAME #

NEWBORN INFORMATION

LAST NAME

FIRST NAME

BIRTH

Month # Day Year HOUR Military Time

DATE DRAWN

Month # Day Year HOUR Military Time

MOTHER

MAIDEN NAME

FIRST NAME

MOM'S DATE OF BIRTH Month # Day Year

ADDRESS AGE

CITY STATE ZIP CODE

PHONE

MEDICAL RECORD NUMBER

OTHER

ETHNICITY RACE

HISPANIC

NON-HISPANIC

ASIAN / PACIFIC ISLANDER

BLACK

WHITE

NATIVE AMERICAN

OTHER

SEX

MALE

FEMALE

ABNORMAL RESULTS

TWINS/MULTIPLE ABC

BIRTHWEIGHT

GRAMS * ONLY *

MEDICAL STATUS

TRANSFUSED DATE

PREMATURE

SICK / I.C.U.

TYPE OF FEEDING

BREAST

PROTEIN IV

FORMULA

NONPROTEIN

1 2 2 3 6 7 5

STATE OF NEW MEXICO

Scientific Laboratory Division

700 Camino de Salud NE / P.O. Box 4700

Albuquerque, NM 87196-4700

Phone (505) 841-2581

Expires: 02/04

SLD 601 2/01

RESULTS WILL NOT BE ISSUED IF THE REQUESTED INFORMATION IS NOT COMPLETED

2

L-6967302

Newborn Screening - Second Specimen Form

SUBMITTER CODE

Prior Transfusion may invalidate results

May Be Used For Repeat Testing

*** LAB USE ONLY ***

SPECIMEN NOT SATISFACTORY Code

NMS LAB ID NUMBER

DATE AND TIME STAMP

HOSPITAL OR LAB SUBMITTING SPECIMEN

SUBMITTER'S NAME

SUBMITTER'S ADDRESS

CITY STATE ZIP CODE

PHONE

DOCTOR

PCP NAME

PHONE

CONTACT NAME #

NEWBORN INFORMATION

LAST NAME

FIRST NAME

BIRTH

Month # Day Year HOUR Military Time

DATE DRAWN

Month # Day Year HOUR Military Time

MOTHER

MAIDEN NAME

FIRST NAME

MOM'S DATE OF BIRTH Month # Day Year

ADDRESS AGE

CITY STATE ZIP CODE

PHONE

MEDICAL RECORD NUMBER

OTHER

ETHNICITY RACE

HISPANIC

NON-HISPANIC

ASIAN / PACIFIC ISLANDER

BLACK

WHITE

NATIVE AMERICAN

OTHER

SEX

MALE

FEMALE

ABNORMAL RESULTS

TWINS/MULTIPLE ABC

BIRTHWEIGHT

GRAMS * ONLY *

MEDICAL STATUS

TRANSFUSED DATE

PREMATURE

SICK / I.C.U.

TYPE OF FEEDING

BREAST

PROTEIN IV

FORMULA

NONPROTEIN

1 2 2 3 6 7 6

STATE OF NEW MEXICO

Scientific Laboratory Division

700 Camino de Salud NE / P.O. Box 4700

Albuquerque, NM 87196-4700

Phone (505) 841-2581

Expires: 02/04

SLD 601 2/01

RESULTS WILL NOT BE ISSUED IF THE REQUESTED INFORMATION IS NOT COMPLETED

■ FIGURE 10-12 ■

Newborn screening specimen forms. **A.** Initial specimen form. **B.** Second specimen form. (Courtesy Daniel Gray, State of New Mexico Scientific Laboratory, Albuquerque, NM.)

11

SPECIAL COLLECTIONS AND POINT-OF-CARE TESTING

REVIEW QUESTIONS

Match the term with the BEST description.

1. ____ ACT
2. ____ aerobic
3. ____ agglutination
4. ____ analyte
5. ____ antimicrobial therapy
6. ____ autologous
7. ____ bacteremia
8. ____ BT
9. ____ chain of custody
10. ____ compatibility
11. ____ ex vivo
12. ____ FUO
13. ____ GTT
14. ____ HMT
15. ____ lookback
16. ____ peak level
17. ____ POCT
18. ____ PP
19. ____ septicemia
20. ____ TDM
21. ____ trough level
22. ____ WBG

a. after a meal
b. bacteria in the blood
c. bedside testing
d. clumping, as in clumping of red blood cells in a transfusion reaction
e. detects carbohydrate metabolism problems
f. fever for which the cause is unknown
g. glucose measured in whole blood
h. high-dose heparin monitoring test
i. highest serum concentration of a drug
j. lowest serum concentration of a drug
k. outside the body
l. pathogenic bacteria in the blood
m. procedure used to manage individual patient drug treatment
n. program that requires notification of recipients of blood products from donors that test positive for a transmissible disease
o. special protocol for collecting, handling, and testing legal specimens
p. substance being measured or detected by analysis
q. suitability to be mixed together with favorable results
r. term used to describe blood donated for one's own use
s. test used to monitor heparin therapy
t. tests platelet plug formation in the capillaries
u. treatment with antibiotics
v. with air

Choose the BEST answer.

23. Eligibility requirements for donating blood include:
   a. age 17–66 years, 110 lb or more.
   b. age 18–75 years, 110 lb or more.
   c. age 21–65 years old, at least 100 lb.
   d. minimum age of 21 years, minimum 100 lb.

24. Identify the condition in which a unit of blood is withdrawn from a patient as a treatment.
   a. ABO and Rh incompatibility
   b. autologous donation
   c. hemochromatosis
   d. leukemia

25. Which specimen requires especially strict identification and labeling procedures?
    a. blood culture
    b. blood type and crossmatch
    c. glucose
    d. therapeutic drug monitoring

26. Before blood salvaged during surgery can be reinfused in the patient it must be tested for:
    a. bacterial contamination.
    b. electrolyte levels.
    c. glucose.
    d. residual free hemoglobin.

27. Donor units of blood are typically collected using needles that are:
    a. 16–18 gauge.
    b. 18–28 gauge.
    c. 20–22 gauge.
    d. 23–25 gauge.

28. A typical unit of donated blood contains approximately:
    a. 250 mL.
    b. 450 mL.
    c. 750 mL.
    d. 1 L.

29. Which of the following tests is collected from patients with a fever of unknown origin (FUO) to rule out septicemia?
    a. blood culture
    b. nasopharyngeal culture
    c. urine culture and sensitivity
    d. wound culture

30. Which type of tube can be used to collect blood for a type and screen?
    a. lavender top EDTA
    b. nonadditive red top
    c. pink top EDTA
    d. any of the above

31. Which of the following tests is collected using special skin decontamination procedures?
    a. blood cultures
    b. blood urea nitrogen

    c. complete blood count
    d. type and crossmatch

32. Which type of test is performed to determine the probability that a specific individual was the father of a particular child?
    a. blood culture
    b. coagulation
    c. paternity
    d. type and crossmatch

33. Why would blood cultures be collected with an antimicrobial adsorbing resin?
    a. the patient has fever spikes
    b. the patient is taking a broad-spectrum antibiotic
    c. to eliminate contaminating normal flora
    d. to remove bacterial contamination

34. Which specimen tubes must contain a 9:1 ratio of blood to anticoagulant to be accepted for testing?
    a. blood bank
    b. chemistry
    c. coagulation
    d. therapeutic drug monitoring (TDM)

35. What type of additive is best for collecting an ethanol specimen?
    a. EDTA
    b. nonadditive red top
    c. sodium citrate
    d. sodium fluoride

36. Which blood culture container is inoculated first when the specimen has been collected by syringe?
    a. aerobic
    b. anaerobic
    c. either
    d. neither

37. The most critical aspect of blood culture collection is:
    a. needle gauge.
    b. skin antisepsis.
    c. specimen handling.
    d. volume of blood collected.

38. A blood culture collection site is typically cleaned using:
   a. 0.5% sodium hypochlorite.
   b. isopropanol and povidone-iodine.
   c. soap and water.
   d. chlorhexidine gluconate.

39. Which of the following additives is sometimes used to collect blood culture specimens?
   a. citrate
   b. EDTA
   c. oxalate
   d. SPS

40. Which type of specimen may require collection of a discard tube before the test specimen is collected?
   a. blood culture
   b. coagulation
   c. paternity
   d. therapeutic drug monitoring (TDM)

41. The abbreviation for a test that assesses platelet plug formation in the capillaries is:
   a. ACT
   b. BT
   c. CBC
   d. PT

42. Which test is used as a screening test for glucose metabolism problems?
   a. 2-hour postprandial (PP)
   b. ethyl alcohol (ETOH)
   c. glucose tolerance test (GTT)
   d. whole blood glucose (WBG)

43. Which of the following activities can affect glucose tolerance test results?
   a. chewing sugarless gum
   b. drinking tea without sugar
   c. smoking low-tar cigarettes
   d. all of the above

44. When does the timing of specimen collection begin during a glucose tolerance test (GTT)?
   a. a GTT is not timed
   b. after the fasting specimen is collected

   c. after the patient finishes the glucose beverage
   d. before the fasting specimen is collected

45. A phlebotomist arrives to collect a 2-hour postprandial glucose specimen on an inpatient and discovers that 2 hours have not elapsed since the patient's meal. What should the phlebotomist do?
   a. ask the patient's nurse to verify the correct time to draw the specimen
   b. come back later at the time the patient says is correct
   c. draw the specimen and write the time collected on the specimen label
   d. fill out an incident report form and return to the laboratory

46. A patient undergoing a glucose tolerance test vomits within 30 minutes of drinking the glucose beverage. What action should the phlebotomist take?
   a. continue the test and note on the lab slip that the patient vomited and at what time
   b. discontinue the test and write on the requisition that the patient vomited the glucose beverage
   c. give the patient another dose of glucose beverage and continue the test
   d. notify the patient's nurse or physician immediately to determine if the test should be continued or rescheduled

47. Increased blood glucose is called:
   a. hyperglycemia.
   b. hyperinsulinism.
   c. hyperkalemia.
   d. hypernatremia.

48. Blood sugar (glucose) levels in normal individuals typically peak within what amount of time after glucose ingestion?
   a. 15–20 minutes
   b. 30–60 minutes
   c. 1–1.5 hours
   d. 2 hours

49. Which statement is true? Glucose tolerance test specimens can be collected by:
    a. a combination of skin puncture and venipuncture.
    b. skin puncture only.
    c. venipuncture.
    d. all of the above

50. Patient preparation before a glucose tolerance test involves:
    a. eating balanced meals containing 150 g of carbohydrate for 3 days before the test.
    b. fasting for at least 12 hours before the test.
    c. no smoking or chewing gum before or during the test.
    d. all of the above

51. Which of the following can be used to clean a site before blood alcohol specimen collection?
    a. isopropanol
    b. methanol
    c. tincture of iodine
    d. benzalkonium chloride

52. Which of the following may require "chain of custody" documentation when collected?
    a. blood culture
    b. crossmatch
    c. drug screen
    d. therapeutic drug monitoring (TDM)

53. The purpose of therapeutic drug monitoring is to:
    a. determine and maintain a beneficial drug dosage for a patient.
    b. maintain peak levels of drug in a patient's system.
    c. maintain trough levels of drug in a patient's system.
    d. screen for illegal drug use.

54. All of the following are drugs subject to therapeutic monitoring EXCEPT:

    a. digoxin
    b. gentamicin
    c. phenylalanine
    d. theophylline

55. A peak drug level has been ordered for 0900 hours (9 AM). You draw the specimen 10 minutes late because of unavoidable circumstances. What additional action does this necessitate?
    a. establish the last dosage time
    b. notify the patient's nurse
    c. record the time change when verifying the specimen
    d. all of the above

56. A trough drug level is collected:
    a. immediately before administration of the next scheduled drug dose.
    b. immediately after administration of the drug.
    c. when the highest serum concentration of the drug is expected.
    d. 30–60 minutes after administration of the drug.

57. Which test requires the collection of multiple specimens?
    a. drug screen
    b. glucose tolerance test
    c. hematocrit
    d. paternity

58. Timing of collection is most critical for drugs with short half-lives such as:
    a. digoxin.
    b. gentamicin.
    c. phenobarbital.
    d. all of the above

59. A bleeding time (BT) test assesses the functioning of which of the following cellular elements?
    a. erythrocytes
    b. leukocytes
    c. neutrophils
    d. thrombocytes

60. The most common reason for glucose monitoring through point-of-care testing is to:
   a. check for glycosuria.
   b. diagnose glucose metabolism problems.
   c. monitor glucose levels in patients with diabetes mellitus.
   d. all of the above

61. A trace-element–free tube is the best choice for collecting a specimen for:
   a. copper.
   b. lead.
   c. zinc.
   d. all of the above

62. Sources of error in point-of-care testing for blood glucose are all of the following EXCEPT:
   a. dehydrated patient.
   b. elevated bilirubin count.
   c. hematocrit between 25% and 60%.
   d. inadequate sample size.

63. Which test typically has the shortest turnaround time?
   a. bleeding time (BT)
   b. glucose tolerance test (GTT)
   c. tuberculosis (TB)
   d. whole blood glucose (WBG)

64. Which of the following is not a point-of-care testing analyzer?
   a. CoaguChek
   b. Hemochron Jr.
   c. I-Stat
   d. BacT/Alert

65. Monitoring blood coagulation through point-of-care testing may be performed during all of the following EXCEPT:
   a. cardiac bypass surgery.
   b. coumadin therapy.
   c. heparin therapy.
   d. lithium therapy.

66. Which of the following is one of the most common bedside or point-of-care testing tests?

   a. activated clotting time
   b. bilirubin
   c. whole blood glucose
   d. rapid plasma reagin

67. Tests used to monitor heparin therapy include:
   a. ACT.
   b. BT.
   c. WBG.
   d. all of the above

68. All of the following equipment is needed for a bleeding time test EXCEPT:
   a. butterfly bandage
   b. standardized incision device
   c. stopwatch
   d. tourniquet

69. At what intervals is the blood blotted during a bleeding time test?
   a. 10 seconds
   b. 20 seconds
   c. 30 seconds
   d. 60 seconds

70. When performing the bleeding time test, a sphygmomanometer is inflated to:
   a. 40 mm Hg.
   b. 60 mm Hg.
   c. 100 mm Hg.
   d. a sphygmomanometer is not needed

71. Which of the following will prolong a bleeding time test?
   a. abnormally low platelet count
   b. recent ingestion of aspirin
   c. touching the incision site with the filter paper
   d. all of the above

72. This test can determine if an individual has developed antibodies to a particular antigen.
   a. glucose tolerance test
   b. skin test
   c. troponin T
   d. whole blood glucose

73. Ionized calcium plays a critical role in:
    a. blood clotting.
    b. cardiac function.
    c. muscular contraction.
    d. all of the above

74. Below normal blood pH is referred to as:
    a. acidosis.
    b. alkalosis.
    c. hypernatremia.
    d. hyperventilation.

75. Which of the following is a protein that is specific to heart muscle?
    a. creatine phosphokinase
    b. low-density lipoprotein
    c. troponin T
    d. none of the above

76. B-type natriuretic peptide (BNP) is a(n):
    a. cardiac antibody.
    b. cardiac hormone.
    c. cardiac enzyme.
    d. protein specific to heart muscle.

77. This test is used to evaluate long-term effectiveness of diabetes therapy.
    a. 2-hour postprandial
    b. glucose tolerance test
    c. hemoglobin A1c
    d. whole blood glucose

78. This test is also referred to as packed cell volume.
    a. erythrocyte sedimentation rate (ESR)
    b. hematocrit (HCT)
    c. hemoglobin (Hgb)
    d. hemoglobin A1c (Hgb A1c)

79. This test detects occult blood.
    a. guaiac
    b. hemoglobin A1c
    c. hematocrit
    d. purified protein derivative

80. Which of the following is a skin test for tuberculosis exposure?
    a. cocci
    b. histo

c. PPD
d. Schick

81. The abbreviation for the hormone detected in urine pregnancy testing is:
    a. HCT.
    b. HCG.
    c. PPD.
    d. TSH.

82. Which point-of-care blood glucose analyzer uses a microcuvette instead of a test strip?
    a. Advantage HQ
    b. HemoCue
    c. I-Stat
    d. ONE TOUCH

83. An uncorrected imbalance of this analyte in a patient can quickly lead to death.
    a. blood urea nitrogen (BUN)
    b. human chorionic gonadotropin (HCG)
    c. iron
    d. potassium

84. What type of specimen is needed for a guaiac test?
    a. amniotic fluid
    b. blood
    c. feces
    d. urine

85. How much antigen is injected when performing a purified protein derivative (PPD) test?
    a. 0.01 mL
    b. 0.1 mL
    c. 1.0 mL
    d. 10 mL

86. Erythema means:
    a. hardness.
    b. inflammation.
    c. redness.
    d. all of the above

87. When reading a patient's tuberculosis test, there is an area of induration and erythema that measures 7 mm in diameter. The result of the test is:
   a. doubtful.
   b. negative.
   c. positive.
   d. unreadable.

88. Point-of-care detection of Group A strep normally requires a:
   a. blood specimen.
   b. nasal swab.
   c. throat swab.
   d. urine specimen.

89. Which of the following can be detected in urine by color reactions that occur on a special reagent strip that is dipped in the urine specimen and then compared visually against color codes on the reagent strip container?
   a. bilirubin
   b. glucose
   c. leukocytes
   d. all of the above

90. New noninvasive technology can be used to measure:
   a. bilirubin.
   b. glucose.
   c. oxygen saturation.
   d. all of the above

ANSWERS AND EXPLANATIONS

1. **s.** activated clotting time, a test used to monitor heparin therapy

2. **v.** with air

3. **d.** clumping, as in clumping of red blood cells in a transfusion reaction

4. **p.** substance being measured or detected by analysis

5. **u.** treatment with antibiotics

6. **r.** term used to describe blood donated for one's own use

7. **b.** bacteria in the blood

8. **t.** bleeding time, tests platelet plug formation in the capillaries

9. **o.** special protocol for collecting, handling, and testing legal specimens

10. **q.** suitability to be mixed together with favorable results

11. **k.** outside the body

12. **f.** fever of unknown origin; fever for which the cause is unknown

13. **e.** glucose tolerance test; detects carbohydrate metabolism problems

14. **h.** heparin management test, a high-dose heparin monitoring test

15. **n.** program that requires notification of recipients of blood products from donors that test positive for a transmissible disease

16. **i.** highest serum concentration of a drug

17. **c.** point-of-care testing, bedside testing

18. **a.** postprandial; after a meal

19. **l.** pathogenic bacteria in the blood

20. **m.** therapeutic drug monitoring, a procedure used to manage individual patient drug treatment

21. **j.** lowest serum concentration of a drug

22. **g.** whole blood glucose; glucose measured in whole blood

23. **a.** To donate blood, an individual must normally be between the ages of 17 and 66 and weigh at least 110 lb.

24. **c.** Hemochromatosis is a disease characterized by excess iron deposits in the tissues. Periodic removal of single units of blood gradually depletes excess iron stores because the body uses iron to make new red blood cells to replace those removed.

25. **b.** Specimens for blood type and crossmatch require especially strict identification and labeling procedures. Misidentification of a blood type and crossmatch specimen can lead to a patient receiving an incompatible unit of blood and having a serious and possibly fatal transfusion reaction. Special blood bank specimen identification systems intended to reduce errors are available. Figure 11-1 shows a phlebotomist comparing information on a blood bank tube containing a label peeled from a special blood bank ID bracelet with the carbon copy of the label on the bracelet attached to the patient's arm.

26. **d.** Blood salvage procedures can lead to hemolysis of red blood cells evidenced by hemoglobin in the blood plasma. If free hemoglobin levels are too high, reinfusing it is of little value and can lead to renal dysfunction.

27. **a.** Large-bore (16- to 18-gauge) needles are used to collect donor units. The large bore helps keep the blood flowing freely and minimizes hemolysis of red blood cells during collection.

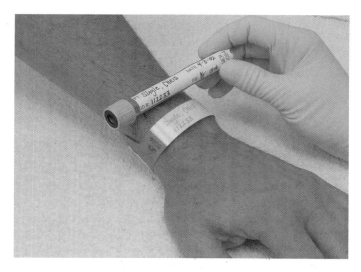

■ FIGURE 11-1 ■

A phlebotomist compares a blood bank tube with a blood bank identification bracelet.

28. **b.** A donor unit is filled by weight, but typically contains approximately 450 mL of blood.

29. **a.** The response of the body to septicemia is to raise body temperature to kill the microorganisms. When a patient experiences fever with no known cause (referred to as fever of unknown origin or FUO), a physician may suspect septicemia and order blood cultures.

30. **d.** A type and screen can be performed on a specimen collected in a nonadditive red top, lavender top EDTA, or special pink top EDTA tube, depending on laboratory preference.

31. **a.** Special skin decontamination procedures are used to collect blood cultures to prevent contamination of the specimen with normal flora of the patient's skin. Figure 11-2

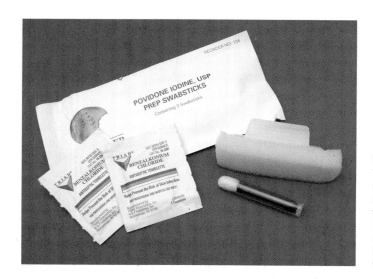

■ FIGURE 11-2 ■

Three types of blood culture cleaning supplies. *Left,* Povidone-iodine swabsticks. (The Purdue Frederick Co., Norwalk, CT.) *Center,* Benzalkonium chloride. (Triad Disposables Inc., Brookfield, WI.) *Right,* Frepp/Sepp povidone-iodine cleaning kit components. (Medi-Flex, Inc., Overland Park, KS.)

shows examples of several types of blood culture site cleaning supplies.

32. c. A paternity test can determine the probability that a specific individual was the father of a particular child. Results of paternity tests can exclude an individual as the father rather than prove that he is the father.

33. b. It is not unusual for patients to be taking antibiotics when a blood culture is collected. Antibiotic present in the blood specimen can inhibit the growth of microorganisms and lead to a false-negative blood culture result. The special resin removes or neutralizes antibiotics. The blood is then cultured by conventional techniques.

34. c. Coagulation specimens must have a 9:1 ratio of blood to anticoagulant or test results on the specimen will not be accurate. If a coagulation tube is not filled completely, this ratio is altered and the lab will not accept the specimen for testing.

35. d. Sodium fluoride prevents the breakdown of alcohol and is the recommended additive for collecting blood alcohol specimens.

36. b. If both aerobic and anaerobic cultures are collected at one time, the anaerobic bottle is inoculated first when filled from a syringe. If a butterfly with tubing is used and blood is collected directly into the bottles, the aerobic bottle is filled first because air from the tubing will be drawn into the bottle ahead of the blood.

37. b. Skin antisepsis is extremely important in blood culture collection. Failure to follow proper antiseptic technique can result in contamination of the blood culture by skin surface bacteria or other microorganisms as well as interfere with interpretation of results.

38. b. A blood culture collection site is typically cleaned (Fig. 11-3) using an alcohol scrub followed by povidone-iodine or tincture of iodine applied in ever-increasing concentric circles (Fig. 11-4).

39. d. As a temporary measure, blood culture specimens are occasionally col-

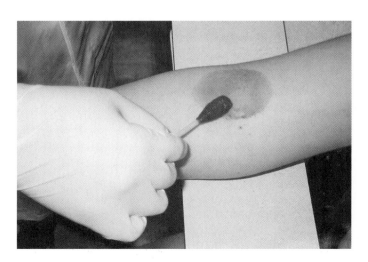

■ FIGURE 11-3 ■

Cleaning a blood culture site using a povidone-iodine swabstick.

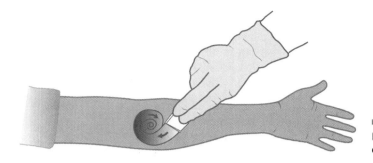

Pattern of concentric circles used when cleaning a blood culture site.

lected in evacuated tubes containing sodium polyanethol sulfonate (SPS) and later transferred into blood culture bottles.

40. **b.** At one time it was customary to draw a "clear" or discard tube before drawing a tube for a coagulation testing. A few milliliters of blood were collected into a plain red top tube to clear the needle of tissue thromboplastin contamination picked up as the needle penetrated the skin. The "clear" tube was discarded if it was not needed for other tests. Although no longer recommended for PT and PTT tests, a discard tube is still recommended for other coagulation tests.

41. **b.** The bleeding time (BT) test is used to assess platelet plug formation in the capillaries.

42. **a.** Carbohydrates break down into glucose. Blood glucose levels rise after ingestion of carbohydrates but return to normal levels within 2 hours in most individuals with normal carbohydrate or glucose metabolism. A 2-hour postprandial (PP) glucose test measures glucose levels 2 hours after ingestion of a special meal containing approximately 100 g of carbohydrate and is an excellent screening test for glucose metabolism problems.

43. **d.** Chewing sugarless gum, drinking sugarless tea, and smoking cigarettes all affect the digestive process and can therefore affect glucose tolerance test results.

44. **c.** The timing of specimen collection during a GTT begins as soon as the patient finishes the glucose beverage. For example, if a patient finishes the glucose beverage at 8:05, the 0.5-hour specimen is collected at 8:35, the 1-hour specimen is collected at 9:05, and so on.

45. **a.** If there is a discrepancy concerning the timing of a 2-hour postprandial specimen, the patient's nurse should be consulted to establish the correct time to draw the specimen. It is not a good idea to ask the patient as he or she may not know the correct time or understand the importance of exact timing. The specimen should not be collected early as glucose levels may still be elevated and lead to misinterpretation of results. Filling out an incident report and returning to the lab does nothing to solve the problem.

46. **d.** If a patient undergoing a glucose tolerance test vomits within 30 minutes of drinking the glucose beverage, his or her nurse or physician should be notified immediately

to determine if the test should be continued or rescheduled.

47. **a.** Increased blood glucose (sugar) is called hyperglycemia. Hyperinsulinism is excessive blood insulin levels. Hyperkalemia is excessive blood potassium levels. Hypernatremia is excess sodium in the blood.

48. **b.** Blood glucose levels in normal individuals typically peak within 30–60 minutes of glucose ingestion and return to normal fasting levels within 2 hours. Glucose tolerance test (GTT) specimen results are plotted on a graph to create what is referred to as a GTT curve. Figure 11-5 shows a graph with examples of normal and abnormal GTT curves.

49. **c.** Blood glucose reference ranges vary according to the method of collection. It is important that the method of collection be consistent for the duration of the test for proper interpretation of results. Consequently, glucose tolerance test blood specimens can be collected by skin puncture or venipuncture, but not a combination of the two methods.

50. **d.** Proper patient preparation before a glucose tolerance test involves eating balanced meals containing 150 g of carbohydrate for 3 days before the test, fasting for at least 12 hours before the test, and no smoking or chewing gum before or during the test.

51. **d.** Alcohol solutions or alcohol-based antiseptics can cause interference in blood alcohol testing and should not be used to clean a site before blood alcohol specimen collection. Isopropyl alcohol (isopropanol), and methanol are types of alcohol. (Methanol is toxic and should never be used as a skin antiseptic). Tincture of iodine cannot be used because tinctures contain alcohol.

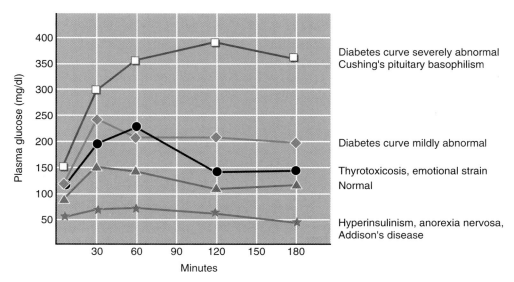

■ FIGURE 11-5 ■

Glucose tolerance test (GTT) curves.

52. c. "Chain of custody" documentation is required for legal or forensic specimens. Whether performed for legal reasons or not, drug screening has legal implications that require use of chain of custody protocol. Figure 11-6 shows an example of a chain of custody requisition form.

53. a. Therapeutic drug monitoring (TDM) is performed to determine and maintain a beneficial drug dosage for a patient. Peak drug levels represent the highest serum concentrations of a drug and are collected during TDM to screen for drug toxicity. Trough drug levels are monitored during TDM to ensure drug levels stay within the therapeutic or effective range. TDM has nothing to do with screening for illegal drug use.

54. c. Phenylalanine is an amino acid, not a drug.

55. c. Timing of therapeutic drug monitoring specimens is extremely important. A pharmacist calculates drug dosages based on blood levels of the drug at specific times. If a specimen is collected late, it is important that the actual time of collection be recorded so that pharmacist is aware of the time change and can calculate values accordingly.

56. a. A trough or minimum drug level is collected when the lowest serum concentration of the drug is expected. A trough drug level is easiest to collect because it is collected immediately before administration of the next scheduled drug dose.

57. b. A glucose tolerance test involves the collection of multiple blood specimens. Blood specimens are serially collected at specific times throughout the duration of the test. Urine specimens are sometimes collected at the same times as the blood specimens.

58. b. A half-life is the time required for the body to metabolize half the amount of the drug. Timing of collection is most critical for aminoglycoside drugs with short half-lives such as gentamicin, amikacin, and tobramycin. Timing is less critical for drugs such as phenobarbital and digoxin, which have longer half-lives.

59. d. Thrombocytes are platelets. A bleeding time (BT) test assesses platelet plug formation in the capillaries. When performing a bleeding time, a standardized incision is made and blood flow is wicked or blotted away without disturbing the incision site, until bleeding stops. The time recorded represents the time it takes for the platelet plug to form. BT equipment is shown in Figure 11-7.

60. c. Glucose monitoring in diabetics (patients with diabetes mellitus) is the most common reason for performing glucose testing through point-of-care testing.

61. d. Traces of elements or minerals such as copper, lead, and zinc can be contaminants in glass and other materials used to make blood collection tubes and stoppers, and can leach from the tube into the specimen. Trace-element–free tubes have the lowest possible contaminating amounts of these elements. Copper, lead, and zinc are all elements or minerals measured in such small quantities that it is best if they are collected in trace-element–free tubes.

ORDERING PHYSICIAN/COMPANY OR FACILITY

SONORA Laboratory Sciences

3401 E. Harbour Dr., Phoenix, Arizona 85034
602 431-5000
800 SONORA-1
800 766-6721

2013AC
SOEHS-T'BIRD SAMARITAN MEDICAL
                    CENTER   2013A

5555 W THUNDERBIRD RD

GLENDALE, AZ   85306
602 588-5555   *RT14

CHAIN OF CUSTODY REQUISITION FORM

Failure to complete form properly could invalidate chain of custody.

D O N O R   I N S T R U C T I O N S   (To be completed by donor)

*************************** IDENTIFICATION IS REQUIRED AT TIME OF COLLECTION ***************************

DONOR AFFIDAVIT

I certify that the specimen identified by the ID number on this form was provided by me on this date and is not adulterated. In my presence, the specimen was sealed with an evidence seal taken from this form. The ID Number on the seal and on this form are identical. I have initialed the seal. By my signature I consent to the release of laboratory test results to the doctor, facility, individual or company shown on this form.

Donor Signature   Donor Name (**Print Clearly**)   Date

Birthdate   Social Security Number   Daytime Phone

You have the right to list any drugs, prescription or non prescription, that you may have taken in the last two weeks or other relevant medical information. Please do so, if desired, in the space provided: _____

C O L L E C T O R   I N S T R U C T I O N S   (To be completed by collector)

1. Check donor identification (**preferably a picture I.D.**)
2. RECORD SPECIMEN TEMP: _____ (90° - 100°)
3. Specimen lid is tight, sealed properly with evidence seal, and initialed by donor.
4. I.D. number on specimen and form must match.
5. Place specimen in tamper-proof bag and seal in the presence of the donor.
6. Form is completed and signed by donor.
7. Collector signs this form, indicates date, time and collection site.

I certify that the specimen identified by this form was collected according to specified procedures, was properly identified and prepared for transport to the laboratory.

Collector Signature   Printed Name   Date   Collection Time

Collection Site   Address   Phone

COMMENTS: _____

LABORATORY USE ONLY

SPECIMEN RECEIVED BY:

SIGNATURE   PRINTED NAME   DATE

SPECIMEN SEAL CONDITION: ☐ INTACT   ☐ NOT INTACT

COMMENTS: _____

Check One Box
☐ Pre-Employment
☐ Post-accident
☐ Random
☐ Reasonable Cause
☐ Periodic
☐ Other_____

TESTS

[X] 2406 (FORENSIC COM-
          PREHENSIVE)

SOCIAL SECURITY NUMBER

_____ _____ _____

DEPT: _____

PHONE: _____

COLLECTION TIME/DATE

_____/_____

*********** SPECIMEN I.D. NUMBER 293012 ***************************

293012 293012   EVIDENCE SEAL   SPECIMEN I.D. NUMBER   EVIDENCE SEAL
                                              293012
293012 293012   Donor Initials
                                                                   EVIDENCE SEAL
293012 293012   EVIDENCE SEAL   ___/___/___
                                              Date

ORIGINAL TO LABORATORY

■ FIGURE 11-6 ■

Chain of custody requisition form. (Courtesy Sonora Laboratory Sciences, Phoenix, AZ.)

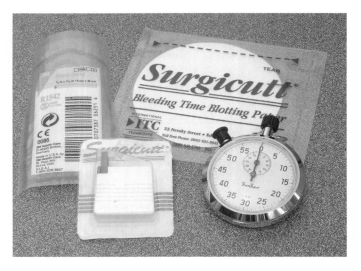

Equipment for bleeding time test, including Surgicutt automated bleeding time device, blotting paper, stopwatch, and Steri-Strips. (ITC, Edison, NJ.)

62. c. For accurate results a patient's hematocrit should be between 25% and 60%. Dehydration causes hemoconcentration of the blood leading to erroneous test results. Elevated bilirubin levels in a specimen interfere with the testing process and lead to erroneous results. Results will be adversely affected if a smaller than normal volume of blood is tested. Consequently, most point-of-care testing instruments will default if an inadequate amount of sample is applied to the testing area.

63. d. Turnaround time in laboratory testing is the amount of time that elapses between when a test is ordered and when the results are returned. WBG results obtained at the bedside using point-of-care testing instruments are available within minutes. A BT is performed at the bedside. However, the test can take from 2–8 minutes, not counting preparation procedures, on a patient with normal platelet function, and much longer if the patient is taking heparin. A GTT is a timed test involving collection of serial specimens over 1–6 hours depending on how it is ordered by the physician. A TB test is performed and results read or interpreted at the bedside; however, interpretation of results takes place approximately 48 hours after the test is administered.

64. d. CoaguChek, Hemochron Jr., and I-Stat are all point-of-care testing analyzers. BacT/Alert is a blood culture collection system.

65. d. Lithium levels are drug levels, and lithium therapy does not involve the coagulation process. Coumadin and heparin are anticoagulants, the effects of which can be closely monitored through point-of-care testing (POCT). POCT is also used to monitor high-dose heparin use during certain surgeries.

66. c. Whole blood glucose (WBG) or bedside glucose monitoring is one of the most common point-of-care-tests. Activated clotting time (ACT)

is a point-of-care test but is not performed nearly as often. Bilirubin is not commonly performed at the bedside. Rapid plasma reagin (RPR) is not a point-of-care test.

67. a. The activated clotting time (ACT) test is used to monitor heparin therapy. The bleeding time (BT) test assesses platelet function. Point-of-care testing for glucose is called whole blood glucose (WBG).

68. d. A butterfly bandage, standardized incision device or lancet, and a stopwatch are all bleeding time (BT) test equipment (see Fig. 11-7). A tourniquet is not used during a BT. A blood pressure cuff is used to provide a standard pressure of 40 mm Hg.

69. c. During a bleeding time test, special filter paper is brought close to the site every 30 seconds to carefully wick or blot the blood away. Care must be taken not to touch the incision site or the platelet plug will be disturbed, and the bleeding time will be falsely prolonged.

70. a. When performing a bleeding time test, a blood pressure cuff is used to provide a uniform pressure of 40 mm Hg.

71. d. A bleeding time (BT) tests platelet plug formation in the capillaries. If the patient has an abnormally low platelet count, it will take longer for the platelet plug to form, resulting in a prolonged BT. Aspirin inhibits platelet function for the life of the platelet. Consequently, if the patient has taken aspirin within 2 weeks of the test, the BT will be prolonged. Touching the incision site disturbs platelet plug formation and also prolongs the test.

72. b. Skin tests involve intradermal injection (Fig. 11-8) of an antigenic substance that causes an allergic response if the patient has an antibody directed against it but does not cause the disease. For example, to perform a tuberculosis (TB) skin test, a modified TB antigen is injected just under the skin on a patient's forearm. (Properly injected antigen forms a temporary wheal or bleb). If the patient has TB antibodies, they will combine with the antigen to cause a visible reaction on the surface of the skin within 48–72 hours.

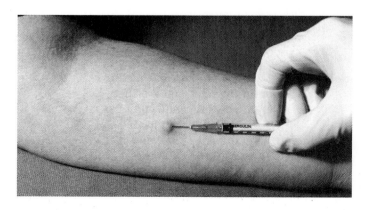

■ FIGURE 11-8 ■

Wheal (bleb) formed by intradermal injection of antigen during skin test procedure.

73. **d.** Ionized calcium makes up approximately 45% of the calcium in the blood. The rest is bound to protein and other substances. Only ionized calcium can be used for critical functions such as blood clotting, cardiac function, and muscular contraction.

74. **a.** Normal arterial blood pH is 7.35–7.45. Below normal blood pH is called acidosis. Above normal pH is called alkalosis. Hypernatremia is excess sodium in the blood. Hyperventilation causes a decrease in carbon dioxide.

75. **c.** Troponin T is a protein that is specific to heart muscle. It is measured in the diagnosis of acute myocardial infarction or heart attack.

76. **b.** BNP is a cardiac hormone produced by the heart in response to ventricular volume expansion and pressure overload.

77. **c.** Hemoglobin A1c is a type of hemoglobin formed by glycosylation (the reaction of glucose with hemoglobin). Glycosylated Hgb levels reflect the average blood glucose level during the preceding 4–6 weeks and therefore can be used to evaluate long-term effectiveness of diabetes therapy.

78. **b.** The HCT test is a measure of the volume of red blood cells in a patient's blood. It is also called packed cell volume because it can be calculated by centrifuging a specific volume of anticoagulated blood to separate the cells from the plasma to determine the proportion of the specimen that is red blood cells.

79. **a.** Occult blood is blood that is hidden or present in such small amounts that it is not apparent on visual examination. The guaiac test detects hidden blood in feces using an alcoholic solution of a tree resin called guaiac. Detection of occult blood in stool (feces) is an important tool in diagnosing gastric ulcer and screening for colon cancer. A number of different companies make occult blood kits containing special cards (Fig. 11-9) on which feces samples are collected and tested.

80. **c.** The test for tuberculosis exposure, the tuberculin (TB) test, is also called a PPD test because of the purified protein derivative (PPD) used in testing. The cocci test is for coccidiodiomycosis, an infectious fungus disease caused by *Coccidiodes immitis;* the histo test detects present or past infection with the fungus *Histoplasma capsulatum;* and the Schick test is for susceptibility to diphtheria.

81. **b.** Most rapid urine pregnancy tests detect human chorionic gonadotropin (HCG), a hormone produced by the placenta that appears in both urine and serum beginning approximately 10 days after conception. Peak urine levels of HCG occur at approximately 10 weeks of gestation.

82. **b.** HemoCue blood glucose analyzer uses a microcuvette instead of a test strip. The Advantage HQ and ONE TOUCH use a reagent strip for testing. The I-Stat uses a special cartridge for testing.

83. **d.** Potassium is an electrolyte. The body maintains electrolytes in specific proportions within narrow ranges, and any uncorrected imbalance can lead to death. Potassium plays a major role in nerve conduction, muscle function, acid-base bal-

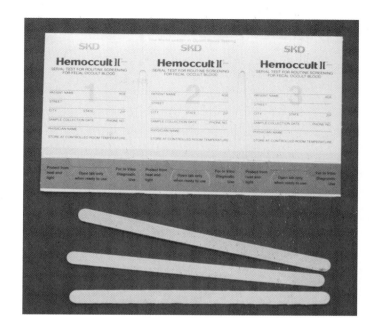

■ FIGURE 11-9 ■

Hemoccult II occult blood collection cards. (Beckman Coulter, Fullerton, CA.)

ance, and osmotic pressure. It influences cardiac output by helping to control the rate and force of heart contraction.

84. c. The guaiac test detects occult or hidden blood in feces. (See explanation of question 79).

85. b. When performing a PPD or tuberculin test, 0.1 mL of diluted antigen is injected under the skin. The antigen injected is purified protein derivative or PPD.

86. c. Erythema means redness.

87. a. Interpretation of a skin test is based on the presence or absence of erythema (redness) and/or induration (hardness) around the injection site. A positive test results when the area of either or both induration and hardness measures 10 mm or greater in diameter. An area between 5 and 9 mm is considered

doubtful. An area less than 5 mm is considered negative.

88. c. Point-of-care detection of Group A strep normally requires a throat swab specimen. Secretions from the swab are tested for the presence of strep A antigen. A number of different companies make special test kits (Fig. 11-10) for rapid detection of strep A.

89. d. Bilirubin, glucose, and leukocytes are all commonly detected in urine by reagent strip methods. Reagent strips also typically detect bacteria, blood, pH, protein, specific gravity, and urobilinogen. A chemical reaction resulting in color changes to the strip take place when the strip is dipped in a urine specimen. Results are determined by visually by comparing color changes on the strip with chart of color codes on the reagent strip container (Fig. 11-11).

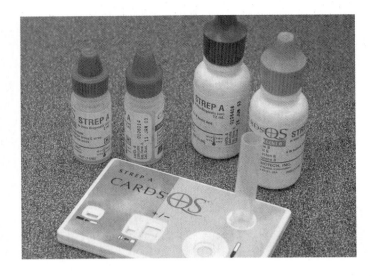

■ FIGURE **11-10** ■
Cards QS Strep A test kit. (Quidel Corp., San Diego, CA.)

90. d. Noninvasive technology can be used to detect glucose, bilirubin, and oxygen saturation. A relatively new device called the GlucoWatch Biographer (Cygnus, Redwood City, CA) is worn like a wristwatch and measures glucose through the skin every 20 minutes. The BiliChek system (SpecRx, Norcross, GA) is a hand-held device that measures bilirubin levels from the skin of newborns, thereby eliminating heel stick serum bilirubin measurements. A special finger cot device can be worn to measure oxygen saturation.

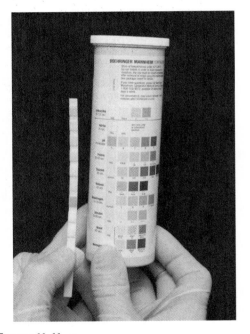

■ FIGURE **11-11** ■
Technician comparing urine reagent strip with chart on reagent strip container.

12

ARTERIAL PUNCTURE PROCEDURES

REVIEW QUESTIONS

Match the term with the BEST description.

1. ____ Allen test
2. ____ ABGs
3. ____ arteriospasm
4. ____ brachial artery
5. ____ collateral circulation
6. ____ femoral artery
7. ____ radial artery
8. ____ steady state
9. ____ thrombus

a. artery located in the thumb side of the wrist; first-choice site for arterial puncture
b. a stable condition; no exercise, suctioning, or respirator changes for 20–30 minutes before obtaining ABGs
c. a way to evaluate collateral blood flow to the hand before arterial puncture
d. blood clot in a blood vessel
e. evaluation of arterial blood to provide information on a patient's oxygenation, ventilation, and acid-base balance
f. main artery of the arm, located in the medial anterior aspect of the antecubital fossa
g. major systemic artery located superficially in the groin, lateral to the pubis bone
h. more than one artery supplies blood to the area
i. reflex constriction of an artery

Choose the BEST answer.

10. Which of the following tests requires an arterial specimen?
    a. ammonia
    b. blood cultures
    c. blood gases
    d. glycohemoglobin

11. All of the following are blood gas components EXCEPT?
    a. pCO_2
    b. pH
    c. pO_2
    d. PO_4

12. Arterial blood gas evaluation would *most* likely be performed on a patient with:
    a. hypothyroidism.
    b. osteochondritis.

    c. pulmonary disease.
    d. viral hepatitis.

13. Training in arterial puncture typically involves:
    a. demonstration of technique.
    b. observation of the actual procedure.
    c. performance of arterial puncture under supervision.
    d. all of the above

14. Arterial puncture site selection is based on:
    a. presence of collateral circulation.
    b. size and accessibility of the artery.
    c. type of tissue surrounding the site.
    d. all of the above

15. All of the following conditions would be reasons to avoid a site as a choice for arterial puncture EXCEPT?
a. edema or inflammation of the extremity
b. presence of collateral circulation
c. recent arterial puncture of the site
d. all of the above

16. The preferred and most common site for arterial puncture is the:
a. brachial artery.
b. femoral artery.
c. radial artery.
d. ulnar artery.

17. Which artery is generally easiest to access during low cardiac output?
a. brachial
b. femoral
c. radial
d. ulnar

18. The *biggest* advantage of choosing the radial artery for arterial blood gas collection is:
a. ability to locate during low cardiac output.
b. ease of compression following puncture.
c. presence of collateral circulation.
d. size and palpability.

19. What are the disadvantages of puncturing the radial artery?
a. it is easy to compress
b. it is small
c. the risk of hematoma formation is greater
d. there is no collateral circulation

20. What are the advantages of using the brachial artery for arterial blood gas collection?
a. it is large and easy to palpate
b. it is not as deep as the radial artery
c. there is less risk of hematoma formation
d. all of the above

21. Disadvantages of puncturing the brachial artery include that it is:
a. close to the basilic vein.
b. harder to compress following puncture.
c. near the median nerve.
d. all of the above

22. Which arterial site poses the greatest risk of infection?
a. brachial
b. femoral
c. radial
d. ulnar

23. Other sites where arterial specimens can be obtained include:
a. dorsal pedis arteries of adults.
b. indwelling arterial lines.
c. scalp and umbilical arteries in infants.
d. all of the above

24. In addition to normal patient identification information, an arterial blood gas requisition typically includes:
a. age at onset of respiratory disease.
b. body temperature and respiratory rate.
c. duration of present symptoms.
d. previous arterial blood gas results.

25. Which of the following is *not* necessary arterial blood gas equipment?
a. antiseptic cleaning solution or wipe
b. proper length needle for the site
c. tourniquet
d. 1 to 5 mL self-filling syringe

26. Arterial blood gas specimens are collected in syringes rather than tubes:
a. because a syringe can hold more blood.
b. because evacuated tube pressure can change results.
c. to guarantee sterility of the specimen.
d. to maintain anaerobic conditions.

27. Personal protective equipment required when collecting arterial specimens includes:
   a. fluid-resistant lab coat.
   b. gloves.
   c. face protection.
   d. all of the above

28. Commercially prepared arterial sampling kits typically contain:
   a. bubble removal caps.
   b. filters that vent residual air.
   c. heparinized syringes.
   d. all of the above

29. Heparin is used in arterial sample collection to:
   a. increase blood flow.
   b. numb the site.
   c. prevent the specimen from clotting.
   d. stabilize oxygen content of the specimen.

30. Lidocaine is sometimes used during arterial puncture to:
   a. help dissolve air bubbles in the specimen.
   b. keep the specimen from clotting.
   c. numb the site.
   d. preserve anaerobic conditions in the specimen.

31. Before an arterial blood gas specimen is collected, a patient should be in a steady state for at least:
   a. 10–15 minutes.
   b. 15–20 minutes.
   c. 20–30 minutes.
   d. 35–45 minutes.

32. Steady state, as in question 31, means that the patient has:
   a. been fasting for at least 8 hours.
   b. been sleeping for at least 1 hour.
   c. had no exercise, suctioning, or respirator changes.
   d. had no oxygen therapy in the past 12 hours.

33. The purpose of performing the modified Allen test before arterial specimen collection is to:
   a. assess patient ventilation status.
   b. determine the presence of collateral circulation.
   c. locate the ulnar artery.
   d. measure pressure in the radial artery.

34. When performing the modified Allen test, which artery is released first?
   a. brachial
   b. femoral
   c. radial
   d. ulnar

35. What constitutes a positive modified Allen test? The
   a. hand flushes pink or normal color within 15 seconds.
   b. hand remains blanched or drained of color for at least 30 seconds.
   c. pressure increases in the radial artery.
   d. ulnar artery pulses irregularly.

36. Which of the following is proper procedure if a patient does *not* have collateral circulation?
   a. check for collateral circulation in the other arm
   b. perform arterial puncture on the radial artery
   c. perform arterial puncture on the ulnar artery
   d. perform arterial puncture on the femoral artery

37. A patient who has collateral circulation:
   a. cannot undergo radial artery puncture.
   b. has normal arterial pressure.
   c. has more than one artery supplying blood to that area of the body.
   d. is well ventilated.

38. Which step in radial arterial blood gas specimen collection is optional?

a. administration of local anesthetic
b. collateral circulation determination
c. steady state assessment
d. none of the above

39. Positioning of the arm for radial arterial blood gas specimen collection includes:
a. arm abducted.
b. palm facing down.
c. wrist flexed 30°.
d. all of the above

40. The radial artery is located in the:
a. antecubital area.
b. groin.
c. little finger side of the wrist.
d. thumb side of the wrist.

41. The thumb should not be used to feel for an artery because it:
a. has a pulse.
b. has collateral circulation.
c. is too big.
d. is too calloused.

42. Proper antiseptic technique before arterial specimen collection would include all of the following EXCEPT:
a. cleaning the phlebotomist's non-dominant finger
b. drying the site with gauze before needle entry
c. maintaining antisepsis of the site
d. using povidone-iodine to clean the site

43. When performing radial arterial puncture, direct the needle:
a. away from the hand, facing the arterial flow.
b. in any way as long as the bevel is up.
c. perpendicular to the wrist.
d. toward the hand, against the blood flow.

44. Which of the following is an acceptable angle of needle insertion for drawing radial arterial blood gases?
a. 15°
b. 20°

c. 45°
d. 90°

45. The proper angle of needle insertion for drawing femoral arterial blood gases is:
a. 15°.
b. 30°.
c. 45°.
d. 90°.

46. The typical needle used to collect blood from a radial artery is:
a. 18-gauge 1 inch.
b. 22-gauge 1 inch.
c. 23-gauge 1.5 inch.
d. 25-gauge 1.5 inch.

47. How do you know when you have "hit" an artery during arterial blood gas collection?
a. a flash of blood appears in syringe hub
b. the artery stops pulsing
c. the syringe starts to vibrate
d. all of the above

48. Which of the following is the best way to tell if a specimen is arterial? As the specimen is collected, the blood:
a. appears bright cherry red.
b. contains air bubbles.
c. looks dark bluish red.
d. pumps into the syringe.

49. As soon as the needle is withdrawn after arterial blood gas specimen collection:
a. the patient should apply pressure to the site for 3–5 minutes.
b. the phlebotomist should apply pressure to the site for 3–5minutes.
c. the phlebotomist should apply a pressure bandage to the site.
d. any of the above

50. Proper arterial blood gas specimen handling immediately after collection includes:
a. ejecting air bubbles from the specimen.
b. gently mixing the specimen to prevent clotting.

c. preventing exposure to air by capping the syringe.

d. all of the above

51. After performing arterial puncture, check the pulse:
    a. distal to the puncture site.
    b. in the ulnar artery.
    c. medial to the puncture site.
    d. proximal to the puncture site.

52. What should the phlebotomist do if the pulse is absent or faint following arterial blood gas collection?
    a. apply a pressure bandage immediately
    b. massage the patient's wrist
    c. notify the patient's nurse or physician
    d. nothing; this is normal after arterial puncture

53. An arterial specimen collected in an appropriate plastic syringe is typically transported:
    a. at room temperature.
    b. in a heat block.
    c. on ice.
    d. protected from light.

54. Specimens for electrolyte testing in addition to arterial blood gas analysis should be:
    a. kept in a heat block.
    b. placed on ice as soon as possible.
    c. transferred to a test tube.
    d. transported at room temperature.

55. If the patient has an elevated white blood cell count, the arterial blood gas specimen should be:
    a. analyzed within 5 minutes of collection.
    b. collected in EDTA.

c. kept in a heat block.
d. placed on ice for transport.

56. Which of the following is a common arterial puncture complication even when proper procedure is used?
    a. arteriospasm
    b. hematoma
    c. infection
    d. thrombus formation

57. Which of the following would be a reason to terminate arterial puncture?
    a. blood spurts into the syringe
    b. the specimen is dark reddish blue
    c. the patient complains of extreme pain
    d. all of the above

58. Sudden fainting during arterial puncture is:
    a. called vasovagal syncope.
    b. caused by a nervous system response to pain.
    c. related to hypotension.
    d. all of the above

59. All of the following could cause erroneous arterial blood gas results EXCEPT?
    a. air bubbles in the specimen
    b. delay in processing longer than 30 minutes
    c. failure to place the syringe on ice
    d. microclots in the specimen

60. Which of the following would cause an arterial blood gas specimen to be rejected for testing by the laboratory?
    a. improper labeling
    b. microclots
    c. quantity not sufficient
    d. all of the above

ANSWERS AND EXPLANATIONS

1. **c.** a way to evaluate collateral blood flow to the hand before arterial puncture

2. **e.** arterial blood gases, evaluation of arterial blood to provide information on a patient's oxygenation, ventilation, and acid-base balance

3. **i.** reflex constriction of an artery

4. **f.** main artery of the arm, located in medial anterior aspect of the antecubital fossa

5. **h.** more than one artery supplies blood to the area

6. **g.** major systemic artery located superficially in the groin, lateral to the pubis bone

7. **a.** artery located in the thumb side of the wrist; first-choice site for arterial puncture

8. **b.** a stable condition; no exercise, suctioning, or respirator changes for 20–30 minutes before obtaining ABGs

9. **d.** blood clot in a blood vessel

10. **c.** The primary reason for performing arterial puncture is to obtain blood for the evaluation of arterial blood gases.

11. **d.** Arterial blood gas components commonly measured include pCO_2, pH, and pO_2. PO_4 is the designation for phosphate, which is not a blood gas component.

12. **c.** Arterial blood gas evaluation is used in the diagnosis and management of respiratory or pulmonary disease to provide information about a patient's oxygenation, ventilation, and acid-base balance.

13. **d.** Personnel who perform arterial blood gas procedures are normally certified by their healthcare institutions after successfully completing training involving theory, demonstration of technique, observation of the actual procedure, and performance of arterial puncture under the supervision of qualified personnel.

14. **d.** Several different sites can be used for arterial puncture. The criteria for site selection include the presence of collateral circulation, how large and accessible is the artery, and the type of tissue surrounding the puncture site.

15. **b.** The presence of collateral circulation is a desirable characteristic of a potential arterial puncture site. Edema, inflammation, or a recent arterial puncture at the site are reasons to avoid a site as a choice for arterial puncture.

16. **c.** The radial artery (Fig. 12-1) located in the thumb side of the wrist is the preferred and therefore the first choice and most common site used for arterial puncture. The brachial artery (Fig. 12-1) located in the medial anterior aspect of the antecubital area near the insertion of the biceps muscle is the second choice. The femoral artery (Fig. 12-2) is located in the groin. Femoral artery puncture is performed primarily by physicians and specially trained emergency room personnel, usually in emergency situations. The ulnar artery (Fig. 12-1) is reserved to provide collateral circulation to the hand in the event the radial artery is damaged and is never used for arterial puncture.

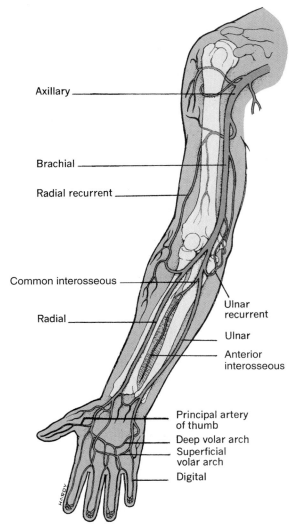

- Axillary
- Brachial
- Radial recurrent
- Common interosseous
- Radial
- Ulnar recurrent
- Ulnar
- Anterior interosseous
- Principal artery of thumb
- Deep volar arch
- Superficial volar arch
- Digital

■ FIGURE 12-1 ■
Arteries of the arm and hand.

lateral circulation. Collateral circulation means that more than one artery supplies blood to the area. If the radial artery were to be inadvertently damaged, the ulnar artery would still supply blood to the area.

19. **b.** One disadvantage of puncturing the radial artery is it requires considerable skill to puncture it successfully because it is so small. The presence of ligaments and bone in the area to aid in compression decreases the chance of hematoma formation and is an advantage, not a disadvantage.

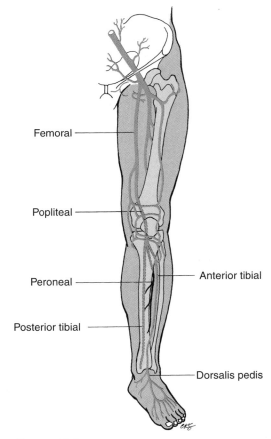

- Femoral
- Popliteal
- Peroneal
- Posterior tibial
- Anterior tibial
- Dorsalis pedis

■ FIGURE 12-2 ■
Arteries of the leg.

17. **b.** The femoral artery is large and easily located and punctured. It is sometimes the only site where arterial sampling is possible on patients with low cardiac output.

18. **c.** The biggest advantage of choosing the radial artery for arterial blood gas collection is the presence of col-

The presence of collateral circulation via the ulnar artery is also an advantage.

20. **a.** One advantage of using the brachial artery is it is large and easily palpated. However, it is located deeper than the radial artery, and there is increased risk of hematoma formation, not less, because it is harder to compress.

21. **d.** Disadvantages of puncturing the brachial artery include the fact that it lies close to the basilic vein and the median nerve, both of which could be inadvertently punctured. In addition, puncture of the brachial artery carries an increased risk of hematoma formation because there are no underlying ligaments or bone to support compression of the artery following the puncture.

22. **b.** The femoral artery (Fig. 12-2) is located superficially in the groin area lateral to the pubis bone. This area poses the greatest risk of infection because the presence of pubic hair makes it difficult to achieve an aseptic site.

23. **d.** In addition to the radial, brachial, and femoral arteries, arterial specimens can be obtained from the dorsal pedis arteries (Fig. 12-2) of adults, scalp and umbilical arteries in infants, and indwelling arterial lines.

24. **b.** An arterial blood gas requisition typically includes the patient's body temperature and respiratory rate in addition to normal patient identification information.

25. **c.** A tourniquet is not used to collect an arterial specimen. An artery is located by feeling its pulse. Arterial blood gas equipment is shown in Figure 12-3.

26. **b.** Arterial blood gas specimens are not collected in evacuated tubes, because tube pressure or vacuum would alter results.

27. **d.** Personal protective equipment required when collecting arterial specimens includes a fluid-resistant lab coat, gloves, and face protection.

28. **d.** Commercially prepared arterial sampling kits are available from

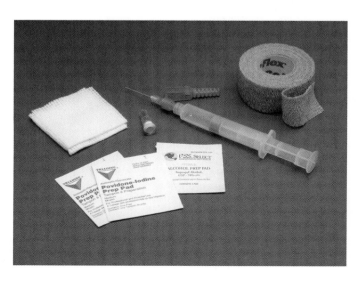

■ FIGURE 12-3 ■
Arterial blood gas equipment.

several manufacturers. A kit typically contains a safety needle or safety needle removal device, a heparinized syringe with a filter that removes residual air, and a bubble or air removal cap.

29. c. Arterial blood gases are performed on whole blood specimens. Therefore, an anticoagulant is needed to keep the specimen from clotting. The anticoagulant of choice is heparin.

30. c. Lidocaine is sometimes used to numb the site before arterial puncture. Although once part of standard arterial puncture procedure, use of local anesthetic is now optional.

31. c. Current body temperature, breathing pattern, and the concentration of oxygen inhaled all affect arterial blood gas results. Consequently, it is best if a patient has been in a steady state (i.e., no exercise, suctioning, or respirator changes) for 20–30 minutes before obtaining blood gases.

32. c. See explanation of question 31.

33. b. The modified Allen test (Fig. 12-4) is performed to determine the presence of collateral circulation. Collateral circulation means that the area of the body receives blood from more than one artery. Collateral circulation is necessary in the event that damage to the artery occurs

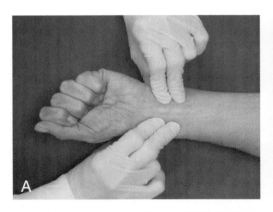
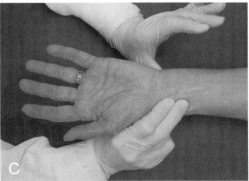
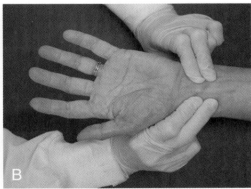

■ FIGURE 12-4 ■

Allen test. **A.** The fingers are used to compress the radial and ulnar arteries while the patient makes a fist. **B.** A blanched appearance to the open hand is observed while both arteries are being pressed. **C.** The patient's hand flushes with color when the ulnar artery is released, signifying a positive Allen test.

during arterial puncture. If the patient has circulation through an alternate artery, the area of the body that is normally fed by the damaged artery will receive blood from the alternate artery.

34. d. The modified Allen test checks for the presence of collateral circulation to the hand via the ulnar artery. Circulation via the ulnar artery is important in the event that the radial artery is damaged during arterial puncture. Consequently, when performing the modified Allen test, the ulnar artery is released first.

35. a. When performing the modified Allen test, both the ulnar and radial arteries are compressed to stop arterial flow to the hand. With both arteries compressed the hand should appear blanched or drained of color. If the patient has collateral circulation, the hand will flush pink or normal color when the ulnar artery is released even though the radial artery is still compressed. The presence of collateral circulation constitutes a positive modified Allen test.

36. a. If the modified Allen test is negative, the patient does not have collateral circulation and arterial puncture cannot be performed on the radial artery of that arm. At this point, the phlebotomist should check for collateral circulation in the other arm. Arterial puncture should never be performed on the ulnar artery.

37. c. A patient who has collateral circulation has more than one artery supplying blood to that area of the body.

38. a. Administration of local anesthetic to numb the site before arterial punc-

ture is optional. Assessment of steady state and determining the presence of collateral circulation are mandatory steps in the procedure.

39. a. Proper arm positioning before puncture of the radial artery includes having the patient's arm abducted (out to the side), with the palm up, and the wrist extended at approximately 30° and supported (e.g., by a rolled towel placed under it).

40. d. The radial artery is located in the thumb side of the wrist. The brachial artery is located in the antecubital area. The femoral artery is located in the groin. The ulnar artery is located in the little finger side of the wrist.

41. a. The thumb should never be used to feel for an artery because it has a pulse that could be misleading when locating the artery.

42. b. Proper antisepsis before arterial specimen collection is important. The site must be cleaned using a suitable antiseptic such as povidone-iodine and allowed to air dry. The phlebotomist's non-dominant index finger should be prepped in the same manner since it will be used to relocate the artery. Antisepsis of the site must be maintained. No non-sterile object should touch the site before puncture.

43. a. During puncture of the radial artery, the needle with the bevel up is directed away from the hand, facing the arterial blood flow, at a 30° to 45° angle (Fig. 12-5).

44. c. An acceptable angle of needle insertion during radial arterial blood gas collection is between 30° and 45°.

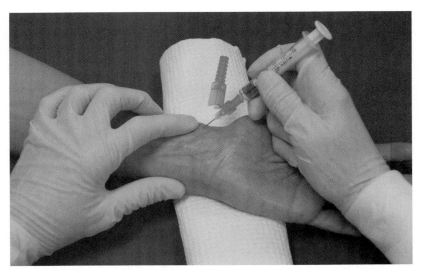

■ FIGURE 12-5 ■
Performing an arterial puncture.

45. d. The proper angle of needle insertion when collecting femoral arterial blood gases is 90° owing to the location of the femoral artery.

46. b. The 20- to 23-gauge and 25-gauge needles can be used for arterial puncture, depending on the collection site. However, a 22-gauge 1-inch needle is most commonly used for radial artery puncture.

47. a. Under normal circumstances, a flash of blood appears in the hub of the syringe when an artery is entered and blood will continue to pump into the syringe under its own power.

48. d. Blood pumping into the syringe under its own power is the best way to be certain that a specimen is arterial. Color is not a reliable indicator of successful arterial puncture. Although normal arterial blood is bright cherry red, arterial blood of patients with abnormal pulmonary function may appear almost as dark as venous blood. Arterial specimens do not normally contain air bubbles. Introduction of air into the specimen causes erroneous results and should be avoided.

49. b. The phlebotomist should manually apply pressure (Fig. 12-6) to the site for 3–5 minutes as soon as the needle is withdrawn following arterial puncture. The patient should never be allowed to hold pressure as he or she may not apply it firmly enough. A pressure bandage should never be used in place of manual pressure over the site. A pressure bandage can be applied after manual pressure has been held for the appropriate amount of time and bleeding has stopped.

50. d. As soon as the arterial blood gas needle is removed from the arm, the needle safety feature is activated or the needle is placed in a safety needle removal device. The

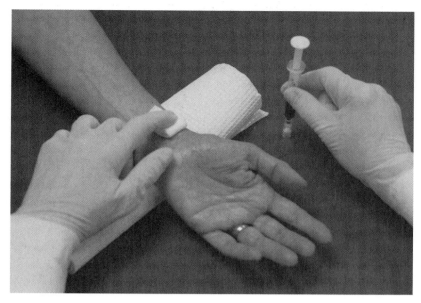

■ FIGURE 12-6 ■

Capping the arterial blood gas syringe while holding pressure over the patient's artery.

needle is removed and air bubbles are ejected from the specimen, or the hub of the syringe is capped (Fig. 12-6) with a bubble removal device to prevent exposing the specimen to air. The specimen is mixed as soon as possible to prevent clotting.

51. **a.** After performing arterial puncture, the pulse is checked distal or below the puncture site to ensure that blood flow is normal and no damage has occurred during the draw. If the pulse is faint or absent, a blood clot or thrombus may be obstructing blood flow and the patient's nurse or physician must be notified immediately so that steps can be taken to restore proper circulation.

52. **c.** An absent or faint pulse following arterial puncture is not normal and indicates blood flow may be partially or completely blocked by a

blood clot or thrombus. The patient's nurse or physician must be notified immediately so that steps can be taken to restore proper circulation.

53. **a.** An arterial specimen should be transported ASAP according to laboratory protocol. At one time it was standard procedure to transport arterial blood gas (ABG) specimens on ice. National Committee for Clinical Laboratory Standards guidelines now call for transporting ABG specimens at room temperature provided they are to be analyzed within 30 minutes of collection. If the patient has an elevated white blood cell count, the specimen should be analyzed within 5 minutes of collection.

54. **d.** Specimens for electrolyte testing in addition to arterial blood gas (ABG) analysis should be transported at room temperature. They should never be placed on ice because cooling affects potassium levels. ABG specimens should never be placed in a heat block.

55. **a.** If the patient has an elevated white blood cell count, an arterial blood gas (ABG) specimen should be transported at room temperature and analyzed within 5 minutes of collection. ABG specimens should never be placed in a heat block or collected in EDTA.

56. **a.** Arteriospasm is a reflex constriction of the artery that can occur even when proper technique is used. It can be caused by patient anxiety, pain during the procedure, or irritation caused by needle penetration of the artery muscle. Although this common complication is transitory, it may make it difficult to obtain a specimen. Hematoma, thrombus formation, and infection are less common complications.

57. **c.** Arterial puncture is typically more painful than venipuncture but should not cause the patient extreme pain. Extreme or significant pain indicates nerve involvement and requires immediate termination of the procedure. It is not unusual for arterial blood to spurt into the syringe during collection. Arterial

blood from a patient with pulmonary function problems may be dark reddish blue (because of reduced oxygen content) rather than the typical bright red of normal arterial blood.

58. **d.** Vasovagal syncope is sudden fainting related to hypotension caused by a nervous system response to abrupt pain or trauma.

59. **c.** Air bubbles or microclots in the specimen or a delay in processing longer than 30 minutes following collection can all cause erroneous arterial blood gas (ABG) results. National Committee for Clinical Laboratory Standards guidelines no longer recommend transporting ABG specimens on ice provided they are processed within 30 minutes of collection.

60. **d.** Improper labeling could lead to misidentification of a patient specimen. Arterial blood gases are performed on whole blood samples, and microclots will cause erroneous results. Quantity not sufficient (QNS) means that there is not enough specimen to perform the test. A specimen that is QNS is also called a "short" draw. Any of the above would cause laboratory personnel to reject the specimen for testing.

13 NONBLOOD SPECIMENS AND TESTS

REVIEW QUESTIONS

Match the term with the BEST description.

1. _____ amniotic fluid
2. _____ antibiotic susceptibility
3. _____ body fluids
4. _____ catheterized
5. _____ CSF
6. _____ clean-catch
7. _____ C&S
8. _____ midstream collection
9. _____ NP
10. _____ occult blood
11. _____ O&P
12. _____ semen analysis
13. _____ suprapubic
14. _____ sweat chloride
15. _____ UA
16. _____ UTI

a. clear, colorless liquid circulating within the cavities surrounding the brain and spinal cord

b. collection of a urine specimen by inserting a needle into the urinary bladder and aspirating urine directly from it

c. describes a urine specimen collected from a sterile catheter inserted through the urethra into the urinary bladder

d. fluid from within the sac that surrounds a fetus

e. laboratory test that includes a physical, chemical, and microscopic analysis of a urine specimen

f. laboratory test to assess fertility and determine effectiveness of sterilization after vasectomy

g. liquid substances found in the body

h. hidden blood such as detected in stool specimens using the guaiac test

i. intestinal parasites and their eggs (ova)

j. method of obtaining a urine sample free of contaminates from the external genital area

k. originating from the nasopharynx as in a sample collected using a special flexible swab inserted gently through the nose into the nasopharynx

l. processes used to grow and identify microorganisms and also identify effective antibiotics to use against them

m. specimen obtained in the middle of urination rather than the beginning or end

n. test performed to determine which antibiotics are effective against a particular microorganism

o. test used to diagnose cystic fibrosis primarily in children and adolescents younger than 20 years of age

p. urinary tract infection

Choose the BEST answer.

17. What special information is required when labeling a nonblood specimen?
    a. biohazard warning
    b. ordering physician's name
    c. special handling needs
    d. type and source of specimen

18. Which type of specimen must be handled and analyzed STAT?
    a. cerebrospinal fluid
    b. gastric fluid
    c. occult blood
    d. urine

19. The most frequently analyzed nonblood specimen is:
    a. cerebrospinal fluid.
    b. feces.
    c. saliva.
    d. urine.

20. What can happen to urine components if not processed in a timely fashion?
    a. bilirubin breaks down
    b. cellular elements decompose
    c. bacteria multiply
    d. all of the above

21. Which specimen is preferred for most urine tests?
    a. fasting
    b. first morning
    c. random
    d. 24-hour

22. Routine urinalysis specimens that cannot be analyzed within 2 hours require:
    a. a preservative.
    b. recollection.
    c. refrigeration.
    d. storage at room temperature.

23. A routine urinalysis typically incudes:
    a. chemical analysis.
    b. microscopic analysis.
    c. physical analysis.
    d. all of the above

24. The most likely reason a culture and sensitivity is ordered is to:
    a. check for glucose in the urine.
    b. diagnose urinary tract infection.
    c. evaluate kidney function.
    d. monitor urine pH levels.

25. Urine cytology studies look for the presence of:
    a. abnormal cells.
    b. crystals.
    c. microorganisms.
    d. all of the above

26. Urine drug screening can be performed to:
    a. detect illegal drug use.
    b. detect prescription drug abuse.
    c. monitor therapeutic drug use.
    d. all of the above

27. Suspected pregnancy can be confirmed by testing for the presence of this hormone in urine.
    a. adrenaline
    b. estrogen
    c. human chorionic gonadotropin
    d. thyroxine

28. Which specimen is preferred for pregnancy testing?
    a. clean-catch
    b. first morning
    c. random
    d. 24-hour

29. Which type of specimen is typically used for routine urinalysis?
    a. double-voided
    b. first morning
    c. random
    d. 24-hour

30. Which urine specimen is the most concentrated?
    a. first morning
    b. fractional
    c. timed
    d. 24-hour

31. This test sometimes requires serial urine specimens collected at specific times.
   a. glucose tolerance test
   b. creatinine clearance
   c. pregnancy test
   d. urine culture and sensitivity

32. What is the recommended procedure for collecting a 24-hour urine specimen?
   a. collect all urine voided in any 24-hour period
   b. collect the first morning specimen and all other urine for 24 hours, including the first specimen the following morning
   c. collect the first morning specimen and all other urine for 24 hours except the first specimen the following morning
   d. void the first morning specimen into the toilet; start the timing; collect all the following specimens including the next morning's specimen

33. All of the following statements are true of urine creatinine clearance specimen collection EXCEPT:
   a. refrigeration is preferred
   b. a 24-hour specimen is required
   c. a blood creatinine is also required
   d. requires a double-voided specimen

34. This type of specimen is sometimes used to compare urine concentrations of glucose and ketones to blood concentrations.
   a. fractional
   b. random
   c. 8-hour
   d. 24-hour

35. Which urine test requires a midstream clean-catch specimen?
   a. culture and sensitivity
   b. creatinine clearance
   c. glucose tolerance test
   d. routine urinalysis

36. Which of the following represents proper midstream urine collection?

   a. void initial urine into the container; interrupt the urine flow momentarily; restart urine flow and void a sufficient amount of urine into the toilet; collect the last urine flow into the container
   b. void initial urine into the container; interrupt the urine flow momentarily; restart urine flow and void a sufficient amount of urine into a second container; void excess urine flow into the toilet
   c. void initial urine into the toilet; interrupt the urine flow momentarily; restart urine flow and collect a sufficient amount of urine into a container; void excess urine flow into the toilet
   d. none of the above

37. Midstream clean-catch urine specimens require:
   a. cleaning of the genital area before specimen collection.
   b. collection in a sterile container.
   c. prompt processing.
   d. all of the above

38. Which urine specimen is obtained by inserting a sterile needle directly into the urinary bladder and aspirating a sample of urine?
   a. catheterized
   b. fractional
   c. pediatric
   d. suprapubic

39. Which of the following tests is sometimes performed on amniotic fluid?
   a. alkaline phosphatase
   b. alpha-fetoprotein
   c. disseminated intravascular coagulation
   d. lactic dehydrogenase

40. Amniotic fluid comes from the:
   a. cavity surrounding the brain and spinal cord.
   b. cavity surrounding the lungs.
   c. sac surrounding a fetus in the uterus.
   d. spaces within the joints.

41. Spinal fluid analysis is used in the diagnosis of:
  a. diabetes.
  b. meningitis.
  c. osteoporosis.
  d. renal failure.

42. Tests commonly performed on spinal fluid include all the following EXCEPT:
  a. cell counts.
  b. glucose.
  c. protein.
  d. hemoglobin.

43. This test requires intervenous administration of histamine or pentagastrin.
  a. gastric analysis
  b. sweat chloride
  c. epinephrine tolerance
  d. glucose tolerance

44. A nasopharyngeal culture swab is sometimes collected to detect the presence of organisms that cause:
  a. genetic defects.
  b. strep throat.
  c. urinary tract infection.
  d. whooping cough.

45. Saliva can be tested to:
  a. detect alcohol abuse.
  b. detect recent drug use.
  c. monitor hormone levels.
  d. all of the above

46. One reason semen analysis is performed is to:
  a. assess fertility.
  b. detect bladder infection.
  c. look for cancerous cells.
  d. identify circumcision candidates.

47. All of the following semen specimens would be acceptable for testing EXCEPT a specimen:
  a. collected in a condom.
  b. delivered in a sterile container.
  c. kept at 37° C.
  d. obtained on site.

48. Which of the following fluids is obtained through lumbar puncture?
  a. peritoneal
  b. pleural
  c. spinal
  d. synovial

49. Serous fluid includes:
  a. pericardial fluid.
  b. peritoneal fluid.
  c. pleural fluid.
  d. all of the above

50. Peritoneal fluid comes from the:
  a. abdominal cavity.
  b. lung cavities.
  c. pericardial sac.
  d. spinal cavity.

51. Fluid from joint cavities is called:
  a. pleural fluid.
  b. pericardial fluid.
  c. peritoneal fluid.
  d. synovial fluid.

52. Pleural fluid is aspirated from the:
  a. abdomen.
  b. lungs.
  c. joints.
  d. all of the above

53. Accumulation of excess fluid in the peritoneal cavity is called:
  a. ascites.
  b. edema.
  c. peritonitis.
  d. sepsis.

54. What is sputum?
  a. gastric fluid
  b. nasal secretions
  c. phlegm
  d. saliva

55. Sputum is collected in the diagnosis and monitoring of:
  a. ascites.
  b. meningitis.
  c. strep throat.
  d. tuberculosis.

56. What test is used to diagnose cystic fibrosis?
    a. cerebrospinal fluid analysis
    b. occult blood
    c. nasopharyngeal culture
    d. sweat chloride

57. Synovial fluid is typically collected in a(n):
    a. EDTA or heparin tube.
    b. nonadditive tube.
    c. sterile tube .
    d. all of the above

58. Synovial fluid can be tested to identify:
    a. arthritis.
    b. gout.
    c. inflammation.
    d. all of the above

59. A process called iontophoresis is used to collect:
    a. amniotic fluid.
    b. semen.
    c. sweat.
    d. tears.

60. Bone marrow is typically aspirated from the:
    a. cranium.
    b. iliac crest.
    c. femur.
    d. wrist bone.

61. Bone marrow is studied to identify:
    a. arthritis.
    b. blood disorders.
    c. diabetes.
    d. osteoporosis.

62. A breath specimen can be used to detect:
    a. cystic fibrosis.
    b. *Helicobacter pylori.*

    c. pertussis.
    d. tuberculosis.

63. Which of the following tests may require a 24-hour stool specimen?
    a. Epstein–Barr virus
    b. thyroxine
    c. tuberculosis
    d. urobilinogen

64. A refrigerated stool specimen would be acceptable for all of the following EXCEPT:
    a. fat analysis.
    b. occult blood.
    c. ova and parasites.
    d. urobilinogen.

65. The guaiac test detects:
    a. cystic fibrosis.
    b. fetal lung maturity.
    c. occult blood.
    d. tuberculosis.

66. Which type of sample can be tested to detect chronic drug abuse?
    a. blood
    b. hair
    c. saliva
    d. urine

67. What type of specimen is required for a "rapid strep" test?
    a. blood sample
    b. throat swab
    c. random urine sample
    d. stool sample

68. What type of specimen is required for a biopsy?
    a. blood
    b. stool
    c. sweat
    d. tissue

ANSWERS AND EXPLANATIONS

1. **d.** fluid from within the sac that surrounds a fetus

2. **n.** test performed to determine which antibiotics are effective against a particular microorganism

3. **g.** liquid substances found in the body

4. **c.** describes a urine specimen collected from a sterile catheter inserted through the urethra into the urinary bladder

5. **a.** cerebrospinal fluids, a clear, colorless liquid circulating within the cavities surrounding the brain and spinal cord

6. **j.** method of obtaining a urine sample free of contaminates from the external genital area

7. **l.** culture and sensitivity, a process used to grow and identify microorganisms and also identify effective antibiotics to use against them

8. **m.** specimen obtained in the middle of urination rather than the beginning or end

9. **k.** originating from the nasopharynx as in a sample collected using a special flexible swab inserted gently through the nose into the nasopharynx

10. **h.** hidden blood such as detected in stool specimens using the guaiac test

11. **i.** intestinal parasites and their eggs (ova)

12. **f.** laboratory test to assess fertility and determine effectiveness of sterilization after vasectomy

13. **b.** collection of a urine specimen by inserting a needle into the urinary bladder and aspirating urine directly from it

14. **o.** test used to diagnose cystic fibrosis primarily in children and adolescents younger than 20 years of age

15. **e.** urinalysis, a laboratory test that includes a physical, chemical, and microscopic analysis of a urine specimen

16. **p.** urinary tract infection

17. **d.** As a minimum, nonblood specimens should be labeled with the same identifying information as blood specimens. Most institutions also require information on the type and source of the specimen

18. **a.** Cerebrospinal fluid is obtained by a physician through lumbar puncture. It should be delivered to the lab STAT and analysis started immediately so that the specimen is not compromised.

19. **d.** Urine is the most frequently analyzed nonblood specimen.

20. **d.** Some components in a urine sample are not stable. If a specimen is not processed in a timely fashion, any bilirubin in the sample will break down to biliverdin, cellular elements will decompose, and bacteria will multiply.

21. **b.** Although not always required, a first morning (also called first voided or 8-hour) specimen is preferred for most urine studies as it is the most concentrated.

22. **c.** Specimens for routine urinalysis that cannot be transported or analyzed promptly can be held at room temperature if protected from light

for up to 2 hours. Specimens held longer should be refrigerated.

23. **d.** A routine urinalysis typically includes a physical, chemical, and microscopic analysis. Physical analysis notes the color, odor, transparency, and specific gravity of the specimen. Chemical analysis typically involves dipping a reagent strip (see Fig. 11-11) into the specimen to detect the presence of bacteria, blood, white blood cells, protein, glucose, and other substances. A microscopic analysis of urine sediment identifies urine components such as casts, cells, and crystals.

24. **b.** The most common reason for ordering a culture and sensitivity (C&S) on a urine specimen is to diagnose urinary tract infection (UTI). A urine C&S can detect the presence of UTI by culturing (growing) and identifying microorganisms present in the urine. When microorganisms are identified, an antibiotic susceptibility is performed to determine which antibiotics are effective against the microorganism.

25. **a.** Urine cytology studies look for the presence of abnormal cells that have been shed from the urinary tract into the urine.

26. **d.** Urine drug screening can be used to detect illegal drug use, abuse or unwarranted use of prescription drugs, and use of performance-enhancing steroids as well as to monitor therapeutic drug use to minimize withdrawal symptoms or confirm drug overdose.

27. **c.** Pregnancy can be confirmed by testing urine for the presence of human chorionic gonadotropin, a hormone produced by cells within the developing placenta that appears in serum and urine approximately 8–10 days after conception or fertilization.

28. **b.** Although a random urine specimen can be used for testing, the first morning specimen is preferred because it is more concentrated and therefore would have the highest human chorionic gonadotropin concentration.

29. **c.** A random urine is typically used for routine urinalysis. Random refers only to the timing of the specimen and not the method of collection.

30. **a.** The first morning specimen is the usually the most concentrated.

31. **a.** The standard glucose tolerance test requires individual urine specimens collected serially at specific times that correspond with the timing of blood collection, such as fasting, 0.5 hour, 1 hour, and so on. A creatinine clearance test requires a 24-hour urine specimen. A pregnancy test requires a single concentrated urine specimen. A urine culture and sensitivity requires a midstream clean-catch specimen collected in a sterile container.

32. **d.** A 24-hour urine specimen is collected to allow quantitative analysis of a urine analyte. Collection of all urine voided in the 24-hour period is critical. A special large collection container (Fig. 13-1) is required. The best time to begin a 24-hour collection is when the patient wakes in the morning, typically between 6 and 8 AM. The first morning specimen is from the previous 24-hours and must be voided and discarded before timing is started. All urine voided over the next 24

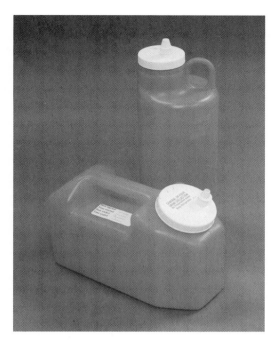

■ Figure 13-1 ■

Two styles of 24-hour urine specimen collection containers.

hours is collected, including the next morning's specimen.

33. d. A double-voided or fractional specimen is collected to compare the urine concentrations of an analyte to its concentration in the blood. It is most commonly used to test urine for glucose and ketones. A urine creatinine clearance requires collection of a 24-hour, refrigerated urine specimen and a blood creatinine specimen.

34. a. A double-voided or fractional specimen is collected to compare the urine concentrations of an analyte to its concentration in the blood. It is most commonly used to test urine for glucose and ketones.

35. a. A urine culture and sensitivity is most often ordered to detect uri-

nary tract infection. It requires collection of a midstream clean-catch specimen into a sterile container. A creatinine clearance requires a 24-hour urine specimen, A glucose tolerance test requires individual urine specimens collected serially at specific times that correspond with the timing of blood collection. A routine urinalysis requires a regular voided random urine specimen.

36. c. A midstream urine collection is performed to obtain a specimen that is free of genital secretions, pubic hair, and bacteria surrounding the urinary opening. To collect a midstream urine specimen, void initial urine into the toilet; interrupt the urine flow momentarily; restart urine flow and collect a sufficient amount of urine into a container; void excess urine flow into the toilet.

37. d. A midstream clean-catch urine collection is typically performed to obtain a specimen for culture and sensitivity testing to detect urinary tract infection. It is important that the specimen is free of genital secretions, pubic hair, and bacteria surrounding the urinary opening. This requires cleaning of the genital area before collecting the specimen midstream into a sterile container (Fig. 13-2) as well as prompt processing to prevent overgrowth of microorganisms present, decomposition of the specimen, and misinterpretation of results.

38. d. A suprapubic urine specimen is collected in a sterile syringe by inserting a needle directly into the urinary bladder and aspirating the urine directly from the bladder. Suprapubic collection is used for

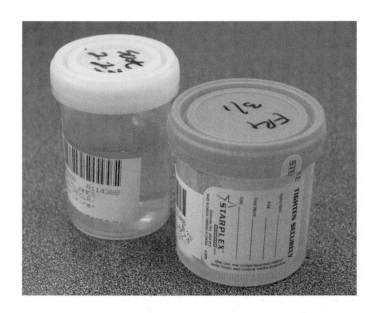

■ FIGURE 13-2 ■
Urine specimens collected in sterile containers for C&S testing.

samples for microbial analysis or cytology studies.

39. b. Alpha-fetoprotein (AFP) is an antigen normally present in the human fetus that is also found in amniotic fluid and maternal serum. Abnormal AFP levels may indicate problems in fetal development such as neural tube defects. AFP testing is initially performed on maternal serum, and abnormal results are confirmed by amniotic fluid AFP testing.

40. c. Amniotic fluid is the clear, almost colorless-to-pale yellow fluid that fills the membrane (amnion or amniotic sac) that contains a fetus within the uterus. It is obtained by transabdominal amniocentesis, a procedure that involves inserting a needle through the mother's abdominal wall into the uterus and aspirating approximately 10 mL of fluid from the amniotic sac.

41. b. The primary reason for collecting spinal fluid is to diagnose meningi-

tis. An increased white blood cell count in spinal fluid is most often associated with bacterial or viral meningitis.

42. d. Routine tests performed on spinal fluid include cell counts, glucose, chloride, and total protein. Other tests are performed if indicated. Hemoglobin, the iron-containing pigment of red blood cells, is not normally found in spinal fluid because red blood cells are not found in spinal fluid unless there is a "traumatic tap" in which blood enters as the lumbar puncture is performed.

43. a. A basal tube gastric analysis involves aspirating a sample of gastric secretions by means of a tube passed through the mouth and throat (oropharynx) or nose and throat (nasopharynx) into the stomach following a period of fasting. This sample is tested to determine acidity before stimulation. After the basal sample has been collected, a gastric stimulant, most commonly histamine or pentagastrin, is administered intravenously and several more samples are collected at timed intervals. Serum gastrin levels may also be collected.

44. **d.** Nasopharyngeal culture swabs are collected to detect the presence of microorganisms that cause diphtheria, meningitis, pneumonia, and whooping cough (pertussis).

45. **d.** Saliva specimens are increasingly being used to monitor hormone levels and detect alcohol and drug abuse because they can be collected quickly and easily in a noninvasive manner. Detection of drugs in saliva is a sign of recent drug use.

46. **a.** Semen analysis is used to assess fertility and also to determine the effectiveness of sterilization after vasectomy.

47. **a.** Semen specimens should be collected in sterile containers, kept warm, and delivered to the lab immediately, which means an on-site collection is ideal. Semen specimens should *never* be collected in a condom. Condoms often contain spermicides, which kill sperm and invalidate test results.

48. **c.** Spinal fluid is obtained through lumbar puncture. Peritoneal fluid is aspirated from the peritoneal cavity; pleural fluid is aspirated from the pleural cavity; and synovial fluid is aspirated from joint cavities.

49. **d.** Serous fluid is a pale yellow, watery fluid found between the double-layered membranes that enclose the pleural, pericardial, and peritoneal cavities and is identified according to the cavity of origin as pleural, pericardial, or peritoneal.

50. **a.** Peritoneal fluid is aspirated from within the membranes lining the abdominal cavity. Pleural fluid comes from the lungs. Pericardial fluid comes from the pericardial sac surrounding the heart. Spinal fluid comes from the cavities surrounding the brain and spinal cord.

51. **d.** Fluid from joint cavities is called synovial fluid. It is a clear, pale yellow, viscous fluid that lubricates and decreases friction in moveable joints. It is normally present in small amounts but increases when inflammation is present. It can be tested to identify or differentiate arthritis, gout, and other inflammatory conditions. Pleural fluid comes from the lungs. Pericardial fluid comes from the pericardial sac surrounding the heart. Peritoneal fluid comes from within the membranes that line the abdominal cavity.

52. **b.** Pleural fluid is aspirated from within the pleural membranes in the lungs. Peritoneal fluid is aspirated from within the membranes that line the abdominal cavity. Synovial fluid is aspirated from joint cavities.

53. **a.** Accumulation of excess fluid in the peritoneal cavity is called ascites (a-si'-tez). Edema is the accumulation of excess fluid in the tissues. Peritonitis is inflammation of the peritoneum, the membranes lining the abdominal cavity. Sepsis is the spread of infection into the blood stream.

54. **c.** Sputum is mucus or phlegm that is ejected from the trachea, bronchi, and lungs through deep coughing.

55. **d.** Sputum specimens are sometimes collected in the diagnosis or moni-

toring of lower respiratory tract infections such as tuberculosis.

56. d. A sweat chloride test analyzes sweat for chloride content in the diagnosis of cystic fibrosis in children and adolescents. Patients with cystic fibrosis have abnormally high (2–5 times normal) levels of chloride in their sweat.

57. d. Synovial fluid is typically collected in three tubes: EDTA or heparin for cell counts, identification of crystals, and smear preparation; a sterile tube for culture and sensitivity; and a nonadditive tube for macroscopic appearance, chemistry, and immunology tests and to observe clot formation.

58. d. Synovial fluid is normally present in small amounts but increases when inflammation is present. It can be tested to identify or differentiate arthritis, gout, and other inflammatory conditions.

59. c. A sweat chloride test involves transporting pilocarpine (a sweat-stimulating drug) into the skin by means of electrical stimulation (iontophoresis) from electrodes placed on the skin. Sweat is collected, weighed to determine the volume, and analyzed for chloride content.

60. b. To obtain bone marrow, a physician inserts a special large-gauge needle into the bone marrow in the iliac crest (hip bone) or sternum (breast bone).

61. b. Because it is the site of blood cell production, bone marrow may be aspirated or withdrawn and examined to detect and identify blood disorders.

62. b. Breath specimens are collected and analyzed in the detection of *Helicobacter pylori,* a type of bacteria that secretes substances that damage the lining of the stomach, causing chronic gastritis and leading to peptic ulcer disease.

63. d. Urobilinogen testing requires a 24-hour refrigerated stool specimen.

64. c. Stool specimens for detection of parasites or their eggs should be kept at body temperature (37° C). Twenty-four-, 48-, or 72-hour stool collections for fat and urobilinogen are refrigerated throughout the collection period. Refrigeration will not affect occult blood testing.

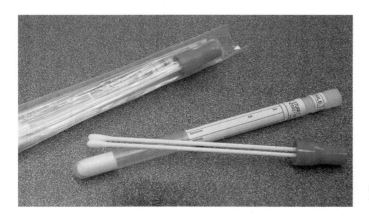

■ Figure 13-3 ■
Throat swab and transport tube.

65. **c.** The guaiac or occult blood test (see Fig. 11-9) detects occult (hidden) blood in feces.

66. **b.** Samples of hair are sometimes analyzed to detect drugs of abuse. Hair can show evidence of chronic drug use rather than recent use. Use of hair samples for drug testing is advantageous because hair cannot easily be altered or tampered with and is easy to obtain. Blood, saliva, and urine drug testing show evidence of recent drug use.

67. **b.** A throat swab (Fig. 13-3) is used for "rapid strep" tests. Results are typically ready in minutes.

68. **d.** A biopsy involves collection of a tissue sample.

14 COMPUTERS AND SPECIMEN HANDLING AND PROCESSING

REVIEW QUESTIONS

Match the term with the BEST description.

1. _____ accession number
2. _____ aerosol
3. _____ aliquot
4. _____ analyte
5. _____ barcode
6. _____ central processing
7. _____ CPU
8. _____ centrifugation
9. _____ cursor
10. _____ data
11. _____ hardware
12. _____ icon
13. _____ ID code
14. _____ impermeable
15. _____ input
16. _____ interface
17. _____ LIS
18. _____ menu
19. _____ mnemonic
20. _____ monitor
21. _____ networking
22. _____ online
23. _____ output
24. _____ password
25. _____ pneumatic tube
26. _____ pre-analytical
27. _____ RAM
28. _____ ROM
29. _____ software
30. _____ storage
31. _____ user manual

a. central processing unit of a computer
b. coded instructions needed to control the hardware that processes computer data
c. computer is connected to the system and operational
d. computer unit containing the display screen
e. connect for the purpose of interaction
f. data entered into a computer
g. does not allow passage of fluids
h. equipment used to process data
i. flashing marker on a computer screen that indicates the starting point for input
j. general term for a substance undergoing analysis
k. image that signifies a computer application (program or document)
l. information collected for analysis or computation
m. laboratory information system
n. linking computers for the purpose of sharing information or resources
o. list of options to choose from
p. location where all specimens are received and prepared for testing
q. handbook containing specimen collection information

r. memory-aiding
s. permanent computer memory that instructs the computer to carry out user-requested operations
t. place for keeping computer data
u. portion of a specimen used for testing
v. before testing
w. processed information generated by the computer
x. secret word or phrase used to enter a computer system
y. separating substances of different densities by spinning them in a special machine at a high number of revolutions per minute
z. series of black bars and white spaces representing a code for numbers or letters
aa. substance released in the form of a fine mist
bb. temporary computer data storage
cc. transportation system that uses pressurized air to move containers of specimens from one location to another through a tube that connects both locations
dd. unique number given to each test request
ee. unique code used to identify a computer user

Choose the BEST answer.

32. To be considered computer literate an individual must be able to:
a. demonstrate a willingness to adapt to changes that computers are making on quality of life.
b. perform basic computer operations to complete required tasks.
c. understand the computer and its functions.
d. all of the above

33. A group of computers linked for the purpose of sharing information is called a:
a. LIS.
b. network.
c. node.
d. any of the above

34. Computer input can come from:
a. barcode scanners.
b. keyboards.
c. light pens.
d. all of the above

35. Computer memory bytes are:
a. peripherals.
b. glitches in memory storage.
c. individual characters of data.
d. data storage disks.

36. All of the following are functions of a computer central processing unit EXCEPT:
a. instructs the computer to carry out user-requested operations
b. manages the processing and completion of user-required tasks
c. performs mathematical processes and logical comparisons of data
d. provides visible display of information being processed

37. Random access memory (RAM):
a. can be lost when the computer is turned off.
b. instructs the computer to carry out user-requested operations.

c. is called firmware.
d. is permanent memory installed by the manufacturer.

38. Computer peripherals include all the following EXCEPT:
a. barcode reader.
b. joystick.
c. modem.
d. central processing unit.

39. Systems software:
a. controls normal computer operation.
b. includes graphics, spreadsheet, and word processing programs.
c. refers to programs from software companies.
d. all of the above

40. The laboratory has a computerized LIS. Once an inpatient specimen has been collected by a phlebotomist and returned to the laboratory, what occurs next?
a. a collection list is generated
b. collection labels are printed
c. patient information is entered into the system
d. specimens are verified

41. A computer terminal is the:
a. computer workstation with a keyboard and monitor as a minimum.
b. monitor on which information is displayed.
c. end of the electrical cord that plugs into the computer.
d. none of the above

42. The unit with a screen that displays text as it is entered into a computer is called a:
a. central processing unit.
b. cursor.
c. modem.
d. monitor.

43. Logging on is the process of:
    a. accessing the internet from a computer station.
    b. entering a password to gain access to a computer system.
    c. turning on the computer.
    d. using icons and menus.

44. To process input data, a computer user must:
    a. log off.
    b. move the cursor.
    c. press the enter key.
    d. select an icon.

45. The process of verifying orders allows the user to:
    a. confirm that the test is appropriate for the patient's condition.
    b. make certain the test was ordered by a physician.
    c. see and review entered information.
    d. all of the above

46. The "order inquiry" function allows the user to:
    a. check the diagnosis of a patient.
    b. delete duplicate test orders.
    c. find errors in patient identification.
    d. retrieve all test orders on a patient.

47. Which of the following is confidential and unique to a single computer user?
    a. icon
    b. password
    c. ID code
    d. all of the above

48. Typical functions of laboratory information systems include:
    a. entering test results.
    b. ordering tests.
    c. printing specimen labels.
    d. all of the above

49. Which of the following does the laboratory use to identify a specimen throughout the testing process?
    a. accession number
    b. hospital number

    c. mnemonic code
    d. tech code

For questions 43 through 45, use the choices indicated by the arrows in Figure 14-1.

50. Which arrow points to the time the specimen is to be collected?

51. Which arrow points to the type of specimen required?

52. Which arrow points to the specimen accession number?

53. Your hospital uses computer-generated specimen labels. What information must be added to the label whenever a specimen is collected?
    a. patient's date of birth
    b. medical record number
    c. patient's full name
    d. phlebotomist's initials

54. A bidirectional computer interface allows:
    a. data to go back and forth between two systems.
    b. the RAM storage capacity of an individual computer to double.
    c. two individuals to use the same computer at the same time.
    d. all of the above

55. All of the following are characteristics of an intranet EXCEPT:
    a. can connect multiple LIS
    b. connects computers within a company
    c. connects LIS with networks outside the company
    d. cannot be connected to the internet

56. In computer language, "hard copy" is:
    a. data printed on paper.
    b. information displayed on the CRT.
    c. information stored on the hard drive.
    d. all of the above

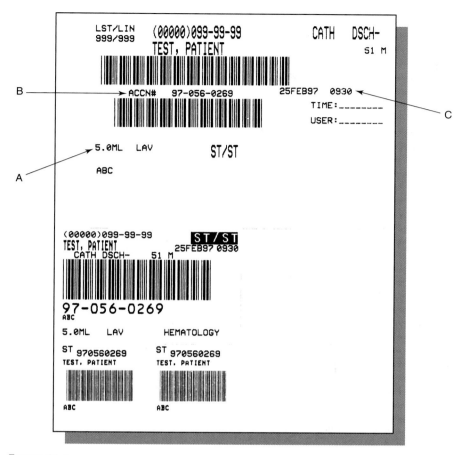

■ FIGURE 14-1 ■

A computerized label generated when the requisition order is entered. (Cerner Corp, Kansas City, MO.)

57. Which of the following describes a current trend in laboratory testing?
   a. microchip laboratory technology is increasing
   b. remote reference laboratory testing is increasing
   c. use of barcode labeling systems is increasing
   d. all of the above

58. Why is specimen handling so important?

   a. effects of improper handling are not always obvious
   b. improper handling can affect quality of results
   c. many lab errors occur in the pre-analytical phase
   d. all of the above

59. Proper specimen handling begins:
   a. as soon as the specimen is collected.
   b. during the venipuncture or skin puncture.
   c. when the patient is identified.
   d. when the test is ordered.

60. You are the only phlebotomist in an outpatient drawing station. A physician orders a test with which you are unfamiliar. What is the appropriate action to take?
    a. call the physician's office for assistance
    b. draw both a serum and a plasma specimen
    c. refer to the user manual for instructions
    d. send the patient to another drawing station

61. The number of tube inversions required during specimen collection depends on the:
    a. difficulty of the draw.
    b. presence or absence of an additive in the tube.
    c. priority of collection status.
    d. all of the above

62. Inadequate mixing of an anticoagulant tube can lead to:
    a. failure of the specimen to clot properly.
    b. hemolysis of the specimen.
    c. lipemia of the specimen.
    d. microclots in the specimen.

63. Which tube does not require mixing?
    a. serum separator tube
    b. plasma separator tube
    c. glass red top
    d. gray top

64. Transporting tubes of blood with the stopper up:
    a. aids clot formation.
    b. minimizes aerosol formation when the tube is opened.
    c. reduces agitation-caused hemolysis.
    d. all of the above

65. The National Committee for Clinical Laboratory Standards (NCCLS) and Occupational Safety and Health Administration (OSHA) guidelines require specimen transport bags to have all of the following EXCEPT:
    a. a biohazard label.
    b. a separate pocket for paperwork.
    c. shock resistance features.
    d. liquid-tight closures.

66. Specimens transported by courier or other air or ground mail systems must follow guidelines defined by the:
    a. Department of Transportation (DOT).
    b. Federal Aviation Administration (FAA).
    c. Occupational Safety and Health Administration (OSHA).
    d. all of the above

67. Which of the following actions will compromise the quality of a specimen?
    a. drawing a blood urea nitrogen level in an amber serum tube
    b. mixing a serum separator tube
    c. partially filling a liquid EDTA tube
    d. transporting a cold agglutinin specimen in a 37° C heat block

68. Which of the following analytes is broken down when exposed to light?
    a. bilirubin
    b. urine porphyrin
    c. vitamin B_{12}
    d. all of the above

69. Some specimens require cooling to:
    a. prevent activation of a cold agglutinin.
    b. prevent clotting.
    c. separate serum more completely.
    d. slow metabolic processes.

70. Chilling can cause erroneous results for this analyte.
    a. ammonia
    b. lactic acid
    c. potassium
    d. renin

71. Which specimen needs to be transported on ice (Fig. 14-2)?
    a. ammonia
    b. bilirubin
    c. complete blood count
    d. cold agglutinin

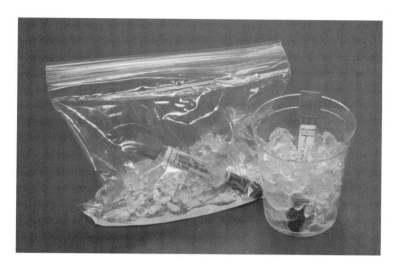

■ FIGURE 14-2 ■
Specimen in ice slurry.

72. The best way to chill a specimen is to:
   a. immerse it in a slurry of ice and water.
   b. place it in a glass of ice cubes.
   c. rubber band it to a large piece of ice.
   d. any of the above

73. How should a cryofibrinogen specimen be transported?
   a. at room temperature
   b. in a 37° C heat block
   c. on ice
   d. protected from light

74. The most likely reason a phlebotomist would wrap a specimen in aluminum foil (Fig. 14-3) would be to:
   a. cool it down quickly.
   b. cover up contamination on the tube.
   c. keep it warm.
   d. protect it from light.

75. A specimen must be transported at or near normal body temperature. Which of the following temperatures meets this requirement?
   a. 25° C
   b. 37° C
   c. 50° C
   d. 98° C

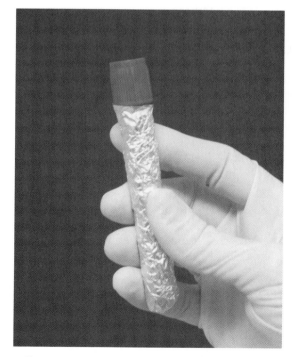

■ FIGURE 14-3 ■
Specimen wrapped in aluminum foil.

76. According to National Committee for Clinical Laboratory Standards (NCCLS), the maximum time limit for separating serum or plasma from cells is:
    a. 15 minutes from the time of collection.
    b. 30 minutes from the time of collection.
    c. 1 hour from the time of collection.
    d. 2 hours from the time of collection.

77. Separator gels prevent glycolysis:
    a. after the specimen has been centrifuged.
    b. as soon as the specimen is collected.
    c. in serum tubes only.
    d. when the specimen is adequately mixed.

78. A glucose specimen collected in a sodium fluoride tube is stable at room temperature for:
    a. 6 hours.
    b. 12 hours.
    c. 24 hours.
    d. 48 hours.

79. Which specimen has processing and testing priority over all other specimens?
    a. ASAP
    b. fasting
    c. STAT
    d. timed

80. All of the following specimens need to be centrifuged EXCEPT:
    a. complete blood count in a lavender top
    b. creatinine collected in a serum separator tube
    c. potassium drawn in a heparin tube
    d. all of the above

81. Slides made from EDTA specimens must be prepared within 1 hour of specimen collection to:

a. ensure they are made before the specimen is fully clotted.
b. minimize platelet clumping on the smear.
c. preserve the integrity of the blood cells and prevent artifact formation.
d. all of the above

82. What protective equipment is required when processing specimens?
    a. face shield
    b. fluid-resistant apron
    c. gloves
    d. all of the above

83. Which of the following conditions would be a reason to reject a specimen for analysis?
    a. incomplete identification
    b. tube is expired
    c. insufficient quantity of specimen
    d. all of the above

84. Reasons to reject a specimen for analysis include all of the following conditions EXCEPT:
    a. a bilirubin specimen that is icteric
    b. a complete blood count specimen that has clots in it
    c. an electrolyte specimen that is hemolyzed
    d. a fasting glucose specimen that is lipemic

85. A delay in processing longer than 2 hours can lead to erroneously decreased results for:
    a. carbon dioxide.
    b. glucose.
    c. ionized calcium.
    d. all of the above

86. An aliquot is a:
    a. filter used to separate serum from cells.
    b. portion of a specimen being tested.
    c. substance being tested.
    d. tube used to balance a centrifuge.

87. Which specimen will be rejected automatically if the tube is not filled until the normal vacuum is exhausted?
    a. complete blood count
    b. electrolytes
    c. glucose
    d. protime

88. Vigorous tube mixing can cause hemolysis, which affects test results of all the following EXCEPT:
    a. hemoglobin.
    b. lactic dehydrogenase.
    c. magnesium.
    d. potassium.

89. Tests performed on plasma are:
    a. collected in anticoagulant tubes.
    b. drawn in green top tubes.
    c. include most hematology tests.
    d. obtained from clotted blood.

90. Chemistry tests are often collected in heparin tubes to:
    a. ensure adequate clotting of the specimen.
    b. minimize effects of hemolysis.
    c. reduce turnaround time.
    d. all of the above

91. It is important to note the type of heparin in a collection tube because:
    a. not all types of heparin prevent coagulation.
    b. some types of heparin can affect results of certain tests.
    c. some types of heparin do not require mixing.
    d. all of the above

92. To avoid airborne infection while processing specimens:
    a. apply the brake when stopping the centrifuge.
    b. "pop" the stoppers when opening tubes.
    c. pour specimens directly into aliquot tubes.
    d. use a stopper remover or cover the stopper with gauze when removing tube stoppers.

93. A nonadditive specimen is spun in a centrifuge (Fig. 14-4) to obtain:
    a. buffy coat.
    b. plasma.
    c. serum.
    d. whole blood.

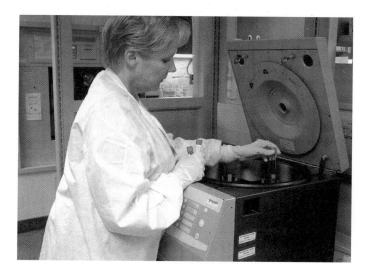

■ FIGURE 14-4 ■
Specimen processor loading a centrifuge.

94. If a serum specimen is not completely clotted before it is centrifuged the:
a. serum may clot.
b. specimen may have to be centrifuged again.
c. specimen may hemolyze.
d. all of the above

95. A serum specimen may take longer than normal to clot completely if the:
a. patient has a high white blood cell count.
b. patient is taking an anticoagulant medication.
c. specimen has been chilled.
d. all of the above

96. Which of the following tests would be most affected by contamination from a drop of perspiration?
a. blood urea nitrogen
b. complete blood count
c. electrolytes
d. glucose

97. Gloves containing powder are:
a. a likely source of specimen contamination.
b. ideal for collecting skin puncture specimens.
c. ideal for use in specimen processing.
d. very difficult to put on.

98. Minimum pre-centrifugation time for specimens drawn in serum separator tubes is:
a. 5 minutes.
b. 10 minutes.
c. 15 minutes.
d. 30 minutes.

99. Repeated centrifugation of a specimen can:
a. alter test results.
b. cause hemolysis.
c. deteriorate an analyte.
d. all of the above

100. Which statement describes proper centrifuge operation?
a. balance specimens by placing tubes of equal volume and size opposite one another
b. centrifuge serum specimens before they have a chance to clot
c. never centrifuge serum specimens in the same centrifuge as plasma specimens
d. remove tube stoppers before placing specimen tubes in the centrifuge

101. If a tube stopper does not have a safety feature to prevent aerosol formation during removal:
a. cover the stopper with a 4 × 4 gauze while removing it.
b. remove stoppers behind a safety shield.
c. use a safety stopper removal device.
d. any of the above

102. Which of the following describes proper aliquot preparation?
a. cap or cover aliquot tubes after transferring the specimen
b. use transfer pipets instead of pouring specimens into aliquot tubes
c. never place serum or plasma from different additive tubes into the same aliquot tube
d. all of the above

ANSWERS AND EXPLANATIONS

1. **dd.** unique number given to each test request

2. **aa.** substance released in the form of a fine mist

3. **u.** portion of a specimen used for testing

4. **j.** general term for substance undergoing analysis

5. **z.** series of black bars and white spaces representing a code for numbers or letters

6. **p.** location where all specimens are received and prepared for testing

7. **a.** central processing unit of a computer

8. **y.** separating substances of different densities by spinning them in a special machine at a high number of revolutions per minute.

9. **i.** flashing marker on a computer screen that indicates the starting point for input

10. **l.** information collected for analysis or computation

11. **h.** equipment used to process data

12. **k.** image that signifies a computer application (program or document)

13. **ee.** unique code used to identify a computer user

14. **g.** does not allow passage of fluids

15. **f.** data entered into a computer

16. **e.** connect for the purpose of interaction

17. **m.** laboratory information system

18. **o.** list of options to choose from

19. **r.** memory-aiding

20. **d.** computer unit containing the display screen

21. **n.** linking computers for the purpose of sharing information or resources

22. **c.** computer is connected to the system and operational

23. **w.** processed information generated by the computer

24. **x.** secret word or phrase used to enter a computer system

25. **cc.** transportation system that uses pressurized air to move containers of specimens from one location to another through a tube that connects both locations

26. **v.** before testing

27. **bb.** random access memory, temporary computer data storage

28. **s.** read-only memory, permanent computer memory that instructs the computer to carry out user-requested operations

29. **b.** coded instructions needed to control hardware that processes computer data

30. **t.** place for keeping computer data

31. **q.** handbook containing specimen collection information

32. **d.** Computer literacy involves (1) the ability to understand a computer and how it functions, (2) the ability to perform basic computer operations, and (3) the willingness to adapt to changes that computers are making on quality of life.

33. **b.** A group of computers linked for the purpose of sharing information is called a computer network. An LIS is

a computer laboratory information system. A node is an individual computer station that is part of a computer network.

34. d. Input is data entered into a computer. Data can be entered in a number of different ways, including the use of barcode scanners, keyboards, and light pens.

35. c. Computer memory bytes are individual characters of data that have been assigned a unique location in random access memory (Fig. 14-5).

36. d. Visible display of data is a function of the computer monitor or display screen, not the central processing unit.

37. a. RAM is temporary storage of data that can be lost if it is not saved to permanent storage before the computer is turned off. Read only mem-

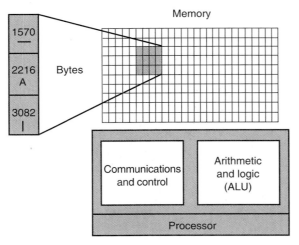

■ FIGURE 14-5 ■
The three elements of the central processing unit, showing memory bytes (characters of data) represented by blocks that have been assigned a unique location in RAM (random access memory). (Adapted from Trainor, D., & Krasnewich, D. (1994). Computers! New York: McGraw-Hill.)

ory (ROM) is permanent memory installed by the manufacturer that instructs the computer to carry out user-requested operations. ROM has characteristics of both hardware and software and is sometimes called firmware to lessen confusion.

38. d. The central processing unit (CPU) is the command center of the computer. Things that attach to the CPU such as barcode readers, joysticks, and modems are referred to as peripherals.

39. a. There are two types of software: systems software and applications software. Systems software controls normal operation of the computer. Applications software refers to programs developed by software companies or computer programmers to perform specific tasks and include graphics, spreadsheet, and word processing programs.

40. d. After returning to the lab with a specimen, the first thing a phlebotomist must do is verify collection of the specimen so that nursing personnel will know that the specimen has been collected and no one else will attempt to collect the specimen. Patient information is entered into the system and labels and collection lists are generated before the specimen is collected.

41. a. As a minimum, a computer terminal (Fig. 14-6) consists of a monitor and a keyboard.

42. d. The unit that contains the screen on which text is displayed is called a monitor. There are two types of monitor display screens: traditional CRTs (cathode ray tubes) and newer LCDs (liquid crystal displays) or flat screen computer monitors.

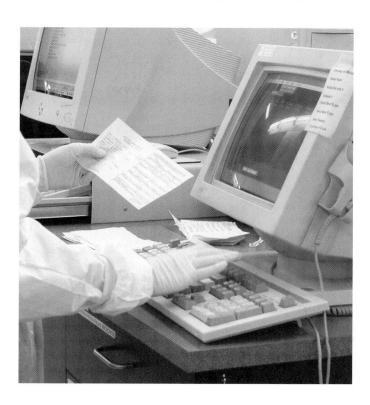

■ FIGURE 14-6 ■

A computer terminal in the specimen-
processing area of the laboratory.

43. **b.** Entering a password to gain access to a computer or computer system is called logging on.

44. **c.** After necessary information has been input or entered into the computer, the enter key must be pressed for information to be processed. When entering patient information in a LIS, the cursor will automatically reset itself at the correct point for data input after the enter key is pressed.

45. **c.** The process of verifying an order allows the user to see and review information that has been entered. It is not a phlebotomist's duty to determine the appropriateness of a physician's order. Confirmation of the test order takes place before the specimen is collected.

46. **d.** The "order inquiry" function allows the user to retrieve any or all test orders on a patient.

47. **b.** A password is confidential and unique to a single user. It allows access to the computer and identifies the user. ID codes are not always confidential. An icon is an image that represents a document or software program. It is the same for all users.

48. **d.** Although specific tasks that LIS perform are defined by and customized for a particular facility, typical tasks that LIS perform include ordering tests, printing specimen labels, and entering test results.

49. **a.** A unique number called an accession number is given to each test order.

This number is used throughout the collection, handling, processing, and testing process to identify a specimen with its test order. Each test order will have a different accession number. A hospital or medical record number is also unique to the patient but remains the same throughout the patient's hospital stay. A mnemonic code is a memory-aiding code or abbreviation. A tech code is used to identify a person entering data into a computer system.

50. **c.** Military or 24-hour time is used on computer-generated labels to eliminate confusion between AM and PM. The specimen in the requisition example in Figure 14-1 should be collected at 0930 or 9:30 AM.

51. **a.** The code on the requisition in Figure 14-1 says 5.0 ML LAV, which indicates that a 5 mL lavender top tube should be collected.

52. **b.** The accession number on the requisition example in Figure 14-1 is 97-056-0269. An accession number is a unique number generated when the test request is entered.

53. **d.** A computer-generated label typically contains the patient's name, medical record number, and patient's date of birth or age. The time of collection and the phlebotomist's initials are added to the label on the collection tube immediately after the specimen is collected.

54. **a.** A bidirectional computer interface allows data to go back and forth between two computer systems.

55. **d.** An intranet is a network of computers within a company. An intranet can be connected to the Internet to connect it with outside companies.

56. **a.** In computer language "hard copy" is data printed on paper.

57. **d.** Current trends in laboratory testing include the increasing use of microchip technology in testing, more and more tests being performed by off-site reference laboratories, and increased use of barcode labeling systems to increase efficiency and minimize errors.

58. **d.** Proper handling of specimens is important for quality results. It has been estimated that 46–68% of all lab errors occur in the pre-analytical phase. Proper handling is important because effects of mishandling are not always obvious, and testing personnel may not be aware that the integrity of a specimen is compromised.

59. **d.** Proper specimen handling begins when a test is ordered and continues throughout the testing process.

60. **c.** Procedures and policies concerning specimen collection can be found in the laboratory user manual. A phlebotomist who is unfamiliar with a requested test should consult the user manual for instructions.

61. **b.** The number of times a specimen tube should be inverted (Fig. 14-7) depends on whether the tube contains an additive and manufacturer instructions. Nonadditive tubes do not require inverting. Additive tubes typically require from 3 to 8 inversions, depending on manufacturer's instructions, to adequately mix the additive with the blood in the tube. The difficulty of the draw and priority of collection have no relationship to the number of tube inversions required.

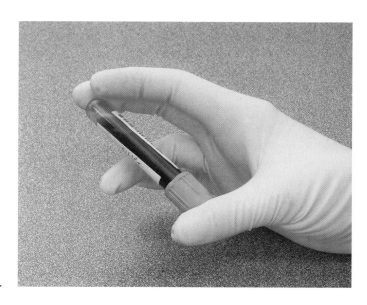

■ FIGURE 14-7 ■
Mixing of anticoagulated tube.

62. d. Inadequate mixing of an anticoagulant tube can lead to microclots in the specimen. An anticoagulant specimen is not supposed to clot. Hemolysis can occur if the specimen is mixed too vigorously. Lipemia is a patient condition that has nothing to do with mixing the specimen.

63. c. A nonadditive or glass red top does not require tube inversions or mixing. A serum separator tube requires mixing to mix the clot activator with the specimen. Both a plasma separator tube and a gray top contain additives that require mixing. Plastic red top tubes typically contain a clot activator additive such as ground glass or silica and do require mixing.

64. d. Transporting tubes with the stopper up aids clotting of serum tubes, allows fluids to drain away from the stopper to minimize aerosol generation when the stopper is removed, and reduces the chance of hemolysis caused by agitation of the tube contents during transportation.

65. c. NCCLS and OSHA guidelines require a specimen transport bag to have a biohazard logo, a liquid-tight closure, and a slip pocket for paperwork. Pneumatic tube system specimen carriers (Fig. 14-8) need to have shock-resistant features to prevent breakage of specimens.

66. d. Specimens transported by courier or other air or ground mail systems must follow guidelines defined by the DOT, FAA, and OSHA.

67. c. The additive in a tube is designed to work most effectively with an amount of blood that fills the tube until the normal vacuum is exhausted. Results of a partially filled tube may be compromised. Although a blood urea nitrogen level does not need to be protected from light, it would not hurt to draw it in an amber serum tube. Serum separator tubes should be mixed. A cold agglutinin specimen should be placed in a 37° C heat block for transport.

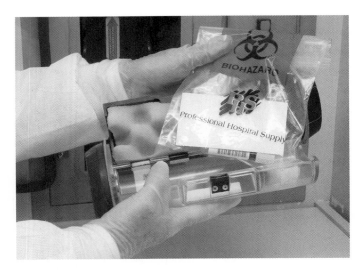

■ FIGURE 14-8 ■
Specimen received in pneumatic tube.

68. **d.** Bilirubin, urine porphyrins, and vitamin B_{12} are all analytes that can be broken down in the presence of light.

69. **d.** Cooling slows certain metabolic processes that continue even after a blood specimen is collected. Some analytes are more affected than others and must be cooled immediately after collection and during transportation. A cold agglutinin is activated when the specimen is cooled and therefore must be transported at body temperature. Cooling may delay clotting; however, it does not prevent it or cause a specimen to separate more completely.

70. **c.** The energy needed to pump potassium into the cells is provided by glycolysis. Cold inhibits glycolysis, causing potassium to leak from the cells, falsely elevating test results. Cooling can also cause hemolysis, which also elevates test results. If a potassium test is ordered along with other tests that require cooling, it must be collected in a separate tube that is not cooled. Ammonia, lactic acid, and renin require cooling for accurate test results.

71. **a.** Ammonia specimens are extremely volatile and must be transported ASAP on ice. Bilirubin specimens require protection from light. A complete blood count does not require special handling. A cold agglutinin must be transported at body temperature.

72. **a.** The best way to chill a specimen is to immerse it in a slurry of ice and water (see Fig. 14-2). Use of ice cubes without water added may prevent adequate cooling of the specimen. Specimens in contact with a solid piece of ice may freeze, resulting in hemolysis and possible breakdown of the analyte.

73. **b.** A cryofibrinogen specimen should be transported at body temperature, which is normally 37° C. Small portable heat blocks that hold a 37° C temperature for approximately 15 minutes are available.

74. **d.** The most likely reason a phlebotomist would wrap a specimen in aluminum foil (see Fig. 14-3) would be to protect it from light. A specimen that needs to be cooled quickly should be placed in an ice slurry. Heat blocks or special warmers are used to keep specimens warm. A contaminated tube should be wiped with disinfectant and placed in secondary bag or container.

75. **b.** Normal body temperature is approximately 37° C (98.6° F).

76. **d.** All specimens should be transported to the laboratory promptly. According to NCCLS guidelines, unless conclusive evidence indicates that longer times do not result in inaccuracy, specimens should be separated from the cells as soon as possible, with a maximum time limit of 2 hours.

77. **a.** Separator gel has a density between that of serum or plasma and cells. During centrifugation it undergoes a change in viscosity and ends up between the liquid portion of the specimen and the cells, becoming a physical barrier between the serum or plasma and the cells that prevents glycolysis. Figure 14-9 shows two SST tubes, one before and the other after centrifugation.

78. **c.** Sodium fluoride can prevent changes in glucose concentration for up to 24 hours at room temperature and up to 48 hours if the tube is refrigerated.

79. **c.** STAT or medical emergency specimens require immediate collection, processing, and testing and have priority over all other specimens.

80. **a.** A complete blood count is performed on whole blood and the specimen should never be centrifuged.

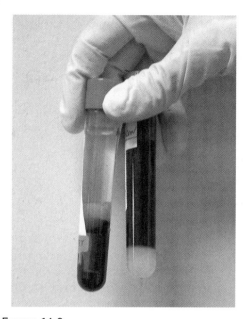

■ Figure 14-9 ■

Hemogard SSTs. (Becton Dickinson, Franklin Lakes, NJ.) *Right,* before being centrifuged. *Left,* after being centrifuged.

81. **c.** Prolonged contact with EDTA can change the staining characteristics of blood cells and result in artifact formation. To preserve the integrity of the blood cells and prevent artifact formation, slides made from EDTA specimens must be prepared within 1 hour of specimen collection.

82. **d.** OSHA regulations require the wearing of protective equipment when processing specimens. Protective equipment includes gloves, fully closed fluid-resistant lab coats or aprons, and protective face gear such as masks and goggles with side shields, or chin length face shields.

83. **d.** Reasons for rejecting a specimen for analysis include missing or incomplete identification, collection in an expired tube, and an insufficient

quantity of specimen (referred to as QNS or quantity not sufficient) to perform the test.

84. **a.** A bilirubin specimen would not be rejected for testing because it was icteric. Specimens with high bilirubin levels typically have an abnormal yellow color described as icteric. A complete blood count specimen with clots in it would be rejected because clots cause low results for cell counts, platelets counts in particular. Hemolysis invalidates electrolyte results, potassium results in particular. When a fasting specimen is lipemic, it is a clue that the specimen was not fasting. A nonfasting specimen may be rejected if a fasting specimen is specifically requested.

85. **d.** A delay in processing longer than 2 hours can lead to erroneously decreased results for carbon dioxide, glucose, and calcium.

86. **b.** An aliquot is a portion a specimen being tested. When several tests are to be performed on the same specimen, portions of the specimen are transferred into separate tubes so that each test has its own tube of specimen. Each portion is called an aliquot, and the tubes containing each portion are called aliquot tubes. Each aliquot tube is labeled with the same identifying information as the original tube.

87. **d.** A protime is a coagulation test collected in a light blue sodium citrate tube. Coagulation tests require a critical 9-to-1 ratio of blood to anticoagulant for test results to be valid. Therefore, an underfilled light blue top for a protime test would not be accepted for testing. All anticoagulant tubes should be filled until the vacuum is exhausted for best results.

However, with the exception of sodium citrate tubes, slightly underfilled anticoagulant tubes are usually accepted for testing. Underfilled serum tubes are almost always accepted for testing provided there is enough specimen to perform the test.

88. **a.** Hemolysis, regardless of the cause, affects lactic dehydrogenase, magnesium, and potassium levels. Hemolysis should not affect hemoglobin levels because the cells must be lysed in the testing process to measure hemoglobin. Other hematology tests, however, are affected by hemolysis and should not be performed on a hemolyzed specimen.

89. **a.** Plasma samples are obtained from blood collected in anticoagulant tubes. A tube containing an anticoagulant must be spun in a centrifuge to obtain plasma for testing. Green top tubes contain the anticoagulant heparin, but not all tests requiring plasma samples are collected in heparin. Hematology specimens are collected in lavender top tubes containing the anticoagulant EDTA, but the tests are performed on whole blood, not plasma. Clotted blood yields serum, not plasma.

90. **c.** The ideal specimen for many chemistry tests is serum. However, to obtain serum, the blood must first be allowed to clot completely before it can be centrifuged and separated. Complete clotting takes anywhere from 15 minutes in an SST to 30 minutes or more in other serum tubes, and even longer if the patient is taking blood thinners. Heparin is an anticoagulant. Anticoagulant specimens do not clot and can be spun in a centrifuge immediately to

obtain plasma for testing. Collecting chemistry specimens in heparin reduces turnaround time, especially for STAT tests.

91. **b.** There are three types of heparin: ammonium, sodium, and lithium heparin. Ammonium heparin is primarily found in capillary tubes for hematocrit determinations; however, sodium heparin and lithium heparin are commonly found in evacuated tubes. It is important to note the type of heparin in a collection tube to prevent interference in test results. For example, sodium heparin must not be used for electrolytes, because sodium is one of the electrolytes measured. Lithium heparin must not be used for lithium levels. All heparin tubes prevent coagulation regardless of the type of heparin they contain provided they are mixed properly, and all heparin tubes require mixing.

92. **d.** Stoppers can be removed using commercially available stopper removal devices or by use of robotics. When not using a stopper removal device the stopper should first be covered with a 4 × 4-inch gauze or tissue to catch any aerosol that may be released. In addition, the tube should be held behind a "splash shield" while the stopper is removed. Applying the break to stop a centrifuge, "popping" stoppers when opening tubes, and pouring specimens directly into aliquot tubes instead of using transfer pipettes are all activities that should be avoided because they can generate aerosols.

93. **c.** Blood in a nonadditive tube will eventually clot. When a clotted specimen is centrifuged, the clear liquid that separates from the cells is called serum. Blood in an anticoagulant tube does not clot. When an anticoagulant tube is centrifuged or allowed to settle, the clear liquid that separates from the cells is called plasma. The red blood cells are heaviest and are at the bottom. The white blood cells and platelets are lighter and form a thin layer on top of the red blood cells called the buffy coat. The plasma is on top. Whole blood is collected with an anticoagulant, but the specimen is not centrifuged.

94. **a.** If a serum specimen is not completely clotted before it is centrifuged the latent fibrin formation may clot the serum. A specimen should never be centrifuged more than once. Repeated centrifugation can cause analyte deterioration and hemolysis. Incomplete clotting does not normally cause hemolysis.

95. **d.** A serum specimen may take longer than normal to clot completely if the patient has a high white blood cell count or is taking anticoagulant medication. Chilling also delays clot formation.

96. **c.** Sweat contains sodium chloride. Sodium and chloride are two of the four electrolytes measured when a set of electrolytes is ordered. The other two electrolytes are potassium and bicarbonate.

97. **a.** Although it does make gloves easier to put on, glove powder is a common source of specimen contamination, especially when collecting skin puncture specimens or processing specimens.

98. **c.** Specimens drawn in serum separator tubes (SSTs) generally clot within 15 minutes. Consequently, to prevent latent fibrin formation in

the serum, the minimum pre-centrifugation time for an SST is 15 minutes.

99. d. A specimen should be centrifuged only once. Repeated centrifugation can cause hemolysis or otherwise deteriorate an analyte and lead to erroneous test results.

100. a. Proper centrifuge operation involves balancing the centrifuge by placing tubes of equal volume and size opposite one another. Specimens should never be centrifuged before they are completely clotted. Specimens should always be centrifuged with the stoppers on to prevent evaporation of the specimen and generation of aerosols. Plasma and serum specimens can be centrifuged at the same time in the same centrifuge.

101. d. If a tube stopper does not have a safety feature to prevent aerosol formation during removal, it should be covered with a 4 × 4 gauze, removed while the specimen is held behind a safety shield, or removed using a safety stopper removal device.

102. d. Proper aliquot preparation involves using transfer pipettes (Fig. 14-10) instead of pouring specimens into aliquot tubes, capping or covering tubes after aliquot preparation, and making separate aliquot tubes for serum or plasma specimens from different additive tubes.

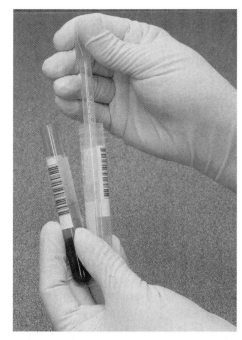

■ FIGURE **14-10** ■
Aliquoting a sample.

APPENDIX D: LISTING OF DEPARTMENTS AND TESTS

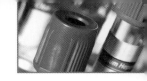

A. Listing of Departments and Tests
1. Department
   a. Tube Types Used
   b. Additives

c. Tests
d. Test Abbreviations
e Sample Considerations
f. Clinical Correlation

REVIEW QUESTIONS

Choose the BEST answer.

1. Another name and abbreviation for alanine transferase (ALT) is:
   a. ALP.
   b. AST.
   c. SGOT.
   d. SGPT.

2. A chemistry test that may require the
   patient to be in an upright position for a
   minimum of 30 minutes before specimen collection is:
   a. aldosterone.
   b. catecholamine.
   c. renin.
   d. Stypven time.

3. Which of the following specimens is collected in a royal blue top?
   a. aluminum
   b. chromium
   c. copper
   d. all of the above

4. A specimen for hemoglobin A1c goes to:
   a. chemistry.
   b. coagulation.
   c. hematology.
   d. microbiology.

5. Which of the following is a chemistry
   test collected in a lavender top tube?

   a. BUN
   b. CO
   c. ESR
   d. GC screen

6. Which of the following is an abbreviation for a type of antibody?
   a. IgA
   b. IgG
   c. IgM
   d. all of the above

7. Most coagulation tests require plasma
   specimens collected in:
   a. gray top tubes.
   b. lavender top tubes.
   c. light blue top tubes.
   d. plasma separator tubes.

8. Which of the following is a drug used in
   the treatment of epilepsy?
   a. carbamazepine
   b. lithium
   c. phenytoin
   d. theophylline

9. Which of the following is a hematology
   test?
   a. A/G ratio
   b. CEA
   c. differential
   d. glycosylated hemoglobin

10. Which test requires a minimum 12-hour fast before specimen collection?
   a. ADH
   b. CK-MB
   c. HDL/LDL
   d. uric acid

11. Which of the following tests is collected in a red top or SST?
   a. ammonia
   b. DIC panel
   c. Hgb A1c
   d. SPEP

12. Gel barrier tubes are not recommended for collection of a(n):
   a. acid phosphatase.
   b. alpha-fetoprotein.
   c. salicylate level.
   d. TSH.

13. Which test is used in the detection of allergies?
   a. CEA
   b. D-dimer
   c. ferritin
   d. RAST

14. Which of the following is a chemistry test performed on either whole blood or serum?
   a. AFB
   b. ANA
   c. cyclosporine
   d. plasminogen

15. Which test requires a whole blood specimen?
   a. CBC
   b. CMV
   c. CRP
   d. EBV

16. Immunology tests are most often performed on:
   a. plasma.
   b. serum.
   c. whole blood.
   d. urine.

17. Which of the following tube types can be used for blood bank tests?
   a. lavender top
   b. non-additive red top
   c. pink top
   d. all of the above

18. This test is used as a tumor marker.
   a. BMP
   b. CA 125
   c. HLA
   d. TIBC & Fe

19. Which tests are used in the diagnosis of pancreatitis?
   a. amylase, lipase
   b. BUN, creatinine
   c. H & H
   d. RPR, FTA

20. Name the type of specimen required and the department that performs the CMV test.
   a. plasma, chemistry
   b. serum, immunology
   c. urine, microbiology
   d. whole blood, hematology

21. This test requires whole blood collected from a stasis-free vein.
   a. C-reactive protein
   b. HBsAb
   c. lactic acid
   d. phosphorous

22. Identify the type of tube required and the department that performs the plasminogen test.
   a. green top, chemistry
   b. light blue top, coagulation
   c. red top or SST, chemistry
   d. yellow top, immunohematology

23. The microbiology department performs tests on:
   a. blood.
   b. sputum.
   c. urine.
   d. all of the above

24. Which of the following tubes is usually required for hematology tests?
    a. green top
    b. lavender top
    c. light blue top
    d. PPT

25. Which of the following is actually a panel of several tests?
    a. BMP
    b. DIC screen
    c. thyroid profile
    d. all of the above

26. An HLA specimen is collected in a tube containing:
    a. ACD.
    b. EDTA.
    c. silica.
    d. thrombin.

27. Which department performs ETOH tests?
    a. chemistry
    b. coagulation
    c. immunology
    d. microbiology

28. Carbamazepine levels are determined in this department.
    a. blood bank
    b. chemistry
    c. hematology
    d. immunology

29. A specimen to be tested for glucose-6-phosphate dehydrogenase deficiency is typically collected in a tube containing:
    a. citrate.
    b. EDTA.
    c. heparin.
    d. SPS.

30. Which of the following is a blood bank test?
    a. AFP
    b. DAT
    c. NH_4
    d. retic

ANSWERS AND EXPLANATIONS

1. **d.** An older name and abbreviation for alanine transferase (ALT) is serum glutamic-pyruvic transaminase (SGPT). ALP is the abbreviation for alkaline phosphatase. Serum glutamic-oxaloacetic transaminase (SGOT) is an older name for aspartate aminotransferase (AST).

2. **a.** Aldosterone is an adrenal hormone that plays a role in the absorption of sodium and water in the renal distal tubules. The test is performed in the chemistry department and typically requires the patient to be in an upright position for a minimum of 30 minutes before specimen collection. Catecholamines are a group of organic compounds that include dopamine, epinephrine, and norepinephrine. Catecholamine plasma specimens are ideally collected after the patient has rested quietly in a recumbent position for 30 minutes following insertion of a venous catheter. Renin is an enzyme that plays a role in hypertension. Renin levels are best collected after the patient has been resting quietly in a supine position for 2 hours. The specimen is typically collected in EDTA and chilled during transportation and centrifugation. The Stypven time test is a coagulation test collected in a light blue top sodium citrate tube. It is also called a Russell viper venom time (RVVT) or lupus anticoagulant test.

3. **d.** Aluminum, chromium, and copper are all metals that can be toxic to humans in elevated amounts. They all require collection in trace-element-free royal blue top tubes.

4. **a.** Hemoglobin A1c (Hgb A1c) is also called glycohemoglobin, glycosylated hemoglobin, and glycated hemoglobin. Glycation is a process in which glucose is bound to hemoglobin. Formation of glycated hemoglobin is irreversible, and the rate of formation is directly proportional to the concentration of glucose in the blood. Hgb A1c concentration therefore reflects the blood glucose concentration over the preceding 6 to 8 weeks. The test is performed in the chemistry department and is ordered to assess long-term glucose control in diabetic patients.

5. **b.** Carbon monoxide (CO) is a chemistry test collected in a lavender top tube. CO more readily binds to hemoglobin than oxygen and can lead to CO poisoning, which can be fatal. CO bound to hemoglobin is called carboxyhemoglobin (HbCO). Blood urea nitrogen (BUN) is a chemistry test typically performed on serum. The erythrocyte sedimentation rate (ESR) is collected in a lavender top tube, but it is a hematology test. GC stands for gonococcus, a microorganism from the species *Neisseria gonorrhoeae* that causes gonorrhea. The GC screen is performed in microbiology.

6. **d.** An antibody is a type of protein molecule called an immunoglobulin (Ig). There are five classes of immunoglobulins: IgA, IgD, IgM, IgG, and IgE.

7. **c.** Most coagulation tests require plasma specimens collected in light blue top sodium citrate tubes.

8. **c.** Phenytoin (Dilantin) is a drug used in the treatment of epilepsy. Lithium is a drug used to treat manic depression. Carbamazepine (Tegretol) is a drug used to treat bipolar affective

disorder. Theophylline is an asthma drug.

9. **c.** A differential (diff) is a hematology test that classifies types of leukocytes, describes erythrocyte morphology, and estimates the platelet count. It can be performed automatically by machine or manually by looking at a stained blood smear under a microscope. Albumin/globulin (A/G) ratio, carcinoembryonic antigen (CEA), and glycosylated hemoglobin are chemistry tests.

10. **c.** Lipids are fats such as cholesterol. Cholesterol is transported throughout the body in complexes with protein called lipoprotein. High-density lipoprotein (HDL) is referred to as *good* cholesterol because it plays a role in removing cholesterol from the arteries and transporting it to the liver where it is removed from the body. Low-density lipoprotein (LDL) is called *bad* cholesterol because it moves cholesterol into the arteries. Accurate measurement of HDL and LDL levels require a 12-hour fast. Antidiuretic hormone (ADH), creatine kinase MB (CK-MB), and uric acid tests do not require fasting specimens.

11. **d.** Serum protein electrophoresis (SPEP or PEP) requires a serum specimen collected in a red top or serum separator tube (SST). An ammonia test requires a plasma specimen collected in green top heparin tube. A disseminated intravascular coagulation (DIC) panel consists of several coagulation tests performed on plasma collected in a light blue sodium citrate tube. Hemoglobin A1c (Hgb A1c) is collected in a lavender EDTA tube.

12. **c.** It is recommended that salicylate (aspirin) levels *not* be collected in gel barrier tubes. It is acceptable to collect acid phosphatase, alpha-fetoprotein, and thyroid stimulating hormone (TSH) specimens in gel barrier tubes.

13. **d.** The radioallergosorbent test (RAST) is used in the detection of allergies. Carcinoembryonic antigen (CEA) is used in diagnosing and monitoring malignancies. D-dimer is a coagulation test. D-dimers are fragments produced by the action of plasmin on fibrin. Ferritin is a reliable indicator of iron stores and is measured in the diagnosis of iron-deficiency anemia and hemochromatosis.

14. **c.** Cyclosporine is an immunosuppressive drug used to suppress organ rejection in transplant recipients. The test can be performed on whole blood or serum. An acid-fast bacillus (AFB) culture is a microbiology test used to diagnose tuberculosis. The antinuclear antibody (ANA) test is a serology/immunology test used in the diagnosis of systemic lupus erythematosus (SLE) and other autoimmune disorders. Plasminogen is a coagulation test performed on patients with disseminated intravascular coagulation (DIC) or thrombosis.

15. **a.** A complete blood count (CBC) is a hematology test performed on a whole blood specimen. Cytomegalovirus (CMV) is a herpes virus that can cause devastating effects in a congenitally infected infant and fatal pneumonia in immunocompromised individuals. C-reactive protein (CRP) is an abnormal protein that appears in the blood during inflammatory illnesses, such as rheumatic fever, rheumatoid arthri-

tis, and acute bacterial or viral infections, and as a response to injurious stimuli, such as myocardial infarction and malignancy. Epstein-Barr virus (EBV) is a herpes virus that is the most common cause of infectious mononucleosis (IM). CMV, CRP, and EBV are serology/immunology tests most commonly performed on serum.

16. **b.** Immunology tests are most often performed on serum specimens.

17. **d.** Although most blood bank tests have been traditionally performed on serum and cells from clotted blood specimens, tests are increasingly being performed on plasma and cells from EDTA anticoagulated specimens obtained in lavender top tubes or special pink top tubes.

18. **b.** A tumor marker is a substance found in blood, other body fluids, and tissues that may indicate the existence of malignancy or cancer. Cancer antigen 125 (CA 125) is an antigen that appears in the blood in increased amounts in the presence of ovarian and endometrial tumors. It is detected using an antibody called OC 125. A basic metabolic panel (BMP) is a designated number of tests covering a certain body system. Antigens that can be detected on white blood cells are called human leukocyte antigens (HLAs). HLA typing is used in tissue typing for parentage determination and transplant compatibility between donor and recipient. Measurement of serum iron (Fe) and total iron-binding capacity (TIBC) aids in the diagnosis of iron deficiency anemia.

19. **a.** Amylase and lipase are enzymes found in greatest concentrations in the pancreas. They are measured in

the diagnosis and treatment of pancreatic disease as well as to differentiate pancreatitis from other abdominal disorders. Urea is an end-product of protein metabolism. In the past it was indirectly measured as blood urea nitrogen (BUN). Most analyzers now measure urea directly, but the term BUN may still be used. Creatinine is a product of creatine metabolism in the muscles. Its formation is related to muscle mass, and values vary according to age and gender. BUN and creatinine are excreted by the kidneys and measured in the assessment of kidney function. Hemoglobin and hematocrit (H & H) are hematology tests used to detect abnormal bleeding and anemia. Rapid plasma regain (RPR) is a nonspecific test used to screen for syphilis antibodies. The fluorescent treponemal antibody (FTA) tests specifically detect antibodies to *Treponema pallidum,* the microorganism that causes syphilis, and are used to confirm positive RPR results.

20. **b.** Cytomegalovirus (CMV) is a herpes virus that can cause devastating effects in a congenitally infected infant and fatal pneumonia in immunocompromised individuals. It is a serology/immunology test most commonly performed on serum.

21. **c.** Lactic acid is a product of carbohydrate metabolism. Excess amounts are produced during hypoxic (oxygen deficiency) states such as shock, hypovolemia (diminished blood volume) and left ventricular failure, and certain metabolic disease states such as diabetes mellitus and drug toxicity. Excess lactic acid in the blood is called lactic acidosis. Strict patient preparation and sample collection and handling procedures must be

followed to ensure accurate testing. Patients should be fasting and at rest for 2 hours before testing. Patients should be instructed not to make a fist before or during specimen collection, and specimens should be obtained without the use of a tourniquet because blood levels are affected by stasis (stoppage of blood flow) and hemoconcentration.

22. **b.** Plasminogen is a coagulation test collected in a light blue top tube. Plasminogen is a precursor of plasmin, an enzyme that dissolves fibrin and fibrinogen. It circulates in the blood until activated and converted to plasmin during fibrin clot formation. Its normal function is to dissolve the fibrin clot when healing has occurred and the clot is no longer needed. Substances called antiplasmins destroy any plasmin released into the blood. When pathologic processes such as thrombosis or disseminated intravascular coagulation (DIC) occur, excess amounts of plasmin are released into the blood and begin destroying other coagulation factors including fibrinogen.

23. **d.** The most common type of testing performed in microbiology is culture and sensitivity (C&S) testing of blood and other body fluids and substances such as urine and sputum.

24. **b.** Most hematology tests are performed on whole blood specimens collected in lavender top tubes containing the anticoagulant ethylenediaminetetraacetate (EDTA). The most common use of heparin-containing green top tubes is to provide plasma for chemistry tests. Light blue top tubes containing sodium citrate are used for coagulation tests. A plasma preparation tube (PPT) is used to provide EDTA plasma for molecular diagnostic tests.

25. **d.** A basic metabolic panel (BMP) includes a designated number of body system chemistry tests. A disseminated intravascular coagulation (DIC) screen, panel, or profile typically includes a platelet count, prothrombin time (protime or PT), activated partial thromboplastin time (APTT), D-dimer assay, and fibrinogen assay. A thyroid profile typically includes measurement of triiodothyronine (T_3), thyroxine (T_4), and thyroid stimulating hormone (TSH).

26. **a.** Human leukocyte antigen (HLA) specimens are typically collected in tubes containing acid citrate dextrose (ACD), although they are sometimes collected in heparin tubes.

27. **a.** Blood alcohol (ethanol or ETOH) tests are performed in the toxicology area of the chemistry department. Specimens are typically collected in gray top sodium fluoride tubes. Alcohol is volatile, and specimens must be kept capped during handling and processing to prevent evaporation of the analyte.

28. **b.** Carbamazepine (trade name, Tegretol) is a drug used to treat seizure disorders. Drug levels are measured in the toxicology area of the chemistry department.

29. **b.** Glucose-6-phosphate dehydrogenase (G-6-PD) is an enzyme that plays a role in glucose metabolism and ultimately in protecting hemoglobin from oxidation. A deficiency of G-6-PD is an inherited sex-linked disorder that can lead to hemolytic anemia. The test for G-6-PD deficiency is commonly performed on a solution of hemolyzed red blood cells ob-

tained from an EDTA specimen. Testing for elevated levels of G-6-PD is performed on serum.

30. b. The direct antiglobulin test (DAT) is a blood bank or immunohematology test that detects antigen antibody complexes on the red blood cells and red blood cell sensitization. It is use-
ful in evaluating hemolytic disease of the newborn (HDN), acquired hemolytic anemias, transfusion reactions, and drug-induced red blood cell sensitization. The alpha-fetoprotein test (AFP) and ammonia (NH_4) are chemistry tests. A reticulocyte (retic) count is a hematology test.

APPENDIX E: LABORATORY MATHEMATICS

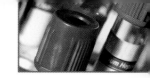

A. Laboratory Mathematics
1. The Metric System
2. Military Time
3. Temperature Measurement
4. Roman Numerals
5. Percent
6. Dilutions
7. Blood Volume
8. Adult Blood Volume
9. Infant Blood Volume

REVIEW QUESTIONS

1. 10 cc of blood equals approximately:
  a. 1 mL of blood.
  b. 5 mL of blood.
  c. 10 mL of blood.
  d. there is no relationship between cc and mL

2. 200 μL is equal to:
  a. 2 mL.
  b. 0.2 mL.
  c. 0.02 mL.
  d. 0.002 mL.

3. Your requisition says that a specimen is to be drawn at 1530. What time would that be in 12-hour time?
  a. 1:30 AM
  b. 3:30 PM
  c. 5:30 AM
  d. 7:30 PM

4. 1:00 PM in 24-hour time is:
  a. 100.
  b. 0100.
  c. 1300.
  d. 01300.

5. Body temperature in centigrade degrees is:
  a. 98.6.
  b. 37.0.
  c. 25.0.
  d. 32.0.

6. If room temperature is 77° F, what is the temperature in centigrade?
  a. 20.
  b. 25.
  c. 32.
  d. 37.

7. A specimen must be transported at body temperature, plus or minus 5° Fahrenheit. Which of the following temperature readings is within that range?
  a. 25° C
  b. 35° C
  c. 37° F
  d. 90° F

8. Your text says that factor VIII is the antihemophilic factor. What common Arabic number is this factor?
  a. four
  b. eight
  c. thirteen
  d. twenty-three

9. How is the number 12 written in Roman numerals?
  a. IIV
  b. VII
  c. IIX
  d. XII

10. Your paper says that you got 45 of 50 questions correct. What is your grade expressed as a percentage?
  a. 45%
  b. 75%

c. 90%
d. 95%

11. What does 2.2 pounds (lb) equal in the metric system?
a. 1 kg
b. 44 g
c. 100 g
d. 454 kg

12. If a red blood cell is 8 μm in diameter, what is its size in millimeters?
a. 0.8
b. 0.08
c. 0.008
d. 0.0008

13. A blood culture bottle containing 45 mL of media requires a 1:10 dilution of specimen. How much blood should be added?
a. 4 mL
b. 5 mL
c. 8 mL
d. 10 mL

14. Normal infant blood volume is 100 mL per kilogram. Calculate the approximate blood volume of a baby who weighs 6 lb.
a. 1.2 L
b. 2.7 L
c. 270 mL
d. 600 mL

15. Normal adult blood volume is 70 mL per kilogram. You weigh 130 lb. What is your blood volume?
a. 1300 mL
b. 1.3 L
c. 59 kg
d. 4.1 L

16. To prepare 100 mL of a 1:10 dilution of bleach, add:
a. 1 mL water to 100 mL bleach.
b. 1 mL bleach to 99 mL water.
c. 10 mL bleach to 90 mL water.
d. 10 mL water to 100 mL bleach.

17. The basic unit of volume in the metric system is the:
a. gram.
b. liter.
c. meter.
d. ounce.

18. In the metric system, a millimeter is:
a. 1/10 meter.
b. 1/100 meter.
c. 1/1000 meter.
d. 1/10,000 meter.

19. 1.2 kg is equal to how many grams?
a. 12
b. 120
c. 1200
d. 12,000

20. One teaspoon is approximately:
a. 1 mL.
b. 5 mL.
c. 10 mL.
d. 15 mL.

21. The basic unit of weight in the metric system is the:
a. gram.
b. liter.
c. meter.
d. ounce.

22. In the metric system the prefix for 1000 is:
a. centi-.
b. deci-.
c. kilo-.
d. milli-.

23. In the metric system a meter is a measure of:
a. mass.
b. density.
c. length.
d. volume.

24. A patient voids 1200 mL of urine for a creatinine clearance test. How much urine is this?

a. less than a liter
b. less than a quart
c. more than a liter
d. more than 2 liters

25. A test requires 3 mL serum. The laboratory requires that the amount of blood collected be 250% of the volume of specimen required to perform the test. Which size tube should you use to collect the specimen?
a. 4 mL
b. 5 mL
c. 10 mL
d. 15 mL

ANSWERS AND EXPLANATIONS

1. **c.** For practical purposes, *mL* and *cc* are equivalent and the terms are often used interchangeably in a laboratory setting. Both are approximately equal to one-thousandth of a liter. The term *milliliter* is used when referring to liquid volume; *cubic centimeter* is used when referring to volume of gas. However, syringes that are used to extract liquid volume are often calibrated in cc rather than in mL.

2. **b.** Microliters are smaller units than milliliters. In the metric system it is possible to convert a smaller unit to a larger unit by moving the decimal point to the left by the amount of the multiple of the unit to which you are converting. One milliliter equals one-thousandth of a liter or 10^{-3} liters. The multiple is minus three. Therefore, to convert 200 microliters to milliliters, move the decimal point three places to the left.

$$200.0 = 0.2 \text{ mL}$$

3. **b.** To change 24-hour time to 12-hour time (Fig. AppE-1) subtract 1200 from any time after 1300. 1530 in 24-hour time less 1200 is 330, which written in 12-hour time is 3:30 PM.

4. **c.** To convert 12-hour time to 24-hour time, add 1200 to the time from 1 PM on; 1:00 without the colon is 100. 100 plus 1200 becomes 1300.

5. **b.** Body temperature in centigrade is 37°. To calculate body temperature in centigrade when given a Fahrenheit reading, subtract 32 from the Fahrenheit temperature and multiply by 5/9. *Note:* A healthcare worker should memorize this centigrade temperature along with a few other temperatures that are common when working in healthcare.

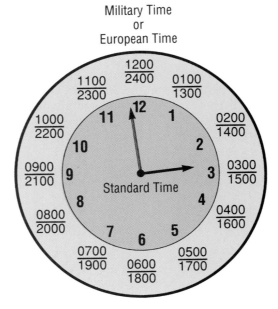

Military Time
or
European Time

■ AppE-1 ■
Clock showing 24-hour (military) time.

6. **b.** To convert 77° Fahrenheit temperature to centigrade or Celsius (Fig. AppE-2) subtract 32 from the Fahrenheit number and multiply the result by 5/9. Healthcare workers should memorize this commonly referenced centigrade temperature.

$$77 - 32 = 45$$
$$5/9 \ (45) = 5/9 \times 45/1$$
$$5/9 \times 45/1 = 225/9$$
$$225/9 = 25° \text{ centigrade}$$

7. **b.** Fahrenheit body temperature is 98.6°. Once we add and subtract 5, we know that we are looking for a temperature that is between 93.6° F and 103.6° F. This eliminates 37° F and 90° F. Celsius and centigrade are the same; 25° Celsius is the same as 77° F. The remaining choice is 35° C. To convert 35° C to Fahrenheit temperature:

$$(9/5 \times 35) + 32 = 63 + 32 = 95° \text{ F}$$

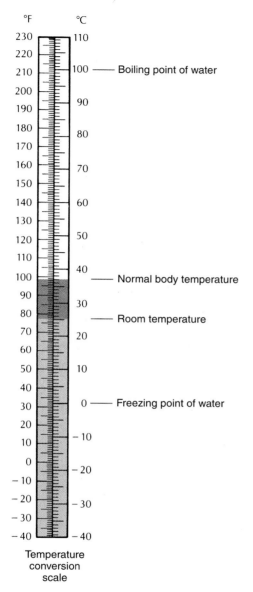

°F / °C

230 / 110
220
210 / 100 —— Boiling point of water
200
190 / 90
180 / 80
170
160 / 70
150
140 / 60
130
120 / 50
110
100 / 40
90 —— Normal body temperature
90 / 30
80
70 —— Room temperature
70 / 20
60
50 / 10
40
30 / 0 —— Freezing point of water
20
10 / −10
0
−10 / −20
−20
−30 / −30
−40 / −40

Temperature
conversion
scale

■ APPE-2 ■

Thermometer showing both Fahrenheit and Celsius degrees (Memmler RI, Cohen BJ, Wood DL).

8. b. If V = 5 and I = 1, then VIII is 5 + 1 + 1 + 1, or 8.

9. d. To write Arabic numbers in Roman numerals, remember the rules. Roman numerals are written from left to right and can never exceed more than three of the same numeral in a sequence. To write the number 12, you should start with a base number such as X = 10 and then add lower value numbers until you reach your desired value, for example, X + I + I = 12.

10. c. To calculate a percentage, a number must be converted to parts per 100. First make the number a fraction. Then multiply the numerator of the fraction by 100, divide by the denominator, and add a percent sign.

$$45/50 \times 100 = 4500/50 = 90\%$$

11. a. One kilogram equals 2.2 lb (Table AppE-1). This is a conversion factor that should be memorized. A helpful hint might be to remember that weight in kilograms is approximately half (divide by 2) the number given in pounds.

12. c. A micrometer (or micron) (Table AppE-2) is equal to one-millionth of a meter and a millimeter is equal to one-thousandth of a meter, which

Table AppE-1

Metric-English Conversion Equivalents			
	Metric		**English**
Distance	Meter (m)	=	3.3 feet/ 39.37 inches
	Centimeter (cm)	=	0.4 inches
	Millimeter (mm)	=	0.04 inches
Weight	Gram (g)	=	0.0022 pounds
	Kilogram (kg)	=	2.2 pounds
Volume	Liter (L)	=	1.06 quarts
	Milliliter (mL)[a]	=	0.03 fluid ounces
	Milliliter (mL)[a]	=	0.20 or 1/5 tsp

[a]A milliliter (mL) is approximately equal to a cubic centimeter (cc) and the two terms are often used interchangeably.

Table AppE-2

English-Metric Conversion Equivalents			
	English	**=**	**Metric**
Distance	Yard (yd)	=	0.9 meters (m)
	Inch (in)	=	2.54 centimeters (cm)
Weight	Pound (lb)	=	0.454 kilograms (kg) or 454 grams (g)
	Ounce (oz)	=	28 grams (g)
Volume	Quart (qt)	=	0.95 liters (L)
	Fluid ounce (fl oz)	=	30 milliliters (mL)
	Tablespoon (tbsp)	=	15 milliliters (mL)
	Teaspoon (tsp)	=	5 milliliters (mL)

means you are converting smaller units to larger units. To do this, the decimal point moves to the left the same number of times as the multiple to which you are converting. A millimeter is 10^{-3} m. The multiple is three, so the decimal point moves three places to the left.

$$008.0 \; \mu m = 0.008 \; mL$$

13. **b.** A blood culture dilution of 1:10 means there is 1 mL of blood and 9 mL of media for every 10 mL of blood culture specimen. Forty-five milliliters of media is five times the original proportion of nine milliliters. To maintain the same 1:10 dilution, you must also have five times the original 1 mL proportion of blood. That means you will need to add 5 mL blood to the 45 mL media.

14. **c.** Normal infant blood volume is approximately 100 mL/kg. If a baby's weight is given in pounds, it must be converted to kilograms by multiplying the pounds by the conversion factor 0.454. Once the weight is es-

tablished in kilograms, multiply that number by 100 because for every kilogram there is 100 mL of blood.

$$6 \; lb \times 0.454 = 2.7 \; kg$$
(rounded to nearest tenth)
$$2.7 \; kg \times 100 \; mL/kg =$$
$$270 \; mL \; or \; 0.27 \; L$$

15. **d.** Normal adult blood volume is approximately 70 mL per kilogram of weight. If the weight is given in pounds, it must be converted to kilograms by multiplying by the conversion factor 0.454 (see Table AppE-2). The weight in kilograms is multiplied by 70 because we know that for every kilogram of weight in an adult there is 70 mL of blood. Divide the result by 1000 because adult blood volume is reported in liters and 1 L equals 1000 mL.

$$130 \; lb \times 0.454 = 59.02 \; kg$$
$$59 \; kg \times 70 \; kg/mL = 4130 \; mL$$
$$4130/1000 = 4.13 \; L$$

16. **c.** A 1:10 dilution of bleach means there is 1 mL of bleach and 9 mL of water for every 10 mL of solution. One hundred milliliters of a 1:10 dilution is 10 times the original 10-mL proportion. That means you will also need 10 times the original amounts of bleach and water; or 10 mL bleach and 90 mL water.

17. **b.** It is easier to remember that the liter is the basic metric unit of volume than to remember other metric measurements, because the soft drink industry in the United States has converted much of their packaging to metric measurements, and we see advertisements for liters of soft drinks all the time.

18. **c.** A millimeter is 1/1000 meter or 10^{-3} m.

Table AppE-3

Commonly Used Measurement Prefixes

		Unit of Measure		
Prefix	Multiple	Meter	Gram	Liter
Kilo- (k)	1000 (10^3)	km	kg	kL
Deci- (d)	1/10 (10^{-1})	dm	dg	dL
Centi- (c)	1/100 (10^{-2})	cm	cg	cL
Milli- (m)	1/1000 (10^{-3})	mm	mg	mL
Micro- (μ)	1/1,000,000 (10^{-6})	μm	μg	μL

19. c. To convert metric units from larger units to smaller units, move the decimal point to the right the appropriate multiple. A kilogram (Table AppE-3) is 1000 or 10^3 g. The multiple, therefore, is 3.

$$1.200 \text{ kg} = 1200 \text{ g.}$$

20. b. By using an English-Metric conversion chart (see Table AppE-2), you can find the right answer or you may choose to memorize certain common conversions, such as 1 tsp = 5 mL.

21. a. The basic unit of weight in the metric system is the gram.

22. c. Kilo-, abbreviated "k," means 1000. It can be used with each of the three basic units of measure in the metric system.

kilogram (kg) = 1000 grams (g)
kiloliter (kL) = 1000 liters (L)
kilometer (km) = 1000 meters (m)

23. c. The metric measurement for length is meter (m).

24. c. A liter is equal to 1000 mL and a quart is equal to 950 mL; therefore, 1200 mL is 200 mL more than a liter and 250 mL more than a quart and 800 mL less than 2 liters.

25. c. The laboratory needs 250% or two and one-half times the 3 mL required for the test. Two times 3 mL is 6 mL. One-half of 3 mL is 1½ mL (or you can multiply 3 times 2.5). You need 7½ mL to do the test. The closest correct size tube is 10 mL.

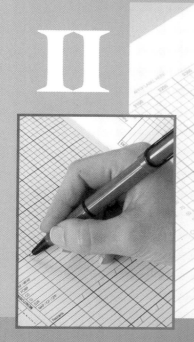

II

Comprehensive Mock Exam

WRITTEN COMPREHENSIVE MOCK EXAM

1. The hematology department performs tests that:
   a. concern the ability of the blood to form and dissolve clots.
   b. deal with the antigen-antibody response of the body to microorganisms that cause disease.
   c. identify abnormalities of the blood and blood forming tissues.
   d. involve the analysis of body fluids and tissues to identify disease-causing microorganisms.

2. A phlebotomist who collects a specimen from an inpatient with this disease would be required to wear an N-95 respirator while in the patient's room.
   a. diabetes mellitus
   b. infectious hepatitis
   c. pulmonary tuberculosis
   d. all of the above

3. Red blood cells are also called:
   a. erythrocytes.
   b. leukocytes.
   c. lymphocytes.
   d. thrombocytes.

4. While organizing your phlebotomy tray, you notice that your latex tourniquet is soiled with blood. What should you do?
   a. autoclave it before reuse
   b. throw it away
   c. wash it with a bleach solution
   d. wipe it with alcohol

5. You have a STAT request to collect an H & H on a post-op patient. Which of the following scenarios best describes the proper response?
   a. go immediately to the surgical recovery room, collect a lavender top on the patient, and deliver it immediately to the laboratory
   b. proceed to post-op as soon as possible, collect one red top on the patient, and return it to the lab as soon as possible
   c. proceed to surgery, scrub and gown, collect a red top and a lavender top on the patient, and call someone from the lab to come and get the specimen while you remove protective clothing and wash up
   d. wait until time for the next sweep, collect that specimen first, and send it down to the lab in the tube system before proceeding to collect the other specimens on your sweep

6. You arrive to collect a specimen on a patient named John Doe in 302B. How do you verify that the patient in 302B is indeed John Doe?
   a. ask the patient, "Are you John Doe?"; if he says yes, collect the specimen
   b. ask the patient to please state his name and date of birth; if it matches your requisition, proceed to check his ID band to see if it matches your requisition
   c. check the patient's ID band; if it matches your requisition, proceed to collect the specimen
   d. any of the above

7. A delay in processing longer than 2 hours can lead to erroneously decreased results for:
   a. carbon dioxide.
   b. glucose.
   c. ionized calcium.
   d. all of the above

8. Which mode of infection transmission occurs from touching contaminated bed linens?
   a. direct contact
   b. droplet contact
   c. indirect contact
   d. vehicle contact

9. Oncology is the medical specialty that treats patients with:
   a. benign and malignant tumors.
   b. kidney disorders.
   c. problems associated with aging.
   d. vision problems.

10. What is the recommended order for removing protective clothing?
    a. gloves, mask, gown
    b. gown, gloves, mask
    c. gown, mask, gloves
    d. mask, gown, gloves

11. All the following could be a cause of hematoma formation during venipuncture EXCEPT:
    a. inadequate pressure is applied to site after needle removal.
    b. the needle bevel is centered in the lumen of the vein.
    c. the needle bevel is only partially inserted in the vein.
    d. the needle has penetrated through the back of the vein.

12. Which of the following is a proper laboratory safety procedure?
    a. keep food and drinks on a separate shelf from laboratory reagents or specimens
    b. keep your mouth closed when you chew gum
    c. tie back hair that is longer than shoulder length
    d. wear your laboratory coat at all times

13. Antiseptics are:
    a. corrosive chemical compounds.
    b. safe to use on human skin.
    c. used to clean surfaces and instruments only.
    d. used to kill pathogenic microorganisms only.

14. A laboratory procedure that requires the use of goggles to prevent exposure from sprays or splashes also requires this protective attire.
    a. earplugs
    b. mask
    c. respirator
    d. sterile gown

15. The respiratory therapy department is responsible for:
    a. administering oxygen treatments.
    b. performing magnetic resonance imaging (MRI).
    c. performing therapeutic drug monitoring (TDM).
    d. providing therapy to restore mobility.

16. Standard precautions should be followed:
    a. if a patient is in isolation.
    b. when a patient is known to be HIV-positive.
    c. when a patient is known to have HBV.
    d. with all patients, at all times.

17. The composition of skin puncture blood more closely resembles:
    a. arterial blood.
    b. lymph fluid.
    c. tissue fluid.
    d. venous blood.

18. You accidentally splash a bleach solution into your eyes while preparing it for cleaning purposes. What is the first thing to do?
    a. dry your eyes with a paper towel
    b. flush your eyes with water for a minimum of 15 minutes
    c. proceed to the emergency room as quickly as possible
    d. put 10-20 drops of saline in your eyes

19. All the following conditions would be reasons to reject a specimen for analysis EXCEPT:
    a. a bilirubin specimen is icteric.
    b. a CBC specimen has clots in it.
    c. a fasting glucose specimen is lipemic.
    d. an electrolyte specimen is hemolyzed.

20. At what interval is the blood blotted during a bleeding time test?
    a. 10 seconds
    b. 20 seconds
    c. 30 seconds
    d. 60 seconds

21. What is the best means of preventing nosocomial infection?
    a. immunization
    b. isolation procedures
    c. proper hand decontamination
    d. wearing gloves

22. The suffix of the term hepatitis means:
    a. condition.
    b. infection.
    c. inflammation.
    d. liver.

23. Symptoms of shock include:
    a. expressionless face and staring eyes.
    b. increased deep breathing.
    c. strong, rapid pulse.
    d. warm, moist skin.

24. You are unfamiliar with a test that has been ordered. The procedure manual says it requires a serum specimen. Which of the following tubes will yield a serum specimen?
    a. green top
    b. lavender top
    c. light blue top
    d. red top

25. Exposure time, distance, and shielding are the main principles involved in:
    a. biohazard safety.
    b. chemical safety.
    c. electrical safety.
    d. radiation safety.

26. When the threshold value of a QA indicator is exceeded and a problem is identified:
    a. a corrective action plan is implemented.
    b. an incident report is filed.
    c. patient specimens must be redrawn.
    d. patients' physicians must be notified.

27. A phlebotomist arrives to collect a 2-hour postprandial glucose specimen on an inpatient and discovers that 2 hours have not elapsed since the patient's meal. What should the phlebotomist do?
    a. ask the patient's nurse to verify the correct time to draw the specimen
    b. come back later at the time the patient says is correct

c. draw the specimen and write the time collected on the specimen label
d. fill out an incident report form and return to the laboratory

28. The delivering chambers of the heart are the:
a. atria.
b. chordae tendineae.
c. vena cavae.
d. ventricles.

29. Which of the following is an example of a work practice control that reduces risk of exposure to bloodborne pathogens?
a. a biohazard symbol
b. an exposure control plan
c. handwashing after glove removal
d. HBV vaccination

30. An inpatient refused to let a phlebotomist collect blood from him one afternoon. Early the next morning, another phlebotomist arrived to collect a specimen on the same patient. The phlebotomist drew the specimen without waking him. The phlebotomist could be charged with:
a. assault and battery.
b. breach of confidentiality.
c. fraud.
d. negligence.

31. A phlebotomist is accidentally punctured on the thumb by a needle that was used to collect a blood specimen from a patient. The first thing he or she should do is:
a. check the patient's medical records.
b. decontaminate the site and fill out an incident report.
c. go to employee health service and get a tetanus booster.
d. leave the area so that the patient does not notice the injury.

32. What should a phlebotomist do if a patient feels faint during a blood draw?

a. immediately discontinue the draw and lower the patient's head
b. lower the patient's head and continue the draw
c. remove the needle and shake the patient to revive him
d. use one hand to hold the patient upright and continue the draw

33. Which of the following is an example of a nosocomial infection? A:
a. catheter site of a patient in ICU becomes infected.
b. drug addict contracts hepatitis from a contaminated needle.
c. patient is admitted with Hantavirus.
d. pediatric patient breaks out with measles the day after admission for a tonsillectomy.

34. All the following are reasons to eliminate a potential venipuncture site EXCEPT:
a. petechiae appear during tourniquet application.
b. massive scarring is present.
c. the arm is edematous.
d. the only vein feels hard and cord-like.

35. The two organizations responsible for the latest Guideline for Isolation Precautions in Hospitals are:
a. CDC and HICPAC.
b. CDC and OSHA.
c. HICPAC and NIOSH.
d. NIOSH and JCAHO.

36. According to laboratory policy, you are required to collect a specimen that will yield 2.5 times the amount of specimen needed to perform the test. If a chemistry test requires 0.5 mL of serum, which of the following tubes is the smallest that can be used?
a. red top microcollection container
b. 3 mL red top
c. 5 mL SST
d. 7 mL PST

37. A short in the wiring of a centrifuge causes a fire. Which type of extinguisher is best for putting it out?
   a. Class A
   b. Class B
   c. Class C
   d. Class D

38. To minimize effects of hemoconcentration caused by blockage of blood flow during venipuncture, the tourniquet should never be left in place longer than:
   a. 30 seconds.
   b. 60 seconds.
   c. 2 minutes.
   d. 4 minutes.

39. Which of the following is an acceptable chemical safety procedure?
   a. familiarize oneself with the MSDS of a new reagent
   b. if mixing acid and water together, add the water to the acid
   c. mix bleach with other cleaners for extra disinfecting power
   d. store chemicals at eye level so the labels are easy to see

40. The minimum qualifications of a clinical laboratory scientist (CLS) are a(n):
   a. advanced degree and experience in the field.
   b. bachelor's degree in medical technology or a chemical or biological science.
   c. high school diploma or equivalent.
   d. 2-year associate's degree or equivalent, or certification from a military or proprietary school.

41. You have just been hired as a phlebotomist but have not been vaccinated against hepatitis B. According to federal law, your employer must offer you hepatitis B vaccination free of charge:
   a. immediately.
   b. once your probationary employment period has ended.

   c. within 1 month of employment.
   d. within 10 working days of assignment to phlebotomy duties.

42. The right to _____ is part of the Patient's Bill of Rights.
   a. decline medical treatment
   b. know the medical status of another patient in the same room
   c. refuse to pay for medical treatment
   d. watch the test being performed in the laboratory

43. NCCLS and OSHA guidelines require specimen transport bags to have all the following EXCEPT:
   a. a biohazard label.
   b. a separate pocket for paperwork.
   c. liquid-tight closures.
   d. shock resistance features.

44. Which of the following needles has the largest diameter?
   a. 18-gauge hypodermic needle
   b. 21-gauge multisample needle
   c. 22-gauge multisample needle
   d. 23-gauge butterfly needle

45. A phlebotomist explains to an inpatient that he has come to collect a blood specimen. The patient extends his arm and pushes up his sleeve. This is an example of:
   a. expressed consent.
   b. refusal of consent.
   c. implied consent.
   d. informed consent.

46. The main difference between serum and plasma is:
   a. plasma contains fibrinogen, serum does not.
   b. plasma is obtained from clotted blood.
   c. serum is clear, plasma is cloudy.
   d. serum is pale yellow, plasma is colorless.

47. While processing blood specimens, you accidentally spill blood on the countertop. What is the best way to clean it up?
a. absorb it with a damp cloth and wash the area with soap and water
b. absorb it with a paper towel or gauze pad and wipe the area with disinfectant
c. wait for it to dry and then scrape it into a biohazard bag
d. wipe it up with an alcohol pad using concentric circles

48. Which statement concerning human anatomy is true?
a. A patient who is supine is lying down on his or her back
b. Phalanges is the medical term for heel bone
c. Sagittal planes divide the body into upper and lower portions
d. The hand is proximal to the wrist

49. Identify the tubes needed to collect a WBC, PT, and STAT calcium by color and in the proper order of collection for a multi-tube draw.
a. gold top, yellow top, light blue top
b. lavender top, SST, royal blue top
c. light blue top, green top, lavender top
d. red top, gray top, light blue top

50. Which type of test is most affected by tissue thromboplastin contamination?
a. chemistry
b. coagulation
c. microbiology
d. serology

51. The silica particles in an SST:
a. enhance coagulation.
b. keep RBCs from sticking to the tube.
c. minimize hemolysis.
d. prevent glycolysis.

52. The best choice of equipment for drawing difficult veins is:
a. butterfly and evacuated tube holder.
b. lancet and microtainer.
c. needle and evacuated tube holder.
d. needle and syringe.

53. A blood smear made from blood collected in EDTA must be prepared within:
a. a few minutes of collection.
b. 30 minutes of collection.
c. 1 hour of collection.
d. 4 hours of collection.

54. Anaerobic conditions must be maintained when collecting and handling this specimen.
a. bilirubin
b. blood gases
c. CBC
d. glucose

55. Some specimens require cooling to:
a. prevent activation of a cold agglutinin.
b. prevent clotting.
c. separate serum more completely.
d. slow metabolic processes.

56. Proper collection and handling of anticoagulant tubes includes:
a. collecting them in the proper order of draw to prevent cross-contamination of other tubes.
b. filling them until the normal vacuum is exhausted to maintain a correct ratio of blood to anticoagulant.
c. mixing them adequately to prevent microclot formation.
d. all of the above

57. You are under a great deal of stress at work. Which of the following is a good way to deal with it?
a. go for long walks on a regular basis
b. prioritize duties at the beginning of the day
c. relax watching a favorite movie
d. all of the above

58. The patient asks if the test you are about to draw is for diabetes. How do you answer?
    a. explain that it is best to discuss the test with the physician
    b. if the test is for glucose, say, "Yes it is"
    c. say that you do not know
    d. tell the patient that it is not, even if it is

59. Which of the following is a safe area for infant heel puncture? The:
    a. area of the arch.
    b. central area.
    c. medial plantar surface.
    d. posterior curvature.

60. Which of the following is a function of the muscular system?
    a. maintain electrolyte balance
    b. produce heat
    c. receive environmental stimuli
    d. secrete hormones

61. The major structural difference between arteries and veins is:
    a. arteries are larger in diameter.
    b. arteries have a different sequence of layers.
    c. veins have a thicker muscle layer.
    d. veins have valves.

62. You arrive to draw a fasting specimen. The patient is just finishing breakfast. What do you do?
    a. check with the patient's nurse first; if the specimen is collected, write "non-fasting" on the lab slip and the specimen label
    b. collect the specimen anyway but write "non-fasting" on the lab slip and the specimen
    c. collect the specimen anyway since the patient had not quite finished eating
    d. refuse to collect the specimen, fill out an incident report, and leave a copy of it at the nurse's station

63. The additive and color code associated with coagulation tests is:
    a. EDTA, lavender.
    b. heparin, green.
    c. sodium citrate, light blue.
    d. thixotropic gel, gold.

64. Povidone-iodine is the recommended solution for cleaning a:
    a. blood culture collection site.
    b. routine venipuncture site.
    c. skin puncture site.
    d. all of the above

65. All the following statements concerning an employee bloodborne pathogen exposure incident are true EXCEPT:
    a. all exposure incidents should be reported to a supervisor.
    b. an exposed employee should have access to a free confidential medical evaluation.
    c. the exposure should be documented on an incident report form.
    d. the source patient must submit to HIV and HBV testing.

66. Which additive prevents coagulation by binding calcium?
    a. EDTA
    b. heparin
    c. sodium fluoride
    d. thixotropic gel

67. Proper electrical safety procedures include:
    a. hiding frayed electrical cords under equipment so no one will touch them.
    b. unplugging electrical equipment before servicing it.
    c. using extension cords for convenient placement of equipment.
    d. all of the above

68. You must collect an ETOH specimen on a patient. Which of the following tubes would be the best choice to collect the specimen?

a. gray top sodium fluoride tube
b. green top plasma separator tube
c. red top clot activator tube
d. royal blue with a lavender-coded label

69. You are the only phlebotomist on the night shift. You receive orders for all the following tests within minutes of one another. Which test has the greatest collection priority?
a. ASAP electrolytes in CCU
b. STAT CBC in labor and delivery
c. STAT electrolytes in the ER
d. timed blood cultures in ICU

70. It is necessary to control the depth of lancet insertion during skin puncture to avoid:
a. bacterial contamination of the specimen.
b. excessive bleeding.
c. injury to the calcaneus.
d. puncturing an artery.

71. Which of the following is the best way to tell if a specimen is arterial? As the specimen is collected, the blood:
a. appears bright cherry red.
b. contains air bubbles.
c. looks dark blue.
d. pumps into the syringe.

72. You must collect a specimen on a 6 year old. The child is a little fearful. Which of the following is the best thing to do?
a. explain what you are going to do in simple terms and ask the child for cooperation
b. have someone restrain the child and go ahead and draw the specimen without explanation
c. tell the child not to worry because it won't hurt
d. tell the child that you will give him a treat if he doesn't cry

73. You must collect a protime specimen from a patient with IVs in both arms. The best place to collect the specimen is:
a. above one of the IVs.
b. below one of the IVs.
c. from an ankle vein.
d. from one of the IVs.

74. What is the meaning of the following symbol?

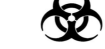

a. biohazard
b. bloodborne pathogen hazard
c. chemical hazard
d. radiation hazard

75. A patient complains of significant pain when you insert the needle. The pain does not subside and radiates down the patient's arm. What should you do?
a. ask the patient if it is all right to continue the draw
b. collect the specimen as quickly as you can
c. discontinue the draw immediately
d. tell the patient to hang in there so that you do not have to stick him again

76. Which of the following microcollection containers should be filled first if collected by skin puncture?
a. gray top
b. green top
c. lavender top
d. red top

77. Quality assurance (QA) procedures include all the following EXCEPT:
a. checking needles for blunt tips and barbs.
b. following strict specimen labeling requirements.
c. keeping track of employee absenteeism.
d. recording results of refrigerator temperature checks.

78. If the phlebotomist makes a blood smear that is too short, he or she should try again and:
    a. decrease the angle of the spreader slide.
    b. exert more pressure with the spreader slide.
    c. increase the angle of the spreader slide.
    d. use a smaller drop of blood.

79. The bleeding time (BT) test assesses:
    a. effectiveness of heparin therapy.
    b. functioning of the red blood cells.
    c. platelet plug formation in the capillaries.
    d. therapeutic action of coumadin.

80. Which of the following diseases can be transmitted through blood and body fluids?
    a. leukemia
    b. rubella
    c. syphilis
    d. thrombocytosis

81. The most common reason for glucose monitoring through POCT is to:
    a. check for glycosuria.
    b. diagnose glucose metabolism problems.
    c. monitor glucose levels in patients with diabetes mellitus.
    d. all of the above

82. Which of the following is an example of possible percutaneous exposure to bloodborne pathogens?
    a. getting stuck with a contaminated needle
    b. handling blood specimens with ungloved, badly chapped hands
    c. having mucous membrane contact with infectious material
    d. ingesting infectious material

83. Which of the following pieces of patient information is typically required on a specimen label?
    a. diagnosis
    b. medical record number
    c. physician's name
    d. room number

84. Which additional identification information is typically required on a non-blood specimen label?
    a. lab accession number
    b. patient diagnosis
    c. physician's name
    d. source of the specimen

85. Which of the following specimens requires protection from light?
    a. bilirubin
    b. urine porphyrin
    c. vitamin B12
    d. all of the above

86. A technologist asks you to collect 5 cc of whole blood for a special test. What volume tube should you use?
    a. 3 mL
    b. 5 mL
    c. 10 mL
    d. 15 mL

87. Your hospital uses computer-generated specimen labels. What information is typically added to the label manually when the specimen is collected?
    a. date of birth
    b. medical record number
    c. patient's full name
    d. phlebotomist's initials

88. You are the only phlebotomist in an outpatient drawing station. A physician orders a test with which you are unfamiliar. What is the appropriate action to take?
    a. call the physician's office for assistance
    b. draw both a serum and a plasma specimen
    c. refer to the user manual for instructions
    d. send the patient to another drawing station

89. Which of the following behaviors play a role in professional ethics?
a. maintaining patient confidentiality
b. presenting a professional appearance
c. promoting positive interpersonal communication
d. all of the above

90. Transporting tubes of blood with the stopper up:
a. aids clot formation.
b. minimizes aerosol formation when the tube is opened.
c. reduces agitation caused by hemolysis.
d. all of the above

91. You are performing a sweat chloride test on a toddler. What infection control precautions must you follow when collecting the specimen?
a. contact precautions
b. droplet precautions
c. no special precautions
d. standard precautions

92. Specimens transported by courier or other air or ground mail systems must follow guidelines defined by the:
a. DOT.
b. FAA.
c. OSHA.
d. all of the above

93. Which of the following is a required characteristic of a sharps container?
a. leak-proof and puncture-resistant
b. locking lid
c. marked with a biohazard symbol
d. all of the above

94. Which statement describes proper centrifuge operation?
a. balance specimens by placing tubes of equal volume and size opposite one another
b. centrifuge serum specimens before they have a chance to clot
c. never centrifuge serum specimens in the same centrifuge as plasma specimens
d. remove tube stoppers before placing specimen tubes in the centrifuge

95. The manufacturer must supply an MSDS for:
a. fluid-resistant laboratory coats.
b. most patient medications.
c. isopropyl alcohol.
d. isotonic saline.

96. Which type of specimen has processing and testing priority over all other specimens?
a. ASAP
b. fasting
c. STAT
d. timed

97. What is the recommended procedure for collecting a 24-hour urine specimen?
a. collect all urine voided in any 24-hour period
b. collect the first morning specimen and all other urine for 24 hours except the first specimen the following morning
c. collect the first morning specimen and all other urine for 24 hours including the first specimen the following morning
d. void the first morning specimen into the toilet; start the timing; collect all the following specimens including the next morning's specimen

98. The abbreviation for the federal agency that instituted and enforces regulations requiring the labeling of hazardous materials is:
a. CDC.
b. JCHAO.
c. NFPA.
d. OSHA.

99. Continuing education units (CEUs) are:
    a. certificates awarded for teaching skills courses.
    b. college credit for taking healthcare courses.
    c. documentation of passing a national certification exam.
    d. proof of participation in workshops to upgrade skills or knowledge.

100. The most common nosocomial infection in the United States is:
    a. hepatitis infection.
    b. respiratory infection.
    c. urinary tract infection.
    d. wound infection.

ANSWERS TO THE WRITTEN COMPREHENSIVE MOCK EXAM

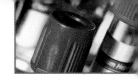

Answers to the Written Comprehensive Mock Exam

1. Ans: **c.**
   Cognitive level: Recall
   Topic: Laboratory Departments
   Chapter: 1

2. Ans: **c.**
   Cognitive level: Application
   Topic: Infection Control
   Chapter: 3

3. Ans: **a.**
   Cognitive level: Recall
   Topic: Circulatory System
   Chapter: 6

4. Ans: **b.**
   Cognitive level: Recall
   Topic: Blood Collection Equipment
   Chapter: 7

5. Ans: **a.**
   Cognitive level: Application
   Topic: Test Priority
   Chapter: 1

6. Ans: **b.**
   Cognitive level: Application
   Topic: Patient Identification
   Chapter: 8

7. Ans: **d.**
   Cognitive level: Recall
   Topic: Specimen Handling
   Chapter: 14

8. Ans: **c.**
   Cognitive level: Recall
   Topic: Infection Control
   Chapter: 3

9. Ans: **a.**
   Cognitive level: Recall
   Topic: Medical Specialties
   Chapter: 1

10. Ans: **a.**
    Cognitive level: Recall
    Topic: Infection Control
    Chapter: 3

11. Ans: **b.**
    Cognitive level: Analysis
    Topic: Complications and Procedural Errors
    Chapter: 9

12. Ans: **c.**
    Cognitive level: Application
    Topic: Safety
    Chapter: 3

13. Ans: **b.**
    Cognitive level: Analysis
    Topic: Blood Collection Equipment
    Chapter: 7

14. Ans: **b.**
    Cognitive level: Recall
    Topic: Safety
    Chapter: 3

15. Ans: **a.**
    Cognitive level: Recall
    Topic: Hospital Service Areas
    Chapter: 1

16. Ans: **d.**
    Cognitive level: Recall
    Topic: Infection Control
    Chapter: 3

17. Ans: **a.**
    Cognitive level: Recall
    Topic: Skin Puncture Principles
    Chapter: 10

18. Ans: **b.**
    Cognitive level: Application
    Topic: Chemical Safety
    Chapter: 3

19. Ans: **a.**
    Cognitive level: Analysis
    Topic: Specimen Handling
    Chapter: 14

20. Ans: **c.**
    Cognitive level: Recall
    Topic: Point-of-Care Testing
    Chapter: 11

21. Ans: **c.**
    Cognitive level: Recall
    Topic: Infection Control
    Chapter: 3

22. Ans: **c.**
    Cognitive level: Recall
    Topic: Medical Terminology
    Chapter: 4

23. Ans: **a.**
    Cognitive level: Analysis
    Topic: First Aid
    Chapter: 3

24. Ans: **d.**
    Cognitive level: Application
    Topic: Evacuated Tubes
    Chapter: 7

25. Ans: **d.**
    Cognitive level: Recall
    Topic: Safety
    Chapter: 3

26. Ans: **a.**
    Cognitive level: Application
    Topic: Quality Assurance
    Chapter: 2

27. Ans: **a.**
    Cognitive level: Application
    Topic: Special Collections
    Chapter: 11

28. Ans: **d.**
    Cognitive level: Recall
    Topic: Heart Structure
    Chapter: 6

29. Ans: **c.**
    Cognitive level: Application
    Topic: Safety
    Chapter: 3

30. Ans: **a.**
    Cognitive level: Analysis
    Topic: Legal Issues
    Chapter: 2

31. Ans: **b.**
    Cognitive level: Application
    Topic: Safety
    Chapter: 3

32. Ans: **a.**
    Cognitive level: Application
    Topic: Blood Collection Complications
    Chapter: 9

33. Ans: **a.**
    Cognitive level: Recall
    Topic: Infection Control
    Chapter: 3

34. Ans: **a.**
    Cognitive level: Application
    Topic: Complications and Procedural
    Errors
    Chapter: 9

35. Ans: **a.**
    Cognitive level: Recall
    Topic: Infection Control
    Chapter: 3

36. Ans: **b.**
    Cognitive level: Application
    Topic: Blood Collection Equipment
    Chapter: 7

37. Ans: **c.**
    Cognitive level: Application
    Topic: Safety
    Chapter: 3

38. Ans: **b.**
    Cognitive level: Recall
    Topic 1: Routine ETS Venipuncture
    Topic 2: Procedural Errors That Affect
    Specimen Quality
    Chapters: 8, 9

39. Ans: **a.**
    Cognitive level: Analysis
    Topic: Safety
    Chapter: 3

40. Ans: **b.**
    Cognitive level: Recall
    Topic: Clinical Laboratory Personnel
    Chapter: 1

41. Ans: **d.**
    Cognitive level: Recall
    Topic: Safety
    Chapter: 3.

42. Ans: **a.**
    Cognitive level: Recall
    Topic: Patient's Rights
    Chapter: 1

43. Ans: **d.**
    Cognitive level: Recall
    Topic: Specimen Handling
    Chapter: 14

44. Ans: **a.**
    Cognitive level: Recall
    Topic: Venipuncture Collection
    Equipment
    Chapter: 7

45. Ans: **c.**
    Cognitive level: Application
    Topic: Legal Issues
    Chapter: 2

46. Ans: **a.**
    Cognitive level: Analysis
    Topic: Circulatory System
    Chapter: 6

47. Ans: **b.**
    Cognitive level: Application
    Topic: Safety
    Chapter: 3

48. Ans: **a.**
    Cognitive level: Analysis
    Topic: Anatomy and Physiology
    Chapter: 5

49. Ans: **c.**
    Cognitive level: Application
    Topic: Blood Collection Equipment
    Chapter: 7

50. Ans: **b.**
    Cognitive level: Recall
    Topic: Special Collections
    Chapter: 11

51. Ans: **a.**
    Cognitive level: Recall
    Topic: Blood Collection Equipment
    Chapter: 7

52. Ans: **a.**
    Cognitive level: Recall
    Topic: Venipuncture Specimen Collection Equipment
    Chapter: 8

53. Ans: **c.**
    Cognitive level: Recall
    Topic: Routine Blood Film Preparation
    Chapter: 10

54. Ans: **b.**
    Cognitive level: Recall
    Topic: Arterial Puncture Procedures
    Chapter: 12

55. Ans: **d.**
    Cognitive level: Recall
    Topic: Specimen Handling
    Chapter: 14

56. Ans: **d.**
    Cognitive level: Analysis
    Topic: Anticoagulants
    Chapter: 7

57. Ans: **d.**
Cognitive level: Application
Topic: Personal Wellness
Chapter: 3

58. Ans: **a.**
Cognitive level: Application
Topic: Venipuncture Collection & Patient Interaction
Chapter: 8

59. Ans: **c.**
Cognitive level: Recall
Topic: Skin Puncture
Chapter: 10

60. Ans: **b.**
Cognitive level: Recall
Topic: Anatomy and Physiology
Chapter: 5

61. Ans: **d.**
Cognitive level: Analysis
Topic: Circulatory System
Chapter: 6

62. Ans: **a.**
Cognitive level: Analysis
Topic: Venipuncture Collection & Patient Interaction
Chapter: 8

63. Ans: **c.**
Cognitive level: Recall
Topic: Blood Collection Additives
Chapter: 7

64. Ans: **a.**
Cognitive level: Recall
Topic: Special Collections
Chapter: 11

65. Ans: **d.**
Cognitive level: Analysis
Topic: Safety
Chapter: 3

66. Ans: **a.**
Cognitive level: Recall
Topic: Tube Additives
Chapter: 7

67. Ans: **b.**
Cognitive level: Application
Topic: Electrical Safety
Chapter: 3

68. Ans: **a.**
Cognitive level: Recall
Topic 1: Blood Collection Equipment
Topic 2: Toxicology Specimens
Chapters: 7, 11

69. Ans: **c.**
Cognitive level: Analysis
Topic: Collection Status & Priority
Chapter: 8

70. Ans: **c.**
Cognitive level: Recall
Topic: Skin Puncture Procedures
Chapter: 10

71. Ans: **d.**
Cognitive level: Recall
Topic: Arterial Puncture Procedures
Chapter: 12

72. Ans: **a.**
Cognitive level: Analysis
Topic: Pediatric Specimen Collection Procedures
Chapter: 8

73. Ans: **b.**
Cognitive level: Application
Topic: Site Selection Variables That Influence Specimen Composition
Chapter: 9

74. Ans: **a.**
Cognitive level: Recall
Topic: Safety
Chapter: 3

75. Ans: **c.**
Cognitive level: Application
Topic: Complications and Procedural Errors That Adversely Affect the Patient
Chapter: 9

76. Ans: **c.**
Cognitive level: Recall
Topic: Skin Puncture Order of Draw
Chapter: 7

77. Ans: **c.**
Cognitive level: Application
Topic: Quality Assurance
Chapter: 2

78. Ans: **a.**
Cognitive level: Analysis
Topic: Routine Blood Film Preparation
Chapter: 10

79. Ans: **c.**
Cognitive level: Analysis
Topic: Point-of-Care Testing
Chapter: 11

80. Ans: **c.**
Cognitive level: Recall
Topic: Infection Control
Chapter: 3

81. Ans: **c.**
Cognitive level: Application
Topic: Point-of-Care Testing
Chapter: 11

82. Ans: **a.**
Cognitive level: Application
Topic: Safety
Chapter: 3

83. Ans: **b.**
Cognitive level: Recall
Topic: Patient Identification
Chapter: 8

84. Ans: **d.**
Cognitive level: Recall
Topic: Nonblood Specimens and Tests
Chapter: 13

85. Ans: **d.**
Cognitive level: Recall
Topic: Specimen Handling
Chapter: 14

86. Ans: **b.**
Cognitive level: Recall
Topic: Math
Chapter: Appendix E

87. Ans: **d.**
Cognitive level: Recall
Topic: Requisitions
Chapter: 8

88. Ans: **c.**
Cognitive level: Application
Topic: Specimen Handling
Chapter: 14

89. Ans: **d.**
Cognitive level: Application
Topic: Professionalism & Client
Interaction
Chapter: 1

90. Ans: **d.**
Cognitive level: Application
Topic: Specimen Handling
Chapter: 14

91. Ans: **c.**
Cognitive level: Application
Topic: Infection Control
Chapter: 3

92. Ans: **d.**
Cognitive level: Recall
Topic: Specimen Handling
Chapter: 14

93. Ans: **d.**
Cognitive level: Recall
Topic: Blood Collection Equipment
Chapter: 7

94. Ans: **a.**
Cognitive level: Application
Topic: Specimen Handling
Chapter: 14

95. Ans: **c.**
Cognitive level: Application
Topic: Safety
Chapter: 3

96. Ans: **c.**
   Cognitive level: Recall
   Topic: Collection Priority
   Chapter: 8

97. Ans: **d.**
   Cognitive level: Application
   Topic: Nonblood Specimens and Tests
   Chapter: 13

98. Ans: **d.**
   Cognitive level: Recall
   Topic: Safety
   Chapter: 3

99. Ans: **d.**
   Cognitive level: Recall
   Topic: Phlebotomy & Professionalism
   Chapter: 1

100. Ans: **c.**
   Cognitive level: Recall
   Topic: Infection Control
   Chapter: 3

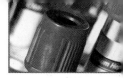

Page numbers followed by *f* indicate figures. Page numbers followed by *t* indicate tables

Timed test, common, 139, 152
Tissue specimen, in biopsy, 244, 251
Tissue thromboplastin contamination, 123, 133
 effects on coagulation test, 296, 305
Toddler(s), sweat chloride test on, infection control for, 300, 307
Tort, 26, 31
 defined, 29, 35
Total quality management (TQM), 27, 31
 principles of, 28, 32
Tourniquet(s)
 application of
  prolonged, 146, 159, 172, 183–184
  site of, 144, 157, 157f
 duration of time worn, 144, 157
 in hand vein drawing, site of, 148, 162
 latex, disposable, 119, 125–126
 properly tied, 144, 157, 157f
 release of, 145, 158
 too tight, results of, 144–145, 157
 during venipuncture, 121, 130
  duration of, 295, 305
  purpose of, 122, 132
  release of, 146, 159
Toxicology, 9, 19
TQM. See Total quality management (TQM)
Trace-element-free tube, in specimen collection, 210, 218
Transfusion(s), blood, disorders transmitted by, 44, 55
Transmission
 droplet contact, 49, 60
 infection, 44, 54, 292, 303
 of syphilis, 299, 307
 of vector infections, 48, 59
 vehicle, 49, 61
Transverse plane, 72, 75f, 85
Tricuspid valve, 88, 88f, 89, 100, 100f, 101
Triglyceride(s), fasting for, 167, 175
Troponin T, 211, 222
Trough drug level
 collection of, 209, 218
 described, 206, 213
Trust, patient's, earning of, 6, 15
Tube inversions, during specimen collection, 258, 266, 267f
Tube stoppers, 122, 123, 130, 133–134
 colors of, 119, 120, 121, 124, 127–129

Tuberculosis (TB), 211, 222
 causes of, 42, 52, 71, 83
 pulmonary, 291, 303
 sputum in, diagnosis of, 243, 249–250
Tuberculosis (TB) test
 interpretation of, 212, 223
 turnaround time for, 210, 218
Tumor(s), lymphoid, malignant, 99, 115
Tumor marker, test used as, 274, 278
Tunica adventitia, 91, 106
Tunica intima, 91, 92, 106, 107, 107f
Tunica media, 91, 106
12-hour fast, 167, 175
24-hour (military) time, 281, 284, 284f
24-hour urine specimen, collection procedure for, 300, 308
2-hour postprandial test, for glucose metabolism problems, 208, 216
Type and screen test, 141, 154
 tube for, 207, 214

UA. See Urinalysis (UA)
Ulnar artery, site of, 231, 232f
Unconscious patients
 blood draw on, 141, 153
 ID of, 142, 154
 laboratory specimens from, identification of, 142, 154
Unit of volume, in metric system, 282, 286
Unit of weight, in metric system, 282, 287
Universal precautions, 41, 51
 history of, 48, 60
Unopette, 189, 196
Uremia, 71, 82
Urinalysis (UA), 10, 12, 20, 22, 241, 245. See also Urine specimens
 described, 240, 245
 routine, 241, 246
 specimens in. See Urine specimens
Urinalysis (UA) department, 11, 22
Urinary system, 69, 78, 79f
 disorder of, 71, 82
 functions of, 69, 76
 test of, 69, 77
Urinary tract infections (UTIs), 43, 53, 301, 308
 C&S test for, 241, 246
 described, 240, 245
Urine, analysis of. See Urinalysis (UA)

Urine creatinine clearance specimen, collection of, 242, 247, 247f
Urine cytology studies, 241, 246
Urine drug screening, 241, 246
Urine porphyrin, 258, 268
 protection against light required for, 299, 307
Urine pregnancy testing, hormone detected in, 211, 222
Urine specimens
 chemical screening tests for, department performing, 11, 22
 components of, time considerations with, 241, 245
 midstream, 242, 247
 midstream clean-catch, 242, 247, 248f
 most concentrated, 241, 246
 preferred specimen, 241, 245
 refrigeration of, 241, 245–246
 suprapubic, 242, 247–248
 24-hour collection procedure for, 242, 246–247, 247f, 300, 308
Urine tests, 242, 247
Urobilinogen testing, 24-hour stool specimen in, 244, 250
User manual, described, 254, 263
UTIs. See Urinary tract infections (UTIs)

Vaccination(s), hepatitis B, 46, 57
 for phlebotomist, 46, 57
Vacuette safety blood collection systems, 132f
VAD. See Vascular access device (VAD)
Value(s)
 reference, described, 188, 195
 threshold, 26, 31
Valve(s), tricuspid, 88, 88f, 89, 100, 100f, 101
Vanishpoint tube holder with needle retracting device, 128f
Vascular access device (VAD)
 described, 166, 174
 subcutaneous, 170, 179–181, 180f
Vascular access pathway, in dialysis, 169, 178–179, 179f
Vascular system, test of, 93, 109
Vasculitis, 94, 110
Vasoconstriction, 98, 114
Vasopressin, 72, 85
Vector, 40, 51
Vector infection transmission, 48, 59
Vehicle transmission, 49, 61